Cancer Targeting Therapies

This volume in the popular series, Drugs and the Pharmaceutical Sciences, begins with the history of cancer treatment, carcinogens, and molecular mechanisms involved in cancer pathogenesis. It includes conventional and advanced cancer therapies ranging from oral and parenteral preparations to advanced fabricated systems such as nanoparticles, liposomes, antibodies, aptamers, poly(amidoamine), and photodynamic therapies. The preparation and mechanisms of molecular targeting of cancer are presented and the authors focus on a diverse audience including undergraduates and research students.

Features

- Timely coverage of changes in process control technology for the phamaceutical industry, a dynamic area in terms of products and manufacturing processes.
- Provides an update on the unique requirements of these industries and how they differ from others, for example, the microelectronics or specialized chemicals industries.
- Draws on the author's vast experience in the field of industrial hygiene and hazardous materials.
- Presents a collection of unique situations in which industrial hygiene was implemented to resolve a variety of scenarios and did not interfere with quality issues.
- Addresses current topics relating to industry evolution such as migration of therapies to higher potency, RiskMAP, new modalities in medicines and treatments, large molecule therapeutics and conjugates.

Drugs and The Pharmaceutical Sciences

A Series of Textbooks and Monographs

Series Editor

Anthony J. Hickey

RTI International, Research Triangle Park, USA

The Drugs and Pharmaceutical Sciences series is designed to enable the pharmaceutical scientist to stay abreast of the changing trends, advances, and innovations associated with therapeutic drugs and that area of expertise and interest that has come to be known as the pharmaceutical sciences. The body of knowledge that those working in the pharmaceutical environment have to work with, and master, has been, and continues, to expand at a rapid pace as new scientific approaches, technologies, instrumentations, clinical advances, economic factors, and social needs arise and influence the discovery, development, manufacture, commercialization, and clinical use of new agents and devices.

Recent Titles in Series

Good Manufacturing Practices for Pharmaceuticals, Seventh Edition, Graham P. Bunn

Pharmaceutical Extrusion Technology, Second Edition, Isaac Ghebre-Sellassie, Charles E. Martin, Feng Zhang, and James Dinunzio

Biosimilar Drug Product Development, Laszlo Endrenyi, Paul Declerck, and Shein-Chung Chow

High Throughput Screening in Drug Discovery, Amancio Carnero

Generic Drug Product Development: International Regulatory Requirements for Bioequivalence, Second Edition, Isadore Kanfer and Leon Shargel

Aqueous Polymeric Coatings for Pharmaceutical Dosage Forms, Fourth Edition, Linda A. Felton

Good Design Practices for GMP Pharmaceutical Facilities, Second Edition, Terry Jacobs and Andrew A. Signore

Handbook of Bioequivalence Testing, Second Edition, Sarfaraz K. Niazi

FDA Good Laboratory Practice Requirements, First Edition, Graham Bunn

Continuous Pharmaceutical Processing and Process Analytical Technology, Ajit Narang and Atul Dubey

Project Management for Drug Developers, Joseph P. Stalder

Emerging Drug Delivery and Biomedical Engineering Technologies: Transforming Therapy, Dimitrios Lamprou

RNA-seq in Drug Discovery and Development, Feng Cheng and Robert Morris

Patient Safety in Developing Countries: Education, Research, Case Studies, Yaser Al-Worafi

Industrial Hygiene in the Pharmaceutical and Consumer Healthcare Industries, Casey Cosner

Cancer Targeting Therapies: Conventional and Advanced Perspectives, Muhammad Yasir Ali, Shazia Anwer Bukhari

For more information about this series, please visit www.crcpress.com/Drugs-and-the-Pharmaceutical-Sciences/book-series/IHCDRUPHASCI

Cancer Targeting Therapies

Conventional and Advanced Perspectives

Edited By

Muhammad Yasir Ali

Department of Pharmaceutics, Faculty of Pharmaceutical Sciences,
GC University Faisalabad, Faisalabad, Pakistan

Shazia Anwer Bukhari

Department of Biochemistry, Faculty of Sciences,
GC University Faisalabad, Faisalabad, Pakistan

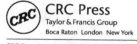

CRC Press
Taylor & Francis Group
Boca Raton London New York

CRC Press is an imprint of the
Taylor & Francis Group, an **informa** business

First edition published 2024
by CRC Press
6000 Broken Sound Parkway NW, Suite 300, Boca Raton, FL 33487-2742

and by CRC Press
4 Park Square, Milton Park, Abingdon, Oxon, OX14 4RN

© 2024 selection and editorial matter, Muhammad Yasir Ali, Shazia Anwer Bukhari; individual chapters, the contributors

CRC Press is an imprint of Taylor & Francis Group, LLC

Library of Congress Cataloging-in-Publication Data
Names: Ali, Muhammad Yasir, editor. | Bukhari, Shazia, editor.
Title: Cancer targeting therapies : conventional and advanced perspectives /
edited by Muhammad Yasir Ali, Shazia Bukhari.
Other titles: Drugs and the pharmaceutical sciences. 0360-2583
Description: First edition. | Boca Raton : CRC Press, 2024. |
Series: Drugs and the pharmaceutical sciences |
Includes bibliographical references and index. |
Identifiers: LCCN 2023020511 (print) | LCCN 2023020512 (ebook) |
ISBN 9781032426259 (hardback) | ISBN 9781032427126 (paperback) |
ISBN 9781003363958 (ebook)
Subjects: MESH: Antineoplastic Agents |
Neoplasms–drug therapy | Drug Delivery Systems
Classification: LCC RC271.C5 (print) | LCC RC271.C5 (ebook) |
NLM QV 269 | DDC 616.99/4061–dc23/eng/20230714
LC record available at https://lccn.loc.gov/2023020511
LC ebook record available at https://lccn.loc.gov/2023020512

ISBN: 978-1-032-4-2625-9 (HB)
ISBN: 978-1-032-4-2712-6 (PB)
ISBN: 978-1-003-3-6395-8 (EB)

DOI: 10.1201/9781003363958

Typeset in Times
by Newgen Publishing UK

Contents

Background

*Isma Iqbal, Daulat Haleem Khan, Maria Manan, Zainab Abdullah,
Muhammad Ali Syed, Sana Hanif, Zeliha Selamoglu, Muhammad Yasir Ali,
and Azhar Rasul*

*Saba Riaz, Azhar Rasul, Muhammad Asif Khalil, Laiba Ameen,
Komal Riaz, Samreen Gul Khan, Sevki Adem, Mudassir Hassan,
Muhammad Javid Iqbal, Muhammad Asrar, and Muhammad Yasir Ali*

*Hafiz Muhammad Irfan, Muhammad Ihtisham Umar, Usman Sabir,
Muhammad Yasir Ali, and Ummaima Shahzad*

*Malik Saadullah, Amna Sehar, Khurram Afzal, Ijaz Ali,
Shams ul Hassan, and Muhammad Yasir Ali*

*Tanzeela Awan, Ghazala Ambreen, Uzma Saher, Saira Afzal,
Muhammad Yasir Ali, and Asia Naz Awan*

Conventional Cancer Therapies

*Ayesha Saeed, Liaqat Hussain, Hua Naranmandura, Qian Qian Wang,
Muhammad Yasir Ali, Ummaima Shahzad, and Ijaz Ali*

*Mishal Fatima, Liaqat Hussain, Yasen Maimaitiyiming, Hua Naranmandura,
Ayesha Saeed, Yang Chang, Muhammad Yasir Ali, and Ummaima Shahzad*

Advanced Cancer Therapies

Preface

Cancer targeting has always been the topic of discussion in the arena of therapeutic choices amongst all other options for tumor treatment. The diversity and poorly determined factors of individual cancer growth, especially enhanced permeation, and retention have posed an ever-lasting threat of treatment failure. This has resulted in continuous ongoing research in the field of chemotherapy, along with discoveries of other treatment options. The resultant extensive and enthusiastic approaches, of researchers, have ended up in the development of different dosage forms along with their further modifications to achieve the required goals. This vast knowledge in the field has always conflated undergraduate students as well as young researchers on treatment options and the making of relevant dosage forms. Consequently, there was a need of time to provide such information out of the box under one title.

The current book provides all the key pieces of information; ranging from the history of cancer therapy to pharmacological choices of the chemotherapeutic agents, from conventional dosage form of table and injections to more sophisticated choices of nanoparticles and from targeting therapies (passive targeting, antibody-based therapies, aptamer based-therapies, etc.) to the recent choice of photodynamic therapy for cancer treatment. While writing about these different options, the reason for excipient selection, methods of fabrication, assessment of these nano-carriers, current research going on, etc. were kept in mind. A chronological model of introduction to the development and assessment has been followed, so that it could become a piece of cake for undergraduate as well as postgraduate students to digest.

All the authors and contributors of the book have been actively engaged in teaching for decades. Therefore, their contribution has resulted in the form of this piece of art comprising all the required information under the umbrella of cancer targeting. Moreover, the active presence of these contributors, in the research over the years, has also influenced the choice of outlines followed in these chapters. Furthermore, their teamwork also inclined the natural flow of information and correlation between various dimensions of cancer targeting, making it easy for students and young researchers to understand. Multicultural and multiorganizational research approaches have also inspired the contributors to provide a book compiled in a sequential fashion.

The editors would like to thank the family members, chapter writers, colleagues, and students for their contribution and support throughout the writing process. Without the care and patience, they demonstrated, we might have faced a lag in meeting our time frame.

Muhammad Yasir Ali
Shazia Anwer Bukhari

Editors

Muhammad Yasir Ali earned a bachelor's and a master's degree in Pharmaceutical Technology in 2009. After earning a degree in Pharmaceutical Technology, he joined the University of Lahore as a faculty member and taught different courses to pharmacy graduates, including pharmaceutical technology. In 2011 after starting his current job, he kept on teaching and conducted research, which is still ongoing. He later earned a doctorate in Pharmaceutical Technology from Philipps University, Marburg, Germany.

He has more than 30 research publications, one research project, practical application of pharmacy knowledge in the form of different marketed products, several book chapters, and one book as editor. He has had the opportunity to present research papers and scientific lectures in different organizations in Germany, the United States, the United Kingdom, and Pakistan.

Shazia Anwer Bukhari completed her undergraduate studies at the Bahuddin Zakariya University, Multan in 2001 and a master's degree in 2003 from the Department of Biochemistry, University of Agriculture, Faisalabad Pakistan. She then continued higher studies at the University of The Punjab, Lahore, Pakistan, and earned a Ph.D. degree in Biochemistry in 2009. Meanwhile, she has worked in different organizations as a research officer and joined GC University Faisalabad, Pakistan, as a faculty member. She has been a professor of biochemistry there since 2019.

Her research interests include the exploration of indigenous flora subjected to the treatment of different diseases. On the molecular level, targeting different signaling mechanisms involved in liver and breast cancer, obesity, diabetes, and other molecular disorders, are her areas of expertise.

She has more than 100 research publications, research projects, several book chapters, research collaborations in different countries (USA, Turkey, UK, South Korea, Egypt, among others), and academic awards in her research profile. Dozens of postgraduate (master's and Ph.D.) students have earned degrees working under the umbrella of her research group, and equally are currently strengthening her laboratory work staff. She has visited various countries to attend and present her research work at international conferences, workshops, and symposia.

Contributors

Sabahat Abdullah
Department of Pharmaceutical Chemistry, Faculty of Pharmacy & Pharmaceutical Sciences, University of Karachi, Karachi, Pakistan.

Zainab Abdullah
Lahore College for Pharmaceutical Sciences, Lahore, Pakistan.

Sevki Adem
Department of Biochemistry, Çankırı Karatekin Üniversitesi, Çankırı, Turkiye.

Khudeja Afroz
Department of Zoology, Faculty of Life Sciences, GC University Faisalabad, Faisalabad, Pakistan.

Khurram Afzal
Department of Human Nutrition, Faculty of Food Science and Nutrition, Bahauddin Zakariya University, Multan, Pakistan.

Saira Afzal
Faculty of Pharmacy, The University of Lahore, Lahore, Pakistan.

Saeed Ahmad
Department of Pharmaceutical Chemistry, Faculty of Pharmacy and Alternative Medicine, The Islamia University of Bahawalpur, Bahawalpur, Pakistan.

Ijaz Ali
Department of Pharmacognosy, Faculty of Pharmaceutical Sciences, GC University Faisalabad, Faisalabad, Pakistan.

Muhammad Yasir Ali
Department of Pharmaceutics, Faculty of Pharmaceutical Sciences, GC University Faisalabad, Faisalabad, Pakistan.

Sajid Ali
Department of Chemistry, Uppsala University, Uppsala, Sweden.

Ghazala Ambreen
Sargodha College of Medical Sciences, Sargodha, Pakistan.

Laiba Ameen
Department of Zoology, Faculty of Life Sciences, GC University Faisalabad, Faisalabad, Pakistan.

Muhammad Umair Amin
Department of Pharmaceutics and Biopharmaceutics, Faculty of Pharmacy, Philipps University Marburg, Marburg, Germany.

Shazia Anwer Bukhari
Department of Biochemistry, Faculty of Sciences, GC University Faisalabad, Faisalabad, Pakistan.

Shumaila Arshad
Doctor Institute of Health Sciences, Sargodha, Pakistan.

Mulazim Hussain Asim
College of Pharmacy, University of Sargodha, Sargodha, Pakistan.

Muhammad Asim Farooq
Monash Institute of Pharmaceutical Sciences, Monash University, Australia.

Nosheen Aslam
Department of Biochemistry, Faculty of Sciences, GC University Faisalabad, Faisalabad, Pakistan.

Muhammad Asrar
Department of Zoology, Faculty of Life Sciences, GC University Faisalabad, Pakistan.

Tanzeela Awan
Department of Pharmacy, The Women University Multan, Multan, Pakistan.

Udo Bakowsky
Department of Pharmaceutics and Biopharmaceutics, Faculty of Pharmacy, Philipps University Marburg, Marburg, Germany.

Yang Chang
School of Medicine and Public Health, Zhejiang University, Hangzhou, China.

Alia Erum
College of Pharmacy, University of Sargodha, Sargodha, Pakistan.

Mishal Fatima
Department of Pharmacology, Faculty of Pharmaceutical Sciences, GC University Faisalabad, Faisalabad, Pakistan.

Sana Hanif
Department of Pharmacy, GC University, Lahore, Pakistan.

Mudassir Hassan
Department of Zoology, Faculty of Life Sciences, GC University Faisalabad, Faisalabad, Pakistan.

Shams ul Hassan
Department of Pharmaceutics, Faculty of Pharmaceutical Sciences, GC University Faisalabad, Faisalabad, Pakistan.

Liaqat Hussain
Department of Pharmacology, Faculty of Pharmaceutical Sciences, GC University Faisalabad, Faisalabad, Pakistan.

Isma Iqbal
Department of Pharmacy, Lahore College of Pharmaceutical Sciences, Lahore, Pakistan.

Muhammad Javid Iqbal
Department of Zoology, Faculty of Life Sciences, GC University Faisalabad, Faisalabad, Pakistan.

Rabia Iqtadar
Department of Pharmaceutical Chemistry, Faculty of Pharmacy & Pharmaceutical Sciences, University of Karachi, Karachi, Pakistan.

Hafiz Muhammad Irfan
College of Pharmacy, University of Sargodha, Sargodha, Pakistan.

Muhammad Asif Khalil
Department of Zoology, Faculty of Life Sciences, GC University Faisalabad, Faisalabad, Pakistan.

Daulat Haleem Khan
Department of Pharmacy, Lahore College of Pharmaceutical Sciences, Lahore, Pakistan.

Gul Bushra Khan
Department of Biotechnology and Bioinformatics, Faculty of Life Sciences, GC University Faisalabad, Faisalabad, Pakistan.

Samreen Gul Khan
Department of Chemistry, Faculty of Physical Sciences, GC University Faisalabad, Faisalabad, Pakistan.

Khatereh Khorsandi
Department of Photodynamic, Medical Laser Research Center, YARA Institute, Tehran University of Medical Sciences (TUMS), Tehran, IRAN.
Department of Biochemistry and Molecular Medicine, School of Medicine and Health Sciences, The George Washington University, Washington, USA.

Maria Manan
Department of Pharmacology, Faculty of Pharmaceutical Sciences, GC University Faisalabad, Faisalabad, Pakistan.

Arshad Mahmood
College of Pharmacy, Al Ain University, Abu Dhabi, United Arab Emirates.

Yasen Maimaitiyiming
School of Medicine and Public Health, Zhejiang University, Hangzhou, China.

Ali Moghadam
Institute of biotechnology, Shiraz University, Shiraz, Iran.

Hua Naranmandura
School of Medicine and Public Health, Zhejiang University, Hangzhou, China.

Ayesha Naseer
Department of Pharmaceutical Chemistry, Faculty of Pharmacy & Pharmaceutical Sciences, University of Karachi, Karachi, Pakistan.

Asia Naz Awan
Department of Pharmaceutical Chemistry, Faculty of Pharmacy & Pharmaceutical Sciences, University of Karachi, Karachi, Pakistan.

Nisar ur Rahman
Department of Pharmacy, COMSATS University, Abbottabad, Pakistan.

Azhar Rasul
Department of Zoology, Faculty of Life Sciences, GC University Faisalabad, Faisalabad, Pakistan.

Syed Atif Raza
University College of Pharmacy, University of the Punjab, Lahore, Pakistan.

Komal Riaz
Department of Zoology, Faculty of Life Sciences, GC University Faisalabad, Faisalabad, Pakistan.

Saba Riaz
Department of Zoology, Faculty of Life Sciences, GC University Faisalabad, Faisalabad, Pakistan.

Mavra Rubab
College of Pharmacy, University of Sargodha, Sargodha, Pakistan.

Malik Saadullah
Department of Pharmaceutical Chemistry, Faculty of Pharmaceutical Sciences, GC University Faisalabad, Faisalabad, Pakistan.

Usman Sabir
College of Pharmacy, University of Sargodha, Sargodha, Pakistan.

Ayesha Sadiqa
Department of Zoology, Faculty of Life Sciences, GC University Faisalabad, Faisalabad, Pakistan.

Ayesha Saeed
Department of Pharmacology, Faculty of Pharmaceutical Sciences, GC University Faisalabad, Pakistan.

Zunaira Saeed
Department of Zoology, Faculty of Life Sciences, GC University, Faisalabad, Faisalabad, Pakistan

Uzma Saleem
Department of Pharmacology, Faculty of Pharmaceutical Sciences, GC University Faisalabad, Faisalabad, Pakistan.

Uzma Saher
Department of Pharmacy, The Women University Multan, Multan, Pakistan.

Amna Sehar
Department of Pharmaceutical Chemistry, Faculty of Pharmaceutical Sciences, GC University Faisalabad, Faisalabad, Pakistan.

Zeliha Selamoglu
Faculty of Medicine, Department of Medical Biology, Nigde Ömer Halisdemir University, Nigde, Turkiye.

Maryam Shabir
Department of Pharmaceutics, Faculty of Pharmaceutical Sciences, GC University Faisalabad, Faisalabad, Pakistan.

Ummaima Shahzad
Department of Pharmaceutics, Faculty of Pharmaceutical Sciences, GC University Faisalabad, Faisalabad, Pakistan.

Rida Siddique
Department of Pharmacology, Faculty of Pharmaceutical Sciences, GC University Faisalabad, Faisalabad, Pakistan.

Muhammad Ali Syed
Faculty of Pharmacy, The University of Lahore, Lahore, Pakistan.
Department of Pharmacy, GC University, Lahore, Pakistan.

Imran Tariq
University College of Pharmacy, University of the Punjab, Lahore, Pakistan.

Hafsa Tariq
Department of Pharmaceutical Chemistry, Faculty of Pharmaceutical Sciences, GC University Faisalabad, Faisalabad, Pakistan.

Muhammad Ihtisham Umar
Department of Pharmacy, COMSATS University Islamabad, Lahore, Pakistan.

Qian Qian Wang
School of Medicine and Public Health, Zhejiang University, Hangzhou, China.

Rabia Zara
Department of Zoology, Faculty of Life Sciences, GC University Faisalabad, Faisalabad, Pakistan.

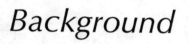

Background

1 History of Cancer Therapies

Isma Iqbal, Daulat Haleem Khan, Maria Manan,
Zainab Abdullah, Muhammad Ali Syed, Sana Hanif,
Zeliha Selamoglu, Muhammad Yasir Ali, and Azhar Rasul

1.1 INTRODUCTION

1.1.1 HIPPOCRATES

Hippocrates was considered to be the first physician with special reference to cancer treatment. The era was betwixt 460–370 BC. His view of treatment for the tumor cells was based on any reason from nature and hence, to establish a better understanding of the disease and ultimately cancer would rely on establishing "wisdom" for identifying the disease and causes of the disease. However, it was systemically based on proper observation, reasoning as well as the experience of "physician" in nature of that era [1]. It was the extract of his old saying that healthcare providers must add wisdom to therapy [2].

1.1.2 POST-HIPPOCRATIC PERIOD

After Hippocrates declined (370 BC), a system was left behind with some of the methodologies but there was no systematized medication or methodology for cancer patients.

1.1.3 GALEN OF PERGAMON

One of the greatest medical physicians of all time, Galen contributed to the principles of autopsy in order to study cancer and disease. He learned cancer treatment and made some advancements in this era (129–199 AD) since his philosophical ideas ruled European medicines for almost 15 centuries. Galen was more specific in disease identification as compared to previous researchers [3]. In cancer pathology, He classified the lumps into different grades, ranging from benign to malignant tumors. His classified "De tumoribus praeter naturam" are deliberated lumps or lesions in modern pathology today [4].

1.1.4 TREATMENT IN LATER ERA

In the later era, there were many remedies and treatments for cancer as compared to the early era. There were handbooks including Oribasios, Aetios (VII C. AD) [5].

1.2 CANCER THERAPY

Nowadays, there are several methods for the treatment of cancer, including surgery, chemotherapy, radiation, targeted drug delivery system (nanoparticles) (Figure 1.1), hormone therapy, and immunotherapy.

DOI: 10.1201/9781003363958-2

1.2.1 SURGICAL TREATMENT

The oldest and most popular method of treating cancer is through surgical operations for the removal of solid malignancies. In contrast to patients from poor or underdeveloped nations, it is clear that the majority of patients in industrialized countries continue to receive their only therapy through surgery. While this is going on, surgical procedures are less popular in developing or underdeveloped nations because of poor treatment options brought on by late cancer diagnosis [6, 7]. However, the procedures may cause metastases, mostly because cancer cells are shed into the bloodstream, anti-tumor immunity is suppressed, allowing circulating cells to survive, and adhesion molecules are upregulated [6, 8]. Therefore, other treatment options are required to be practiced.

1.2.2 RADIATION THERAPY

The usage of x-rays in the treatment of cancer increased after its discovery. The DNA of cancer cells is harmed when these rays are used carefully. Radiation does damage both healthy and malignant cells, however, healthy cells can usually repair these damages and continue to function normally. Also, the radiotherapy is administered at the highest dose tolerable for the nearby normal tissues. As a result, it is now a crucial therapy choice in cancer care programs [9–11]. The face of cancer treatment approaches has changed as a result of the combination of this with chemotherapy and surgery [12, 13]. Radiation therapy's efficiency has improved the overall survival rate of cancer patients, but the unintended tissue damage raises concerns about the patient's quality of life. This problem is worse in the case of young patients, where the late effect of radiation in normal cells may cause uncontrolled damage.

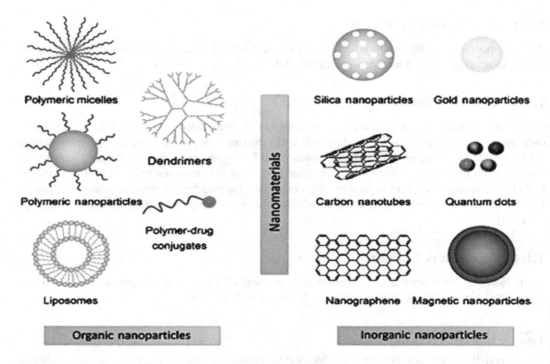

FIGURE 1.1   Different delivery agents for chemotherapy including organic and inorganic sources [14].

1.2.3 CHEMOTHERAPEUTICS

Chemotherapy is the old conventional method of cancer treatment along with surgery and radiation. Chemotherapy usually involves the infusion of a small amount of chemotherapeutic drug that interacts with the DNA molecules, modifies them, and leads to the death of the cancer cells [15].

1.2.3.1 Evolution of Chemotherapy

Radiotherapy, surgery, and chemotherapy are the therapies available for treating tumors these days. The history of chemotherapy was initiated in the 20th century; however, its utilization for cancer therapy was initiated in the 1930s. The word chemotherapy was used by Paul Ehrlich who showed specific curiosity in alkylating agents and who appeared with the word to express the chemical therapy of disorder.

After the discovery of x-rays for the therapy of cancers, a remarkable turn to the therapy of cancers and the development of a number of drugs happened during the Second World War with the accidental discovery of nitrogen mustard that exhibited a reduced number of leukocytes. This gave rise to the usage of nitrogen mustard as an initial chemotherapeutic drug for treating lymphomas [16]. The era of chemotherapy started in the 1940s with the use of nitrogen mustard as an effective treatment for cancer. Lious Goodman and Alfred Gilman, in 1942, used, for the first time, nitrogen mustard gas for the treatment of non-Hodgkin's lymphoma and gave the concept that it can reduce cancer regression. After this alkylating drugs like chlorambucil and cyclophosphamide were prepared for treating tumors [17].

In 1948, Sydney Farber used antifolates to successfully induce remissions in children with acute lymphoblastic leukemia. Heidelberger designed a drug 5-fluorouracil for solid cancers, which is a crucial chemotherapeutic drug until now for treating neck, head, and colorectal tumors [18]. George Hitchings and Gertrude Elion, in 1948, synthesized the purine analog 6-mercaptopurine. The 1950s experienced the development of corticosteroids in addition to the formation of a cancer chemotherapy national service center, which was used to analyze antitumor drugs.

Drugs used as monotherapy attained small responses in some tumor types [19]. The National Cancer Institute (NCI) was formulated in 1954, which was a systematic program for cancer screening. Roy Hertz and Min Chiu Li in 1958 demonstrated that methotrexate as a single agent could cure choriocarcinoma, the first solid tumor to be cured with chemotherapy. The Food and Drug Administration (FDA) in 1959 approved cyclophosphamide as a chemotherapeutic agent. In the 1960s and 1970s novel combined treatments utilizing many chemotherapeutic medicines with various mechanisms initiated to be suggested clinically [20].

The trend of combined anti-cancer therapy has described a pivotal moment of decision for the therapy of cancers, due to the achievement of therapeutic effect as compared to single anticancer therapy. In particular, combination treatment kills a greater number of cancer cells with a greater dose of every medicine, which is why remaining within the tolerated doses of these medicines is important [20]. Moreover, it allows greater interaction between drug and tumor cells with many genetic disorders. It also inhibits the succeeding rise in drug resistance [21]. During the 1960s the prime focus was hematologic tumors. Better therapies were designed from vinca alkaloids to treat Hodgkin's disorder and leukemia [22].

1.2.3.2 Drugs used in Cancer Treatment

A few commonly used anti-cancer drugs against different types of tumors have been listed in Table 1.1.

1.2.3.3 Combination Therapy

In 1965 combination chemotherapy was introduced, which had shown long-term remissions. Hodgkin's disease was treated utilizing MOMP guidelines, which used vincristine, methotrexate, and prednisone in combination with nitrogen mustard and using MOPP guidelines consisting of procarbazine, not methotrexate [43].

Vincent DeVita and others in 1970 cured lymphomas with combination chemotherapy. Emil Frei with colleagues in 1972 demonstrated that chemotherapy after surgical removal of osteosarcoma can improve the cure rate (adjuvant chemotherapy). Gianni Bonadonna and Umberto Veronesi in 1972 suggested a study to analyze the effectiveness of adjuvant treatment after surgery, utilizing the medicines: fluorouracil, cyclophosphamide, and methotrexate, which ameliorated the likelihood of survival of tumor patients [44].

Bonadonna in 1973 suggested a novel combination of medicines dacarbazine, bleomycin vinblastine, and adriamycin called ABCD for treating Hodgkin's lymphoma. The outcomes showed that this combination cured many patients and was better tolerated with fewer adverse effects [45]. Large B-cell lymphoma was treated utilizing C-MOPP guidelines, which replaced nitrogen mustard with cyclophosphamide [43].

In 1975 a combination of cyclophosphamide, methotrexate, and fluorouracil (CMF) was shown to be effective as adjuvant therapy for node-positive chemotherapy. In 1978, the FDA approved cisplatin for the treatment of ovarian cancer, a drug that would prove to have broad-spectrum activity [20].

1.3 RECENT ADVANCES IN CANCER TREATMENT

In the treatment of cancer, the major challenge is to deliver the drug effectively at the cancer site while minimizing the side effects at the same time. The use of nanocarriers as drug delivery systems can improve pharmacokinetic properties. Among the many nano drug delivery systems micelles, liposomes, nano/microspheres, and nanoparticles have gained popularity with special reference to the treatment of cancer. Many drugs have gained approval while a number of drugs are in the trial phase. The nanoparticles lead the treatment of cancer to a new level.

TABLE 1.1
List of Some Frontline Drugs for Different Types of Cancers

Sr. No.	Drug	Type of Cancer	Reference
1.	Cyclophosphamide	Breast cancer	[23]
2.	Cisplatin	Lymphomas, cervical, ovarian, lung, bladder, melanoma	[24]
3.	5-fluorouracil	Broad-spectrum activity against solid tumors, e.g., breast, liver, GIT etc	[25]
4.	Doxorubicin	Pancreatic cancer, metastatic adenocarcinoma	[26]
5.	Camptothecin	Colon, breast, ovarian, brain, and lung cancers	[27]
6.	Paclitaxel	Breast, pancreatic ovarian, and brain tumors	[28, 29]
7.	Mitomycin C	Bladder	[30]
8.	Mitoxantrone	Neuromyelitis optical spectrum disorder (second line agent)	[31]
9.	Mitomycin C	Adenocarcinoma of the stomach, breast, pancreas	[32, 33]
10.	Etoposide	Testicular, prostate, bladder, stomach, and lung	[34, 35]
11.	Carboplatin	Breast cancer	[36, 37]
12.	Irinotecan	Colorectal cancer	[38]
13.	Gemcitabine	Pancreatic cancer	[39, 40]
14.	Floxuridine	Colorectal liver metastases	[41]
15.	Melphalan	Ovarian, breast cancers, and multiple myelomas	[42]

1.3.1 Micelles

The micelles are small colloidal suspensions that range in size from 5–100 nm and are amphiphilic in nature, i.e., having both hydrophilic and hydrophobic properties. The hydrophobic core of micelles allows chemotherapeutic drug delivery.

1.3.2 Liposomes

They consist of a totally encircling lipid bilayer that completely encases the interior water core employed for drug encapsulation [46]. They can be categorized based on a variety of factors, including phospholipid content (Table 1.2), number of bilayers (uni, oligo, or multilamellar), and size (small, large, or huge) (cation, anionic, or neutral). Both hydrophilic medications (in the center watery core) and hydrophobic pharmaceuticals can be trapped by them (in the lipid bilayer). To achieve specific goals, such as lengthy systemic circulation, greater tumor accumulation via active targeting, and enhanced cellular internalization, liposomal surface can be altered using a variety of techniques [47, 48].

1.3.3 Nanoparticles

The conventional chemotherapeutics agents are administered systemically, which are associated with a number of side effects, including hair loss, nausea, vomiting, liver toxicity, kidney toxicity, and bone marrow suppression. These aspects determine the dose of chemotherapeutic agents and the limit to which these affect the tumor cells. In recent years, new products with more specificity were designed called nanoparticles. The nanoparticles are more specific in targeting and these have fewer side effects as compared to the conventional dosage forms [50].

Over the past few years, nanoparticles are in increased use for cancer treatment. They aim to provide the sustained release effect by directly targeting the infected cells and providing the

TABLE 1.2
Examples of Some Commonly Used Lipids for Liposomes [49]

Sr. No.	Name	Abbreviation
1.	1,2-dipalmitoyl-sn-glycero-3-phosphocholine)	DPPC
2.	1,2-distearoyl-sn-glycero-3-phosphocholine	DSPC
3.	1,2-distearoyl-sn-glycero-3-phosphoethanolamine	DSPE
4.	1,2-distearoyl-sn-glycero-3-phosphoethanolamine-N-[amino(polyethylene glycol)-2000]	DSPE-PEG(2000) Amine
5.	1,2-distearoyl-sn-glycero-3-phosphoethanolamine-N-[amino(polyethylene glycol)-2000]	DSPE-PEG(5000) Amine
6.	1,2-distearoyl-sn-glycero-3-phosphoethanolamine-N-[cyanur(polyethylene glycol)-2000]	DSPE-PEG(2000) Cyanur
7.	1,2-distearoyl-sn-glycero-3-phosphoethanolamine-N-[maleimide(polyethylene glycol)-5000]	DSPE-PEG(5000) Maleimide
8.	1,2-dipalmitoyl-sn-glycero-3-phosphoethanolamine	DPPE
9.	1,2-dipalmitoyl-sn-glycero-3-phosphoethanolamine-N-[azido(polyethylene glycol)-2000]	DPPE-PEG(2000) Azide
10.	1,2-dioleoyl-sn-glycero-3-phosphoethanolamine	DOPE
11.	1,2-dioleoyl-sn-glycero-3-phosphoethanolamine-N-[amino(polyethylene glycol)-2000]	DOPE-PEG(2000) Amine
12.	1,2-dioleoyl-sn-glycero-3-phosphoethanolamine-N-[carboxy(polyethylene glycol)-2000]	DOPE-PEG(2000) Carboxylic Acid

sustained release of drugs [51]. In the mid-1980s, the first nanoparticle came for the clinical trial (liposome with encapsulated doxorubicin). In 1995, the first nanoparticle-based drug came into the market [52].

In general, the nanoparticles are polymeric and lipid in nature colloidal particles (Table 1.3), which may be embedded in lipid or polymeric nanomatrix or may be absorbed/entrapped on the surface of the matrix. The nanoparticles can increase the half-life ($t_{1/2}$) up to 10 times hence leading towards less frequency of dose administration leading towards patient compliance and improved quality of life. For example, for the treatment of lymphocytic leukemia, the half-life of L-asparaginase is short between 8–10 hours. But with polyethylene glycol (PEG)-L-asparaginase conjugate the half-life is almost 14 days, hence only one infusion administration is required after every 2 weeks.

The nanoparticles not only target the tumor cells but also reach the cell surface and deep inside the cell organelles. The nanoparticles provide better treatment by providing the specific site drug targeting plus the controlled release of the drug [53].

The nanoparticles are sub-micron-sized colloidal particles with an encapsulated therapeutic agent within the polymeric complex conjugated or absorbed onto the surface. These can deliver the drug at the specific targeted site by crossing different biological barriers, including the blood–brain barrier. By coating the nanoparticles with polysorbates, the drug-loaded nanoparticles can cross the blood–brain barrier [54].

The nanoparticles can be formulated from different materials and a variety of materials like proteins, nucleic acids, chemotherapeutics can be encapsulated in them [55].

Natural polymers are biopolymers obtained from different proteins and polysaccharides and due to their biodegradability and biocompatibility properties, suitable for targeted drug deliveries. The semi-synthetic polymers can be produced by the combination of natural polymers with synthetic polymers. In a controlled drug delivery system, the semi-synthetic polymer types gain more attention because of their higher ability to incorporate the drugs. The polymeric nanoparticles can be assembled by three following methods, i.e., entrapment method, encapsulation, and conjugation [56, 57].

The nanoparticles as a chemotherapeutic agent have so many advantages over conventional drugs, e.g., size tuning, solubility improvement, lesser adverse events, better compliance, etc.

The nanoparticles show the improved intracellular concentrations of the drugs in both active and passive targeting while bypassing the toxicity in the normal cells. There are specific challenges associated with targeted nanoparticles in cancer treatment. Among these, one challenge is that

TABLE 1.3

Classification of the Most Commonly Used Polymers for Nanoparticles [49]

Sr. No.	Class	Polymer	Abbreviation
1.	Natural Polymers	Albumin	
		Alignate	
		Chitosan	
2.	Synthetic Homo-polymers	Poly(epsilon-caprolactone)	PCL
		Poly(lactide)	PLA
		Poly(lactide-co-glycolide)	PLGA
3.	Co-polymers	Poly(lactide)-poly(ethylene glycol)	PLA-PEG
		Poly(lactide)-poly(ethylene glycol)	PLGA-PEG
		Poly(epsilon-caprolactone)-poly(ethylene glycol)	PCL-PEG
4.	Colloidal Stabilizers	All co-polymers	PVA
		Dextran	
		Poly(vinyl alcohol)	

the nanoparticles may become changed in stability, pharmacokinetic properties, and solubility of the carried drug. The other limitations of nanoparticles are their shelf life, leakage, and toxicity of the material. There are some materials such as Poly (lactic-co-glycolic acid PLGA) that have low toxicity but also less stability because it degrades very quickly.

1.3.3.1 Types of Nanoparticles

1.3.3.1.1   Metal Oxide Nanoparticles

The metal nanoparticles play an important role in cancer therapy by providing better targeting and drug deliveries. These are thought to maybe overcome the problems associated with conventional dosage forms. In addition to therapy, these are used in the diagnosis and imaging of cancer cells. These provide the controlled and targeted release of drugs [58]. Metal nanoparticles possess anti-bacterial and anti-oxidant properties. Copper nanoparticles contain anti-bacterial properties [59]. Arsenic is a metal/metalloid where arsenical-based cancer drugs are the modern approach for treating cancer [60]. Zirconium and silver nanoparticles are in use nowadays for the preparation of nanoparticles. Silver (Ag) nanoparticles are extensively in use with respect to the treatment of cancer [61].

1.3.3.1.2   Cation Nanoparticles

The cationic polymers are completely soluble in water. There is a number of cationic polymers that are in use for targeted drug delivery.

Chitosan: Chitosan is a natural polymer of cationic nature. The chitosans are made through side chain grafting and deacetylation for targeting the phenomenon. Chitosan shows the anti-cancer effect after oral absorption and hence is suitable with respect to patient compliance.

Polyethylene imine: It is the most studied, effective, and easily available cationic polymer used in the manufacturing of cancer-treating drugs.

Poly-L-lysine: This is the biodegradable polymer that forms nanosize complexes (<100 nm). It is obtained through the polymerization of N-carboxy-anhydride of lysine.

Polymethacrylate: These are cationic polymers with vinyl-base. This type of cationic polymer has a wide range of chemical structures and molecular masses.

1.3.3.1.3   Cationic Dendrimers

These are synthetic molecules with average protein size and are branched proteins in nature. These have a large surface area, which favors adsorption or encapsulation [62].

1.3.3.1.4   Protein Nanoparticles

Albumin is the protein present in the blood plasma. Albumin is the most widely used protein in the preparation of nanoparticles because of its good compatibility and very low cytotoxic effect. Drug deliveries with protein-based nanoparticles are widely in use as drug carriers.

Different polymeric and proteinous nanoparticles have been prepared by different formulation techniques and a few examples are mentioned in Table 1.4.

1.4 RECENT INNOVATIONS AND TARGETED THERAPY

George Köhler and César Milstein's work in 1975 has lead off the formation of many hybrid mono-clonal antibodies for various antigens or cellular targets, achieved by the awareness of hybridomas, coming from the combination of human myeloma cells and murine B lymphocytes, making massive monoclonal antibodies [75]. Nadler in 1980 used murine monoclonal antibody AB89 to treat a patient suffering from non-Hodgkin lymphoma, but the therapy did not produce a remarkable clinical response [76].

TABLE 1.4
Cancer Treatment Loaded with Nanoparticles

Drug	Formulation Technique	Polymeric Material	Reference
Cyclophosphamide	Electrospray deposition system	Gliadin-gelatin nanoparticles	[23]
Cisplatin		PCL-PEG nanoparticles	[63]
Paclitaxel	Solvent evaporation, emulsification	Chitosan	[64]
Paclitaxel	Nanoprecipitation	Cyclodextrin	[65]
Paclitaxel	Entrapment method	Emulsifying wax	[66]
Camptothecin	Entrapment method	PEG-PCL	[27]
Paclitaxel	Encapsulation method	PCL-PEG-PCL	[28]
Paclitaxel	Encapsulation method	PLGA-PEG	[29]
Doxorubicin	Encapsulation method	PLGA-TPGS	[67]
Metformin			
Cisplatin	Encapsulation method	PEG-PGlu	[68]
Doxorubicin	Encapsulation method	m-PEG-PLGA-PGlu	[69]
Doxorubicin	Entrapment	PEO-b-PAsp	[26]
Doxorubicin	Encapsulation method	PEO-PPO-PEO	[70, 71]
Doxorubicin	Encapsulation method	PCLLA-PEG-PCLLA	[72]
Paclitaxel	Entrapment method	PEI-PLA	[73]
Paclitaxel	Co-polymer drug conjugation	HPMA	[74]

Nonetheless, this was the first try at targeted treatment by utilizing a monoclonal antibody to target cancer, and resulted in cell death by direct and indirect pathways. These pathways are defined as the prevention of a pathway participating in cancer progression or the improvement of defense pathways via stimulation of cytotoxic mechanisms and complement-mediated cytotoxicity [77].

The revolutions in the subject of molecular biology established the development of novel targeted treatments and selective medicines specific to various cancers. These discoveries gave rise to a new revolution in cancer treatment, which started in the 1980s with the designing of selective kinase inhibitors and monoclonal antibodies [16]. Increased cure rates for germ cancer and cisplatin were attained by using bleomycin, vincristine, and cisplatin in combination [78].

Many drugs with different mechanisms were developed in the 1980s. Succeeding developments gave rise to liposomal therapy, which puts medicines inside it reducing some adverse effects of chemotherapy like cardiotoxicity. In 1989, the NCI introduced a disease-oriented screening using 60 cell lines derived from different types of human tumors [16].

Targeted chemotherapy was started in the 1990s by analyzing important targets. This was possible due to research work carried out on transcriptomics, genomics, and the human genome. This is also due to the awareness in molecular and cellular areas and improvement in drug discovery techniques. We observed the growth of targeted therapy [79].

In 1989, the NCI introduced a disease-oriented screening using 60 cell lines derived from different types of human tumors. In 1992, the FDA approved paclitaxel (Taxol), which became the first highly effective oncology drug. Studies by Brian Druker in 2001 led to FDA approval of imatinib mesylate for chronic myelogenous leukemia, a new drug in targeted chemotherapy [20].

In 2004, the FDA approved bevacizumab, the first clinically proven anti-angiogenic agent for the treatment of colon cancer. Researchers at Harvard University in 2004 defined mutations in the epidermal growth factor receptor that conferred selective responses to the targeted agent gefitinib, indicating that conferred selective responsiveness to the targeted agent gefitinib, showing that molecular testing might be able to prospectively identify subsets of patients that would respond to targeted agents [80].

1.4.1 MONOCLONAL ANTIBODIES IN TUMOR TREATMENT

After the discovery of trastuzumab in 1992 many monoclonal antibodies were introduced clinically for tumor. In 1975 Köhler and Milstein reorganized tumor therapeutics with hybridoma technology, utilized to form monoclonal antibodies. Succeeding due to genetic engineering technologies many kinds of monoclonal antibodies were obtained for the therapy of hematological and solid tumors [81].

A combination regimen consisting CHOP chemotherapy (cyclophosphamide, doxorubicin, vincristine, prednisone) and rituximab was suggested in 2002. This regimen has revealed a remarkable result improvement in patients suffering from non-Hodgkin lymphomas. Genentech discovered pertuzumab, accepted by the FDA in 2012 [82].

In succeeding years, panitumumab was discovered and accepted for the therapy of metastatic colorectal tumors obstinate to standard chemotherapeutic drugs. The development of bevacizumab was started in 1983. Bevacizumab, used as a single drug, was well tolerated by patients and when administered with other anti-tumor drugs did not cause a rise in systemic adverse effects. Nivolumab and pembrolizumab were the antibodies designed in 2012 [83].

1.4.2 SELECTIVE TYROSINE KINASE AND SERINE/THREONINE-PROTEIN KINASE SMALL MOLECULES INHIBITORS

Imatinib mesylate, a tyrosine kinase blocker that was developed in the early 1990s, is a competitive blocker of ATP. It was an important event in the development of targeted therapy. Imatinib was found effective for treating gastrointestinal stromal tumors. Gefitinib, accepted for the treatment of NSCLC in 2001, exhibited anti-cancer activity in many cancers like ovarian, colon, lung, and breast cancers [84].

Erlotinib is approved for the treatment of NSCLC (non-small cell lung cancer) and for advanced and/or metastatic pancreatic carcinoma, in association with gemcitabine. Lapatinib is an inhibitor of HER1 (epidermal growth factor receptor 1) and HER2 (epidermal growth factor receptor 2) accepted in 2007, inhibits cancer cell growth. Lapatinib is utilized in combination with many chemotherapeutic drugs like trastuzumab and capecitabine in patients with HER2-positive breast tumors. In 2006, the FDA accepted sunitinib malate for the therapy of advanced renal cell carcinoma [85].

Other selective blockers were designed for treating hematological malignancies like multiple myeloma and mantle cell lymphoma. Among these blockers, carfilzomib and bortezomib are used clinically nowadays. All these targeted drugs are presently utilized for treating cancers, frequently in association with other anti-cancer drugs or with monoclonal antibodies [86]. Erlotinib was approved for the therapy of NSCLC and metastatic pancreatic carcinoma.

These developments and research on genetics played an important role in the decline in mortality rates. Details from genome sequence revealed that various disorders linked with tumors might be due to the irregular functioning of a few protein kinases. The present pharmacological drift has been to design kinase inhibitors [87]. Initial cancers treated by medicines accepted by the FDA was renal tumor, gastrointestinal stromal cancer, and hepatocellular cancer.

In present years, many tumors have been analyzed with many kinase inhibitors and there is a swing towards combination treatment with these novel targeted medicines. Since 1990 the occurrence and death due to tumors have been reducing and notwithstanding the rise in the aged population, the death rate decreased from 2005 to 2007 in the United States.

In 2004, the FDA approved bevacizumab, the first clinically proven anti-angiogenic agent for the treatment of colon cancer. Researchers at Harvard University in 2004 defined mutations in the epidermal growth factor receptor that conferred selective responses to the targeted agent gefitinib, indicating that conferred selective responsiveness to the targeted agent gefitinib, showing that molecular testing might be able to prospectively identify subsets of patients that would respond to targeted agents [80].

1.4.3 Immune Checkpoint Inhibitors for Tumor Therapy

A new strategy for the tumor treatment was the first accepted immune checkpoint blocker, ipilimumab, developed in 2011. Ipilimumab is a human IgG1 antibody, which activates the immune system against tumors. Ipilimumab is used alone or in combination with nivolumab for the therapy of metastatic melanoma [88].

Currently, nivolumab and pembrolizumab are two antibodies accepted for the therapy of metastatic melanoma, urothelial carcinoma, and NSCLC. Durvalumab is a monoclonal antibody accepted therapeutically for metastatic urothelial carcinoma. Immune checkpoint inhibitors are used in association with other anti-cancer drugs for making regimens as efficacious as possible [89].

1.4.4 Molecular Radiotherapy in Tumor

Molecular radiotherapy is a therapeutic strategy used in clinical practice for many decades based on the usage of radiopharmaceuticals like sodium iodide, 89Sr-strontium chloride, 32P-sodium phosphate, phosphorus-32, yttrium-90, and yttrium-90. These are ingested or injected. Radiopharmaceuticals were first used in 1942 when iodine-131 was used for treating Basedow-Graves' disease [90]. Nowadays, radiotherapy is used for treating tumors like thyroid cancers, bone metastasis, phaeochromocytoma, neuroblastoma, colorectal liver metastasis, and neuroendocrine tumors [91].

Drug discovery is a continuously evolving field and many new strategies and approaches are suggested every year. Parallel to the rise in the number of drugs and the effectiveness of therapies, remarkable improvement was noticed in the survival of patients.

The chemotherapeutics act through different mechanisms, including nucleic acid synthesis inhibiting alteration in DNA structure. Chemotherapy can damage normal cells and can lead to body damage, including hair loss, and gastrointestinal toxicity [80]. The word chemotherapy comes from two words chemical and therapy and these agents tend to damage the parasitic cells without damaging the host cells. However, the selection and effectiveness of chemotherapeutic drugs depend upon the growth, area, location, and type of cancer and to how much extent the cancer is spread to the body tissues.

Several factors affect chemotherapy including the apparent condition of the patient, the stage of cancer at which the chemotherapy was started, and the interaction of the drugs. The mode of chemotherapeutics depends upon understanding the cellular mechanisms. The human cell cycle is the same by which both the normal and cancerous cells pass. During the cell division process, the cell undergoes five different phases namely G1, S, G2, M, and G_0 (Figure 1.2).

G1: The cell prepares for division, post-mitotic gap.
S: DNA synthesis takes place in this step for cell division (most of the chemotherapeutics act on this step to cause the death of cancerous cells).
G2: In this step, specialized protein and RNA are synthesized for cell division normally refers to as pre-mitotic gap.
M: The 'M' refers to the mitotic phase in which the cell divides into identical cells.
Go: This is the resting phase; the cells remain alive but are unable to divide.

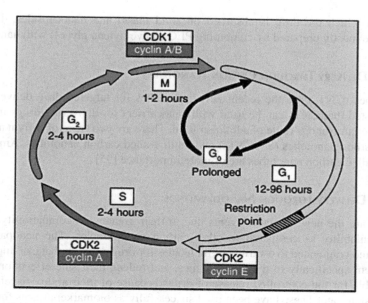

FIGURE 1.2 Different phases of the cell cycle [92].

Chemotherapy usually involves a properly planned treatment (course) within a specific time, which may last for up to 6 months. The course of chemotherapy involves fixed treatment days over the week and then the cycle is repeated for another few weeks. The reason for the repeated treatment plan is that some cells that are in the resting phase during the first treatment cycle will be destroyed during the next and the gap between the cycle helps the human body to recover from the side effects [93].

The side effects due to chemotherapy can be of various intensities varying from mild to moderate, severe, etc. The long-term side effects lead to the damage in bone marrow, blood, nephrotoxicity, etc. [94].

1.4.5 Use of Nanotechnology in Cancer Treatment Through Gene Therapy

Gene therapy is the transfer of genetic material to the human cells, to ensure the targeted molecular intervention and to achieve the desired higher level action at the specific site than the usual cytotoxic chemotherapy. Despite the promising factors, there are a number of difficulties associated with gene therapy.

In recent years, gene silencing technology has gained popularity. There are three main types of nucleic acid-based gene silencing, i.e., antisense oligodeoxyribonucleic acids, siRNA, and micro RNA. The success of gene therapy depends largely upon the activity produced by targeted genes and the route used for drug delivery.

1.4.6 Polymeric Nanoparticles as the Targeted Drug Delivery Systems

The polymeric nanoparticles give a promising means of targeted drug delivery systems for the chemotherapeutic agents with higher efficacy, controlled and long-term drug release, fewer side effects, increased patient compliance, and ability to cod-liver more than one drug with synergistic effects at the same site.

The protective covering of polymeric nanoparticles on the chemotherapeutic drugs refrains them to interact with healthy cells. Polymeric nanoparticles are available in different forms including nanospheres (in which the drug is absorbed on solid mass) and nanocapsules. The polymeric nanoparticles are mostly prepared by combining PEG (polyethylene glycol) with nanoparticles.

1.4.7 Drug Delivery Through Carbon Nanotubes

Carbon nanotubes (CNTs) are the recent new approaches for targeted drug delivery systems. It has been suggested that CNTs can be used with nanocarriers for delivering drugs into the human body through the intravenous route of administration. There are two types of carbon nanotubes, i.e., single-walled carbon nanotubes (SWCNTs) and multi-walled carbon nanotubes. Among these two types, single-walled carbon nanotubes are of more importance [95].

1.4.8 Drug Delivery Through Nanodiamonds

Nanodiamonds are the new attractive agents due to their greater bio-compatibility, stability, and commercial availability as compared to other carbon nanoparticles. The nanoparticles can be functionalized and conjugated to a variety of molecules for drug delivery that can improve the solubility, direct them specifically to the targeted sites, and reduce their side effects on normal cells. These are suitable for the controlled release of drugs because of their ability to release the drugs slowly at a constant rate. These have been used successfully as biomarkers/traces for the treatment of lung cancers [96].

1.4.9 Radiomics and Patronymics

Currently, the radiomics and pathomics are two innovative and promising fields based on collecting the quantitative imaging features from pathology and radiology screening as therapeutic and prognostic indicators. Effective cancer therapy relies on surgery and in almost 50% of patients it relies on radiotherapy that can be delivered by using an external beam source of a radioactive compound or by locally inserting a radioactive source. The localization of the beam is facilitated by image-guided radiotherapy (IGRT), in which the images of the patients are required during the session of treatment to allow the best amount of radiation to be set. With the invention of intensity-modulated radiotherapy (IMRT), radiation fields with different intensities can be created, which helps to receive lower doses to the healthy tissues thus preventing the healthy tissues from much damage. In this type of treatment, radioactivity resistance may arise during the treatment session leading to its lower efficacy. The patronymics rely on the generation and characterization of the high resolution of tissue imaging.

1.4.10 Thermal Ablation and Magnetic Hyperthermia

Thermal ablation includes hyperthermia or hypothermia (exploit heat or cold) for the destruction of neoplastic tissues. In this method, cell necrosis occurs at higher temperatures (60°C) or low-temperature values (–40°C). Long exposure to a temperature between 41–55°C shows effectiveness in tumor necrosis. In studies, it has been recorded that cancerous cells are more sensitive to heat than healthy cells.

The hypothermic destructions are because of the formation of ice crystals, upon cooling, which leads to the destruction of the cell membrane leading to cell death. Argon gas is the preferred cooling agent that can be used (as it can cool down up to –160°C).

Hyperthermic ablation uses radiofrequency, microwave, and laser ablation. Radiofrequency ablation is mostly used in clinics, which are applied to a target zone with the help of an insulated electrode tip while the second electrode is needed to close the circuit, and is placed on the skin surface. This interaction with skin leads to the rotation of the ions in the extracellular fluids leading towards heat production.

TABLE 1.5
Different Cancer Treatments with Merits and Demerits

Sr. No.	Type of Treatment	Advantages	Disadvantages
1.	Nanoparticles	1: good biocompatibility and bioavailability 2: more specificity and more stability	1: depends upon the particular nanoparticle
2.	Natural antioxidants	1: easily available in higher quantities 2: exploitation of intrinsic properties	1: low bioavailability 2: toxicity
3.	Targeted therapy	1: low side effects 2: higher specificity	1: lack of information regarding long-term side effects
4.	Gene therapy	1: expression of pro-apoptotic and chemosensitizing genes 2: expression of genes able to solicit a specific anti-tumour immune response 3: targeted silencing of oncogenes and safety.	1: limited efficacy in a specific subset of patients 2: genome integration. 3: Inflammation 4: off-target side effects
5.	Thermal ablation Magnetic hyperthermia	1: precise treatment in the specific area 2: the possibility of more accurate treatment along with magnetic hyperthermia (MRI imaging).	1: high efficiency only for localized areas 2: less penetration access
6.	Pathomics / Radiomics	1: therapeutic and prognostic indicators of disease outcome	1: many factors are undefined up to now 2: need more precision in work

Microwave ablation is based upon the electromagnetic interaction betwixt the polar molecules and microwaves in the tissues like water leading towards the increase in temperature (Table 1.5). A new way to treat tumors is through magnetic hyperthermia. This technology uses ferromagnetic or super-para-magnetic nanoparticles that can produce heat after stimulation with an alternating magnetic field. Magnetic hyperthermia can reach any part of the body. The most studied systems in nanoparticles are SPIONs. To date, a formulation of 15 nm iron oxide nanoparticles coated with aminosilane has gotten approval for the treatment of glioblastoma [97].

1.5 CONCLUSION

History of cancer treatment ranges from chemotherapy, radiotherapy, and surgery to more advanced techniques like nanotechnologies (micelles, liposomes, microspheres, nanospheres, nanoparticles, polymeric nanoparticles, carbon nanotubes, nanodiamonds), photodynamic therapy, hyperthermia, immunotherapy, etc. Nanotechnology is offering novel techniques, which are either utilized alone or in association with other anti-cancer drugs and could be utilized to target tumor cells. Nanoparticles lead the treatment of cancer to a new level. Many tumors resist standard therapies, and a combination of different therapeutic choices is the only solution to destroy the cancerous tissues. In short, it is evident that tumor therapies are continually developing. Since the Second World War, there has been a rise in the number of new medicines and treatments available for treating solid and hematological cancers, which have caused a remarkable decrease in tumor death rates. More research work is needed because these chemotherapeutic agents along with other novel ways of therapy are opening doors for the successful treatment of cancer.

REFERENCES

1. Galmarini, C.M., *Lessons from Hippocrates: Time to change the cancer paradigm. International Journal of Chronic Diseases*, 2020. **2020**: 4715426.

2. Grammaticos, P.C. and A. Diamantis, *Useful known and unknown views of the father of modern medicine, Hippocrates and his teacher Democritus. Hellenic Journal of Nuclear Medicine*, 2008. **11**(1): pp. 2–4.

3. Faguet, G.B., *A brief history of cancer: Age-old milestones underlying our current knowledge database. International Journal of Cancer*, 2015. **136**(9): pp. 2022–2036.

4. Nutton, V., *Galen, On my own opinions: Edition, Translation and Commentary, CMG V 3, 2*. 1999, Akademie Verlag: Berlin.

5. Karpozilos, A. and N. Pavlidis, *The treatment of cancer in Greek antiquity. European Journal of Cancer*, 2004. **40**(14): pp. 2033–2040.

6. Benjamin, D.J., *The efficacy of surgical treatment of cancer–20 years later. Medical Hypotheses*, 2014. **82**(4): pp. 412–420.

7. McCrate, F., et al., *Surgical treatment choices for breast cancer in Newfoundland and Labrador: A retrospective cohort study. Canadian Journal of Surgery*, 2018. **61**(6): p. 377.

8. Tohme, S., R.L. Simmons, and A. Tsung, *Surgery for cancer: A trigger for metastases. Cancer Research*, 2017. **77**(7): pp. 1548–1552.

9. Baskar, R., et al., *Cancer and radiation therapy: current advances and future directions. International Journal of Medical Sciences*, 2012. **9**(3): p. 193.

10. Jackson, S.P. and J. Bartek, *The DNA-damage response in human biology and disease. Nature*, 2009. **461**(7267): pp. 1071–1078.

11. Chen, H.H. and M.T. Kuo, *Improving radiotherapy in cancer treatment: Promises and challenges. Oncotarget*, 2017. **8**(37): p. 62742.

12. Barton, M.B., et al., *Estimating the demand for radiotherapy from the evidence: A review of changes from 2003 to 2012. Radiotherapy and Oncology*, 2014. **112**(1): pp. 140–144.

13. Baskar, R., et al., *Biological response of cancer cells to radiation treatment. Frontiers in Molecular Biosciences*, 2014. **1**: p. 24.

14. Zhou, Q., L. Zhang, and H. Wu, *Nanomaterials for cancer therapies. Nanotechnology Reviews*, 2017. **6**(5): pp. 473–496.

15. Shields, M., *Chemotherapeutics*. In *Pharmacognosy*. 2017, Elsevier: Amsterdam. pp. 295–313.

16. Falzone, L., S. Salomone, and M. Libra, *Evolution of cancer pharmacological treatments at the turn of the third millennium. Frontiers in Pharmacology*, 2018. **9**: p. 1300.

17. Gilman, A. *Therapeutic applications of chemical warfare agents*. In *Federation Proceedings*. 1946. **5**: pp. 285–292.

18. Heidelberger, C., et al., *Fluorinated pyrimidines, a new class of tumour-inhibitory compounds. Nature*, 1957. **179**(4561): pp. 663–666.

19. Pearson, O., et al., *Acth- and cortisone-induced regression of lymphoid tumors in man. A preliminary report. Cancer*, 1949. **2**(6): pp. 943–945.

20. Arruebo, M., et al., *Assessment of the evolution of cancer treatment therapies. Cancers*, 2011. **3**(3): pp. 3279–3330.

21. Lilenbaum, R.C., et al., *Single-agent versus combination chemotherapy in advanced non–small-cell lung cancer: The Cancer and Leukemia Group B (study 9730). Journal of Clinical Oncology*, 2005. **23**(1): pp. 190–196.

22. DeVita, V.T., A. Serpick, and P.P. Carbone, *Preliminary clinical studies with ibenzmethyzin. Clinical Pharmacology & Therapeutics*, 1966. **7**(4): pp. 542–546.

23. Gulfam, M., et al., *Anticancer drug-loaded gliadin nanoparticles induce apoptosis in breast cancer cells. Langmuir*, 2012. **28**(21): pp. 8216–8223.

24. Ghosh, S., *Cisplatin: The first metal based anticancer drug. Bioorganic Chemistry*, 2019. **88**: p. 102925.

25. Ciaffaglione, V., et al., *Mutual prodrugs of 5-fluorouracil: From a classic chemotherapeutic agent to novel potential anticancer drugs. ChemMedChem*, 2021. **16**(23): pp. 3496–3512.

26. Vilar, G., J. Tulla-Puche, and F. Albericio, *Polymers and drug delivery systems. Current Drug Delivery*, 2012. **9**(4): pp. 367–394.

27. Çırpanlı, Y., et al., *Antitumoral activity of camptothecin-loaded nanoparticles in 9L rat glioma model. International Journal of Pharmaceutics*, 2011. **403**(1–2): pp. 201–206.

28. Hu, J., et al., *Paclitaxel-loaded polymeric nanoparticles combined with chronomodulated chemotherapy on lung cancer: In vitro and in vivo evaluation. International Journal of Pharmaceutics*, 2017. **516**(1–2): pp. 313–322.

29. Guo, J., et al., *Aptamer-functionalized PEG–PLGA nanoparticles for enhanced anti-glioma drug delivery. Biomaterials*, 2011. **32**(31): pp. 8010–8020.

30. Qi, L., et al., *Development of mitomycin C-loaded nanoparticles prepared using the micellar assembly driven by the combined effect of hydrogen bonding and π–π stacking and its therapeutic application in bladder cancer. Pharmaceutics*, 2021. **13**(11): p. 1776.

31. Enriquez, C.A.G., A.I. Espiritu, and P.M.D. Pasco, *Efficacy and tolerability of mitoxantrone for neuromyelitis optica spectrum disorder: A systematic review. Journal of Neuroimmunology*, 2019. **332**: pp. 126–134.

32. Bradner, W., *Mitomycin C: A clinical update. Cancer Treatment Reviews*, 2001. **27**(1): pp. 35–50.

33. Crooke, S.T. and W.T. Bradner, *Mitomycin C: A review. Cancer Treatment Reviews*, 1976. **3**(3): pp. 121–139.

34. Reyhanoglu, G. and P. Tadi, *Etoposide.* In StatPearls [Internet]. 2020, Treasure Island: StatPearls Publishing: USA.

35. Wen, Q., et al., *Real-world evidence of ABVD-like regimens compared with ABVD in classical Hodgkin lymphoma: a 10-year study from China. Journal of Cancer Research and Clinical Oncology*, 2023: **149**(7): pp. 3989–4003.

36. Perez, E.A., *Carboplatin in combination therapy for metastatic breast cancer. The Oncologist*, 2004. **9**(5): pp. 518–527.

37. Chen, X., et al., *Weekly paclitaxel plus carboplatin is an effective nonanthracycline-containing regimen as neoadjuvant chemotherapy for breast cancer. Annals of Oncology*, 2010. **21**(5): pp. 961–967.

38. Fuchs, C., E.P. Mitchell, and P.M. Hoff, *Irinotecan in the treatment of colorectal cancer. Cancer Treatment Reviews*, 2006. **32**(7): pp. 491–503.

39. Carmichael, J., et al., *Phase II study of gemcitabine in patients with advanced pancreatic cancer. British Journal of Cancer*, 1996. **73**(1): pp. 101–105.

40. Epelbaum, R., et al., *Curcumin and gemcitabine in patients with advanced pancreatic cancer. Nutrition and Cancer*, 2010. **62**(8): pp. 1137–1141.

41. Allen-Mersh, T., et al., *Quality of life and survival with continuous hepatic-artery floxuridine infusion for colorectal liver metastases. The Lancet*, 1994. **344**(8932): pp. 1255–1260.

42. Sarosy, G., et al., *The systemic administration of intravenous melphalan. Journal of Clinical Oncology*, 1988. **6**(11): pp. 1768–1782.

43. DeVita Jr, V.T., A.A. Serpick, and P.P. Carbone, *Combination chemotherapy in the treatment of advanced Hodgkin's disease. Annals of Internal Medicine*, 1970. **73**(6): pp. 881–895.

44. De Lena, M., et al., *Treatment of metastatic breast cancer with cyclophosphamide, methotrexate, vincristine and fluorouracil. Tumori Journal*, 1973. **59**(1): pp. 11–24.

45. Bonadonna, G., et al., *Combination chemotherapy of Hodgkin's disease with adriamycin, bleomycin, vinblastine, and imidazole carboxamide versus MOPP. Cancer*, 1975. **36**(1): pp. 252–259.

46. Cukierman, E. and D.R. Khan, *The benefits and challenges associated with the use of drug delivery systems in cancer therapy. Biochemical Pharmacology*, 2010. **80**(5): pp. 762–770.

47. Deshpande, P.P., S. Biswas, and V.P. Torchilin, *Current trends in the use of liposomes for tumor targeting. Nanomedicine*, 2013. **8**(9): pp. 1509–1528.

48. Patil, Y.P. and S. Jadhav, *Novel methods for liposome preparation. Chemistry and Physics of Lipids*, 2014. **177**: pp. 8–18.

49. Ali, M.Y., *Advanced Colloidal Systems for Targeted Chemotherapy.* 2019, Philipps-Universität Marburg.

50. Dürr, S., et al., *Magnetic nanoparticles for cancer therapy. Nanotechnology Reviews*, 2013. **2**(4): pp. 395–409.

51. Gu, F.X., et al., *Targeted nanoparticles for cancer therapy. Nano Today*, 2007. **2**(3): pp. 14–21.

52. Nguyen, K.T., *Targeted nanoparticles for cancer therapy: Promises and challenges. Journal of Nanomedicine and Nanotechnology* 2011. **2**(5).

53. Saha, R.N., et al., *Nanoparticulate drug delivery systems for cancer chemotherapy. Molecular Membrane Biology*, 2010. **27**(7): pp. 215–231.

54. Misra, R., S. Acharya, and S.K. Sahoo, *Cancer nanotechnology: Application of nanotechnology in cancer therapy. Drug Discovery Today*, 2010. **15**(19–20): pp. 842–850.

55. Guo, X., et al., *Polymer-based drug delivery systems for cancer treatment. Journal of Polymer Science Part A: Polymer Chemistry*, 2016. **54**(22): pp. 3525–3550.

56. Dreaden, E.C., et al., *Size matters: Gold nanoparticles in targeted cancer drug delivery. Therapeutic Delivery*, 2012. **3**(4): pp. 457–478.

57. Fukumori, Y. and H. Ichikawa, *Nanoparticles for cancer therapy and diagnosis. Advanced Powder Technology*, 2006. **17**(1): pp. 1–28.

58. Sharma, A., A.K. Goyal, and G. Rath, *Recent advances in metal nanoparticles in cancer therapy. Journal of Drug Targeting*, 2018. **26**(8): pp. 617–632.

59. Chompunut, L., et al., *Synthesis of copper nanoparticles from the aqueous extract of Cynodon dactylon and evaluation of its antimicrobial and photocatalytic properties. Food and Chemical Toxicology*, 2022. **166**: p. 113245.

60. Dilda, P.J. and P.J. Hogg, *Arsenical-based cancer drugs. Cancer Treatment Reviews*, 2007. **33**(6): pp. 542–564.

61. Kuppusamy, P., et al., *In vitro anticancer activity of Au, Ag nanoparticles synthesized using Commelina nudiflora L. aqueous extract against HCT-116 colon cancer cells. Biological Trace Element Research*, 2016. **173**: pp. 297–305.

62. Bilensoy, E., *Cationic nanoparticles for cancer therapy. Expert Opinion on Drug Delivery*, 2010. **7**(7): pp. 795–809.

63. Eatemadi, A., et al., *Comparison, synthesis and evaluation of anticancer drug-loaded polymeric nanoparticles on breast cancer cell lines. Artificial Cells, Nanomedicine, and Biotechnology*, 2016. **44**(3): pp. 1008–1017.

64. Li, F., et al., *Anti-tumor activity of paclitaxel-loaded chitosan nanoparticles: An in vitro study. Materials Science and Engineering: C*, 2009. **29**(8): pp. 2392–2397.

65. Bilensoy, E., et al., *Development of nonsurfactant cyclodextrin nanoparticles loaded with anticancer drug paclitaxel. Journal of Pharmaceutical Sciences*, 2008. **97**(4): pp. 1519–1529.

66. Koziara, J.M., et al., *In-vivo efficacy of novel paclitaxel nanoparticles in paclitaxel-resistant human colorectal tumors. Journal of Controlled Release*, 2006. **112**(3): pp. 312–319.

67. Shafiei-Irannejad, V., et al., *Reversion of multidrug resistance by co-encapsulation of doxorubicin and metformin in poly (lactide-co-glycolide)-d-α-tocopheryl polyethylene glycol 1000 succinate nanoparticles. Pharmaceutical Research*, 2018. **35**: pp. 1–13.

68. Plummer, R., et al., *A phase I clinical study of cisplatin-incorporated polymeric micelles (NC-6004) in patients with solid tumours. British Journal of Cancer*, 2011. **104**(4): pp. 593–598.

69. Yuan, J.-D., et al., *pH-sensitive polymeric nanoparticles of mPEG-PLGA-PGlu with hybrid core for simultaneous encapsulation of curcumin and doxorubicin to kill the heterogeneous tumour cells in breast cancer. Artificial Cells, Nanomedicine, and Biotechnology*, 2018. **46**(sup1): pp. 302–313.

70. Venne, A., et al., *Hypersensitizing effect of pluronic L61 on cytotoxic activity, transport, and subcellular distribution of doxorubicin in multiple drug-resistant cells. Cancer Research*, 1996. **56**(16): pp. 3626–3629.

71. Valle, J.W., et al., *A phase 2 study of SP1049C, doxorubicin in P-glycoprotein-targeting pluronics, in patients with advanced adenocarcinoma of the esophagus and gastroesophageal junction. Investigational New Drugs*, 2011. **29**: pp. 1029–1037.

72. Hu, D., et al., *Oxygen-generating hybrid polymeric nanoparticles with encapsulated doxorubicin and chlorin e6 for trimodal imaging-guided combined chemo-photodynamic therapy. Theranostics*, 2018. **8**(6): p. 1558.

73. Jin, M., et al., *Smart polymeric nanoparticles with pH-responsive and PEG-detachable properties for co-delivering paclitaxel and survivin siRNA to enhance antitumor outcomes. International Journal of Nanomedicine*, 2018. **13**: p. 2405.

74. Terwogt, J.M.M., et al., *Phase I clinical and pharmacokinetic study of PNU166945, a novel water-soluble polymer-conjugated prodrug of paclitaxel. Anti-Cancer Drugs*, 2001. **12**(4): pp. 315–323.

75. Köhler, G. and C. Milstein, *Continuous cultures of fused cells secreting antibody of predefined specificity. Nature*, 1975. **256**(5517): pp. 495–497.

76. Nadler, L.M., et al., *Serotherapy of a patient with a monoclonal antibody directed against a human lymphoma-associated antigen. Cancer Research*, 1980. **40**(9): pp. 3147–3154.

77. O'Mahony, D. and M.R. Bishop, *Monoclonal antibody therapy. Frontiers in Bioscience-Landmark*, 2006. **11**(2): pp. 1620–1635.

78. Einhorn, L.H., *Testicular cancer as a model for a curable neoplasm: The Richard and Hinda Rosenthal Foundation Award Lecture. Cancer Research*, 1981. **41**(9_Part_1): pp. 3275–3280.

79. Tsimberidou, A.-M., *Targeted therapy in cancer. Cancer Chemotherapy and Pharmacology*, 2015. **76**: pp. 1113–1132.

80. Chabner, B.A. and T.G. Roberts Jr, *Chemotherapy and the war on cancer. Nature Reviews Cancer*, 2005. **5**(1): pp. 65–72.

81. Pento, J.T., *Monoclonal antibodies for the treatment of cancer. Anticancer Research*, 2017. **37**(11): pp. 5935–5939.

82. Harbeck, N., et al., *HER2 dimerization inhibitor pertuzumab-mode of action and clinical data in breast cancer. Breast Care*, 2013. **8**(1): pp. 49–55.

83. Gordon, M., et al., *Phase I safety and pharmacokinetic study of recombinant human anti-vascular endothelial growth factor in patients with advanced cancer. Journal of Clinical Oncology*, 2001. **19**(3): pp. 843–850.

84. Ciardiello, F., et al., *Antitumor effect and potentiation of cytotoxic drugs activity in human cancer cells by ZD-1839 (Iressa), an epidermal growth factor receptor-selective tyrosine kinase inhibitor. Clinical Cancer Research*, 2000. **6**(5): pp. 2053–2063.

85. Adams, V.R. and M. Leggas, *Sunitinib malate for the treatment of metastatic renal cell carcinoma and gastrointestinal stromal tumors. Clinical Therapeutics*, 2007. **29**(7): pp. 1338–1353.

86. Vanneman, M. and G. Dranoff, *Combining immunotherapy and targeted therapies in cancer treatment. Nature Reviews Cancer*, 2012. **12**(4): pp. 237–251.

87. Manning, G., et al., *The protein kinase complement of the human genome. Science*, 2002. **298**(5600): pp. 1912–1934.

88. Sakamuri, D., et al., *Phase I dose-escalation study of anti–CTLA-4 antibody ipilimumab and lenalidomide in patients with advanced cancers ipilimumab and lenalidomide in advanced malignancies. Molecular Cancer Therapeutics*, 2018. **17**(3): pp. 671–676.

89. Faiena, I., et al., *Durvalumab: An investigational anti-PD-L1 monoclonal antibody for the treatment of urothelial carcinoma. Drug Design, Development and Therapy*, 2018. **12**: pp. 209–215.

90. Hertz, S., A. Roberts, and W. Salter, *Radioactive iodine as an indicator in thyroid physiology. IV. The metabolism of iodine in Graves'disease. The Journal of Clinical Investigation*, 1942. **21**(1): pp. 25–29.

91. Cheng, Y., et al., *Phosphorus-32, a clinically available drug, inhibits cancer growth by inducing DNA double-strand breakage. PLoS One*, 2015. **10**(6): p. e0128152.

92. Israels, E. and L. Israels, *The cell cycle. The Oncologist*, 2000. **5**(6): pp. 510–513.

93. Dua, P., V. Dua, and E.N. Pistikopoulos, *Optimal delivery of chemotherapeutic agents in cancer. Computers & Chemical Engineering*, 2008. **32**(1–2): pp. 99–107.

94. Schirrmacher, V., *From chemotherapy to biological therapy: A review of novel concepts to reduce the side effects of systemic cancer treatment. International Journal of Oncology*, 2019. **54**(2): pp. 407–419.

95. Elhissi, A., et al., *Carbon nanotubes in cancer therapy and drug delivery. Journal of Drug Delivery*, 2012. **2012**: 837327.

96. Jabir, N.R., et al., *Nanotechnology-based approaches in anticancer research. International Journal of Nanomedicine*, 2012. **7**: pp. 4391–4408.

97. Pucci, C., C. Martinelli, and G. Ciofani, *Innovative approaches for cancer treatment: Current perspectives and new challenges. Ecancermedicalscience*, 2019. **13**: p. 961.

2 Cancer and Carcinogens

*Saba Riaz, Azhar Rasul, Muhammad Asif Khalil,
Laiba Ameen, Komal Riaz, Samreen Gul Khan,
Sevki Adem, Mudassir Hassan, Muhammad Javid Iqbal,
Muhammad Asrar, and Muhammad Yasir Ali*

2.1 INTRODUCTION

Cancer is characterized by a condition in which tissues grow abnormally and spread throughout the body and all the cells of our body are equally susceptible to it. The phenomenon by which normal cells become cancerous is called carcinogenesis [1]. Skin cancer is the most common cause of cancer, among other cancers, with increased prevalence worldwide [2]. Other types include cancer of the prostate, breast, lungs, and colon (the latter type is often combined with the cancer of the rectum and termed colorectal cancer) [3].

Carcinogen is defined as "any substance, radionuclide, radiation, chemical, or combination of chemical substances that promotes carcinogenesis, at any level of dose or through any exposure route in animals". The word "carcinogen" derived from the Greek word, karkinos, meaning "crab" [4]. The term "complete carcinogen" refers to a substance that works as both an initiator and a promoter of tumor growth since tumor development can take place without the addition of another substance [5].

Although it is difficult to measure the number of cancer-related mortalities, an incredible 70–95% of the cases may be attributed to recognizing the risk factors, which include food (30–35%), cigarettes (25–30%), infections (15–20%), obesity (10–20%), alcohol (4–6%), and others (10–15%), such as pollution and radiation [6, 7]. In vivo study, cancer epidemiology studies and clinical research is necessary to demonstrate a link between chemical and human cancer [8].

2.1.1 TYPES OF CARCINOGENS

There are mainly three types of carcinogens (1) physical carcinogens, (2) chemical carcinogens, and (3) biological carcinogens as shown in Figure 2.1. Moreover, six broad categories can be used to group these carcinogens: (I) biological agents, (II) pharmaceuticals, (III) arsenic, fibers, metals, and dust, (IV) personal habits and indoor combustions' radiation (V) and chemicals, (VI) and associated fields of work [9].

2.1.2 CHARACTERISTICS OF CARCINOGENS

Human carcinogens are categorized by ten key characteristics (Figure 2.2), which include (1) change cell death, cell proliferation, and angiogenesis, (2) genotoxic, (3) change DNA repair, (4) cause epigenetic alterations, (5) cause oxidative stress, (6) induce chronic inflammation, (7) immunosuppression, (8) trigger receptor-mediated signaling, (9) induce cell immortalization, and (10) electrophilic or metabolically active [10, 11].

DOI: 10.1201/9781003363958-3

These essential properties of the carcinogens offer a mechanistic foundation for assessing their activity [12]. Many carcinogens display a number of these ten characteristics on average of four characteristics per agent [9]. Although carcinogens may not be immediately genotoxic, they can destroy DNA by inducing inflammation. Palladium, arsenic, cadmium, aluminum, titanium, chromium, cobalt, and nickel are heavy metals that cause serious problems by releasing cytokines that promote inflammation and oxidative stress (Figure 2.3) [13]. The primary features of carcinogens, for example, perfluoroalkyl and poly-fluoroalkyl substances (PFAS), are immunosuppression, oxidative

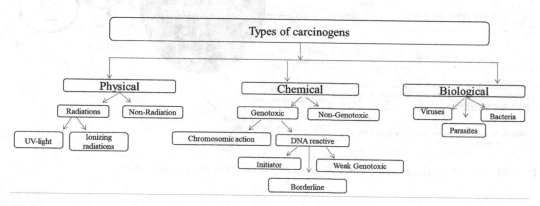

FIGURE 2.1 Types of carcinogens: (1) physical carcinogens, (2) chemical carcinogens, and (3) biological carcinogens.

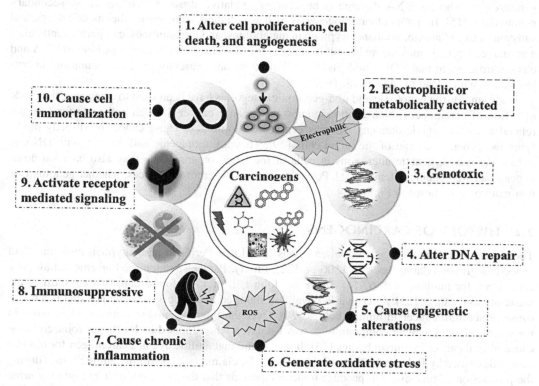

FIGURE 2.2 Schematic representation of different characteristics of carcinogens.

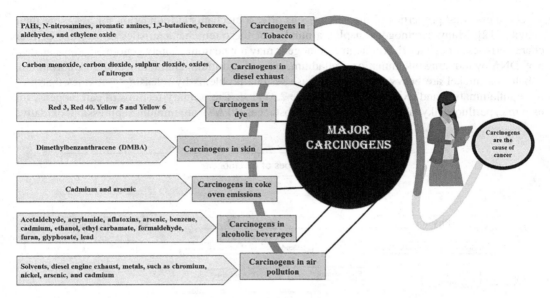

FIGURE 2.3   Major carcinogens, which we encounter in our daily life are elaborated.

stress, and receptor-mediated action. PFAS is responsible for cancer in animals and raises the risk of cancer [14].

Particle-induced carcinogens, such as polycyclic aromatic hydrocarbons can cause primary genotoxicity, whereas DNA damage is brought by oxidative stress, which can cause secondary genotoxicity [15]. Initiators of carcinogenesis, such as radiation, some chemotherapeutic drugs, and substances like aflatoxin, urethane, tryptophan metabolites, and nitrosamines, can permanently alter a normal cell genetic makeup and result in cancer [16, 17]. These carcinogens can bind to DNA and change structure to make DNA adducts. In the initiation stage, carcinogens cause mutations in critical genes, which lead to cancer [18, 19].

Traditionally, the genotoxic and non-genotoxic categories have been used to categorize the mode of action of carcinogens. Non-genotoxic substances cause cancer through pathways that are not related to direct genetic damage, whereas genotoxic carcinogens cause cancer by directly modifying the genetic material of the target cells [20]. They are mutagenic and interact with DNA to induce permanent genetic alterations in cells of the target organs. They may also have no dose-dependent carcinogenic potential [21]. Possible action of different substances, whether genotoxic or non-genotoxic is shown in Figure 2.4.

2.2   HISTORY OF CARCINOGENS

The history of carcinogens started when it was found that Peruvian and Egyptian mummies had cancerous growths dating back to 1500 BC [22]. Firstly, Paracelsus identified arsenic sulfide as a carcinogen for humans in 1567 [4]. Later on, John Hill in 1775 found that tobacco snuff is the cause of nasal cancer [23]. After that Percival Pott reported that soot is a carcinogen that is a major cause of scrotum cancer in human beings [24]. Over the time, scientists continued their work in the search of carcinogenic compounds. It was Bouisson who reported in 1859, that tobacco is the cause of oral cancer in human beings [25]. It was found that aniline dye is a carcinogen for bladder cancer described by Rehn in 1895. In his hypothesis, he claimed that breathing aniline fumes during the production of fuchsine that produce toxic compounds that the kidneys discharge into the urine and that prolonged urine stagnation in the ureters cause tumor growth. He found cases of bladder

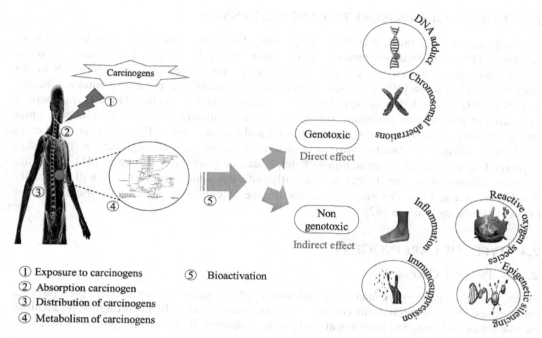

FIGURE 2.4 Genotoxic and non-genotoxic substances affect the body either directly or indirectly and result in DNA adduct formation, chromosomal aberrations, inflammation, immunosuppression, and so on.

cancer in 1906 [26]. After 5 years of experiments, the mutation theory of carcinogenesis was given by Boveri during the 1900s. After that radium was found as a carcinogen for skin cancer by Marie, Clunet, and Raulot-Lapointe in 1910–1912. By having exposure to paraffin, coal tar and different types of petroleum products increased the risk of skin cancer [27]. Along with research on human carcinogens, the first chemical induction of cancer in laboratory animals was given by Yamagiwa and Ichikawa in 1915 [28].

Later on, the first pure carcinogen,1,2,5,6-dibenzanthracene was reported by Kenneway and Cook in 1929 and the 1930s [29]. In the 1940s and 1960s, many experiments were conducted in laboratories and it was found that asbestos is a carcinogen that is the cause of mesothelioma [30]. Then, radon was also found as a carcinogen by the International Agency for Research on Cancer (IARC) in 1988 [31]. It was reported that indoor radon is a cause of lung cancer and is found to be the main cause of lung cancer among people who had never smoked [32]. Along with conducting experiments on radon, the IARC also found that alcoholic beverages are carcinogenic for human beings in 1988. There are about 18 carcinogenic compounds (cadmium, acetaldehyde, aflatoxins, furan, acrylamide, arsenic, benzene, 4-methylimidazole, ethanol, ochratoxin A, safrole, ethyl carbamate, formaldehyde, glyphosate, lead, N-nitroso dimethylamine, pulegone, 3-MCPD) in alcoholic beverages, which are identified by the IARC [33].

Later on, IARC categorized diesel exhaust as a human carcinogen in 2012 based on its carcinogenicity to the lungs [34]. After one year on October 17, 2013, an announcement was made by the World Health Organization (WHO) that outdoor air pollution can cause cancer in human beings [35]. It was also reported that the Basic Red 9 dye is also carcinogenic for humans [36].

Recently, according to the 15th report on carcinogens given by The National Toxicology Program (NTP), persistent *Helicobacter pylori* infection has been linked to human cancer [37]. Many new compounds are also found as human carcinogens, like exposure to aflatoxins is associated with an increased risk of liver cancer [38].

2.3   ROUTES OF EXPOSURE TO CARCINOGENS

Carcinogens can enter into the body by the process of dermal contact, ingestion, inhalation, or injection. The most common pathway is ingestion. Many heavy metals like arsenic, polycyclic aromatic hydrocarbons, and nitrosamines in preserved and smoked food enter in the body through ingestion [39]. The route of exposure to carcinogens present in smoke, tobacco, and air pollutants is inhalation [40]. The largest organ in the body is the skin, and transdermal exposures to carcinogens constitute another significant pathway to cancer. Carcinogens enter into the blood system by crossing the skin barrier and causing cancer. Eyes are peculiarly more sensitive to chemicals. Another way of exposure to carcinogens is by injection. If the skin is pierced or penetrated by contaminated items, carcinogens enter the body [41]. Exposure route of carcinogen is crucial since it frequently indicates which organ system will eventually develop neoplasia [39]. The risk for the occurrence of cancer increases with the amount of exposure to the carcinogen [42].

2.4   TYPES OF CARCINOGENS

2.4.1   Physical Carcinogens

Fibers, particle debris, gels, and hard and soft synthetic materials are examples of physical carcinogens. Physical carcinogens can be either man-made or naturally occurring. Non-radiations include asbestos, burns, and mechanical, and surgical implants. Radiations include ultraviolet light or ionizing radiation [43].

2.4.1.1   Fibers

Wollastonite, an asbestiform fiber, found in commercial talc and other fibrous silicates, is an example of natural fiber. Additional synthetic fibers include glass wool, rock wool and slag wool (produced by blowing, centrifuging, and dragging molten rock or slag), and ceramic fibers [44, 45]. "Several studies demonstrate biologically plausible and statistically significant increases in the incidence of lung cancer and mesothelioma in rats and hamsters exposed to glass wool by various routes using standard scientific methods: intrapleural injection, intrapleural implantation, intraperitoneal injection, and intratracheal instillation [46–48]". Glass wool fibers contribute to the elevated risk of lung cancer seen among employees [49].

2.4.1.2   Non-Fibrous Particulate Material

Metallic cobalt, crystalline silica, and nickel powders are examples of non-fibrous particles [50]. Following intrafemoral or subcutaneous insertion, pure metallic nickel particles with sizes between 2 and 50 m have been demonstrated to produce sarcomas of various histotypes in roughly 28% of implanted rats [51].

2.4.1.3   Particulate Air Pollution

Particulate matter is the conventional name for a concoction of solid and liquid droplets in the air. Diesel trucks, wood stoves, and industrial activities are some of the sources of particulate matter. Burning fuel in household fireplaces, wood stoves, and industrial processes produce fine particles that are released into the air. In the atmosphere, gases including sulfur dioxide, and nitrogen oxides can also produce fine particles [52].

Electromagnetic fields: The topic of extremely low-frequency electromagnetic fields (ELFEMF) has generated a lot of debate [53]. According to studies done in the 1980s and the early 1990s, leukemia, brain tumors, and male breast cancer may all be more common in ELFEMF-exposed employees [54].

2.4.1.3.1 Mechanism of Physical Carcinogens

Physical carcinogens employ different mechanisms, which are followed by cascades of reactions during which different proteins and enzymes are upregulated or downregulated and cause cell proliferation and neoplasia (Figure 2.5). The idea that solid carcinogens are inert leads to the physical theory. Exogenous DNA can generate mutations in eukaryotic cells in a variety of ways, which can aid in the development of asbestos-induced cancer [55].

2.4.2 BIOLOGICAL CARCINOGENS

When pathogenic bacteria interact with mammalian cells, a wide range of reactions occur in infected cells, like the internalization or phagocytosis of the bacteria, the release of cytokines, and the creation of oxygen radicals. Research, however, revealed that many bacteria are capable of inducing apoptosis in the host cells. Bacteria can upregulate endogenous receptors, which causes apoptosis on the upper surface of the infected cells, or to activate various pro-apoptotic proteins, such as caspases, and to inactivate anti-apoptotic proteins, such as NF kappa B or MAP-kinases [56]. The increased infections caused by bacteria, viruses [57, 58], and parasites [59] can either cause or inhibit apoptosis [60, 61]. There are some bacteria that may cause apoptosis; these are given below.

2.4.2.1 Shigella flexneri

Shigella flexneri is a model for bacterially caused apoptosis. *Shigella flexneri* secretes several proteins into the host cells or macrophages, using its type III secretions system. A number of proteins that make up different type III secretion systems [62] and eventually forms a needle-like structure out of rings or necks that span the inner and outer bacterial membranes. The type III secretion system can "inject" bacterial protein into the host cells when they come into contact with the membrane, which causes internalization of the bacteria and causes apoptosis. IpaB protein is one of the components that *Shigella flexneri* injects into macrophages [63]. Caspase 1 is activated when IpaB binds to it [63–66].

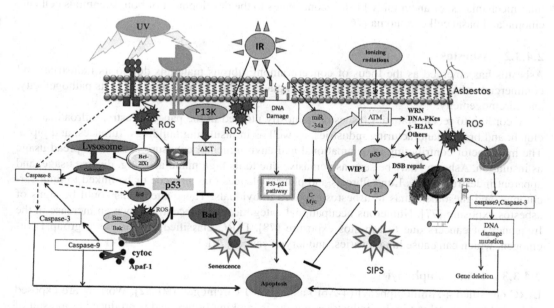

FIGURE 2.5 A cascade of changes takes place in different pathways during the action of carcinogens and ultimately results in cancer.

Studies have indicated that *Staphylococcus aureus* causes infection. *S. aureus* causes apoptosis by activating caspase 3 and 8, acid sphingomyelinase, and JUN-N-terminal kinases (JNK) [67]. *S. aureus* transfers some proteins into the host cells in connection with the induction of death by *Salmonella* or *Shigella*. These proteins either directly or indirectly activate caspases and the acid sphingomyelinase and JNK act as downstream targets of caspases. Toxins cause apoptosis by activating JNK, caspases, and sphingomyelinases. Two proteins necessary for induction of apoptosis in host cell macrophage are expressed by Yersinia species YopP in *Yersinia enterocolitica* and YopJ in Yersinia pestis and pseudotuberculosis [68]. The type III secretion system is used to transport the Yop proteins inside the infected cell. The fact that apoptosis-deficient YopJ mutants are less pathogenic than wild-type bacteria, which suggests the importance of YopJ's ability to induce apoptosis [69].

2.4.3 CHEMICAL CARCINOGENS

Chemicals play a significant role in the development of human malignancies among recognized carcinogenic agents (viruses, UV light, and ionizing radiation). The final forms of carcinogens are electrophilic reactants, which emerge through in vivo metabolism. Chemical carcinogenesis is a multi-stage process [70]. There are many types of chemical carcinogens that employ different mechanisms causing various biological changes in a multistep process of cancer development [71]. Some well-known chemical carcinogens are given in the following.

2.4.3.1 Arsenic

Arsenic imposes various biological effects when exposed to human tissues. Arsenic contributes to the development of various human disorders including hepatobiliary, respiratory, and urinary systems [72]. It enters the body through respiration, skin absorption, or oral ingestion [73, 74]. Contaminated water is one of the major sources of exposure to arsenic [73]. IARC classified arsenic as a class 1 carcinogen and its carcinogenicity may be attributed to the abnormal DNA repair, cellular mechanisms, or aneuploidy [75]. It contributes to the development of both squamous cell carcinoma and basal cell carcinoma [76].

2.4.3.2 Asbestos

Asbestos has emerged as the focus of concern among fibrous materials due to its industrial, and commercial value, widespread usage in the workplace, and early identification of its pathogenicity, and carcinogenicity.

According to recent statistics, asbestos is mostly utilized in the paper industry, railroad carrier, clutch, and brake manufacturing industries, as well as in insulating buildings, furnaces, and pipes. The main factor contributing to occupational and environmental exposure is its widespread usage as insulation. Asbestos may be seen as pervasive due to its high manufacturing, diverse usage, and apparent indestructibility. Lung fibrosis and pleural plaques may precede or be linked to lung carcinomas and mesotheliomas in asbestos-exposed individuals. These alterations could be signs of asbestos exposure [77]. Numerous occupational categories have recently shown an increase in the frequency of cancers due to asbestos exposure [78]. IARC classified asbestos as a group I carcinogen, which can cause lung, ovaries, and larynx cancer [79].

2.4.3.3 4-Aminobiphenyl

IARC classified 4-Aminobiphenyl (4-AbP) as a class 1 carcinogen [80–82]. Workers are exposed to 4-ABP while working in dye industries, present in cooking fumes, and is produced as a result of the combustion of nitrogen-containing organic compounds [82]. It is believed that this chemical has the mode of action through the formation of aromatic amines adducts in the DNA of the bladder epithelium [83].

2.4.3.4 Benzene

Industrial effluents, chemical industries, printing industries, petrochemicals used in cars, and combustion of gasoline are the major sources of benzene in our environment. Studies also suggest smoke is a major source of indoor benzene exposure [84–86]. The general public and workers can be exposed to benzene in the vehicular exhaust and gasoline vapors [87]. Various studies show that benzene is responsible for the development of various cancers, including bone marrow hypoplasia, non-Hodgkin lymphoma, aplastic anemia, and lung cancer [86–88].

2.4.3.5 2-Chloroethyl Sulfide

2-chloroethyl sulfide, commonly known as mustard gas. It is a colorless, odorless, and oily liquid having high stability in the environment [89]. Sulfur mustard was largely developed during World War 1 and larger stockpiles are still present in several countries [90]. Most recently, Iraqi Government used sulfur mustard as a weapon during the Iran–Iraq conflict [91]. Respiratory tracts provide enormous surface area to the chemical mustard vapor that are absorbed through the mucous. Chemically it reacts with proteins, which cause massive damage to all the tissues [92] and contributes to the development of pulmonary fibrosis [93].

2.4.3.6 Cigarette Smoke

According to assessments by IARC, among 400 identified chemicals in cigarette smoke IDE so far, more than 60 are considered carcinogens [94]. These are the main cause of cancer from cigarette smoke. Among these 400 chemical carcinogens, the strongest carcinogens in smoke are N-nitrosamines, polycyclic aromatic hydrocarbons (PAH), and aromatic amine. These chemicals are present in very small quantities. The most prevalent carcinogens are volatile organic compounds like butadiene, benzene, and aldehydes, which constitute almost 10–1000 µg/cigarette. When we are concerned with lung cancer, the most important carcinogens are polycyclic aromatic hydrocarbons (PAH) and nicotine-derived nitrosamine ketone (NAK) present in cigarette smoke [95].

Tobacco use accounts for about one-third of all cancer deaths annually and is leading preventable cause of cancer and cancer mortalities worldwide [96]. There is sufficient data to draw a conclusion that smoking causes cancers of the lungs [95, 97–110], larynx [111–121], oral cavity [122–131], pharynx [132–137], esophagus [138, 139], pancreas [140–142], urinary bladder [104, 143–147], kidney [104, 140, 148, 149], cervix [140, 150–153], and stomach [140, 154]. Additional evidence also suggests a connection between colorectal [140, 155, 156] and liver cancer and tobacco consumption [104, 157].

2.4.3.6.1 Association of Cigarette Smoke with Major Types of Cancers
Cigarette smoke affects humans from head to toe in a myriad way and causes several cancers [158]. Some of the well-known cancers are briefly explained.

2.4.3.6.1.1 Cigarette Smoke and Lung Cancer Tobacco smoking has been linked to every lung cancer histological subtype and is now considered the primary risk factor for this disease [159]. The first conclusive proof of a direct link between lung cancer and smoking came from human studies carried out in Germany between 1930 and 1940 [159]. Compared to big cell lung cancer or squamous cell carcinoma, adenocarcinoma is more common in women whereas squamous cell carcinoma is more common in males [160–163]. Scientists estimate that smoking causes more than

85% of lung cancers, with the remaining portion in non-smokers being brought on by secondhand smoking [164].

2.4.3.6.1.2 Cigarette Smoke and Bladder Cancer   Cigarette smoking is the major cause of bladder cancer [165–167]. Recent research showed that there is a threefold chance of bladder cancer in a smoker as compared to non-smokers [168]. The chances of bladder cancer are associated with several compounds found in smoke, including 2-Nepthylamine and 4-Aminobiphenyl, which are primary candidates for the specific causative agents [169].

2.4.3.6.1.3 Cigarette Smoke and Oral Cancer   Several factors contribute to the development of oral cancer. The most established and common factor is tobacco smoking [122]. Oral squamous cell carcinoma (OSCC) is a serious health issue mainly caused by cigarette smoke (CS) [170, 171]. Smoking increases a person's risk of oral cancer by three to five times [172, 173]. When tobacco is consumed in association with alcohol, it has a synergic effect and increases the risk of OSCC 10 to 15 times [125]. OSCC accounts for almost 90% of oral cancers [174]. Chemical carcinogens in smoke can alter the epigenetic makeup of oral epithelial cells, interfere with several host's immune system processes by the use of toxic metabolites, and generate oxidative

TABLE 2.1
Summarizing Structures, Sources, Target Organs, and Route of Exposure of Different Genotoxic Chemical Carcinogens

Carcinogens	Source	Target Organs	Route of Exposure	References
Arsenic	Drinking water, industries,	Lungs, urinary bladder, skin, liver, kidneys, integument,	Ingestion, inhalation, dermal contact	[72–74] [176–178]
Asbestos	Industries, mines, rockwool, talcum powders	Prostate, lungs, larynx, ovary, mesothelium, stomach	Ingestion, inhalation	[179–182]
4-Aminobiphenyl	Dyes industries, tobacco smoke	Urinary bladder	Inhalation, dermal contact,	[82, 183]
Benzene	Rubber industries, oil refineries, oil shipping, shoe making industries	Hematopoietic stem cells, lungs, non-Hodgkin lymphoma, lips	Inhalation, ingestion	[184–188]
Tobacco smoke	Tobacco	Esophagus, larynx, oral cavity, stomach, intestine, liver, lungs, kidneys, prostate, pancreases, urinary bladder, cervix, colorectal	Inhalation	[95, 97–151, 153–157]
Bis(2chloroethyl) Sulfide (Sulfur Mustard) Or (Mustard gas)	Chemical weapon	Lungs, liver, stomach cancer, larynx, trachea,	Inhalation	[89, 189–194]
2-Nepthylamine	Dyes industries	Urinary bladder	Inhalation, ingestion, dermal contact	[195–197]
Nickel compounds	Industries, volcanic eruption, soil, oceanic floor and water	Lungs, nasal sinuses, rectum, kidney	Inhalation, ingestion, dermal contact	[198–202]
Chromium compound	Metallurgical industries	Lungs, nose, nasal sinuses, digestive organs, CNS	Ingestion, inhalation, dermal contact	[203–207]
Benzidine	Industries, laboratories	Urinary bladder, liver, kidneys	Inhalation, ingestion, dermal contact	[208, 209]

stress in tissues leading to OSCC [175]. Some of the genotoxic chemical carcinogens are listed in Table 2.1.

2.4.4 ENVIRONMENTAL CARCINOGENS

In addition to some lifestyle choices, environmental carcinogens include a wide spectrum of chemical, physical, and biological agents. Despite the low absolute risk of developing cancer from exposure to environmental carcinogens, attributable risks might be very substantial due to the widespread exposure [210].

Additionally, environmental chemicals such as PAHs, NOCs, AAs, and aflatoxins may be present in food at low concentrations and cause cancer. According to the World Health Organization (WHO), environmental risks including air pollution, chemical management, radiation, and worker protection, are responsible for 20% of cancer cases globally [211]. The level of industrialization affects the burden of cancer caused by environmental factors [212].

The Integrated Risk Information System (IRIS) program, developed by the EPA in 1985, assesses and categorizes risks to human health connected to environmental contaminants. More than 150 of these substances have been classified by the IRIS as carcinogenic [213].

2.5 METABOLISM OF CARCINOGENS

Procarcinogens can enter the body through a number of different pathways. The majority of chemical carcinogens need to be metabolically activated in vivo before they cause cancer [214]. Approximately 75% of the various carcinogens to which individuals are often exposed have metabolic enzymes that are CYPs [215]. These are primary enzymes involved in the metabolism of the carcinogens [216]. The CYP (P450s) enzymes can metabolize several carcinogens including heterocyclic amines, polycyclic aromatic hydrocarbons, azo-dyes, nitrosamines, and alkylating compounds [217]. Steps involved in the metabolism of carcinogens are classified into two phases, phase I and phase II. Phase I enzymes contain cytochrome P450 families and epoxide hydroxylases, which instigate reactive groups into carcinogens to increase hydrophilicity and to produce reactive intermediates for the subsequent conjugation reaction [218].

Phase II reactions contain N-acetyltransferases, Glutathione-S-transferases, and sulfotransferases enzymes that conjugate water-soluble moieties and then render reactive intermediates harmless [219]. As a result of the reactive intermediate's interactions with DNA, DNA adducts may result in somatic mutations and start the carcinogenesis process. A larger risk of DNA damage may thus exist in those with low phase II activity and high phase I activity [220].

Some discrepancies in the metabolism of carcinogens are attributed to variations in chromosomal DNA sequences. An enzyme can produce a mutant form with amino acid substitution as a consequence of a single base alteration, or "single nucleotide polymorphism (SNP)", which might have a significant impact on the enzyme's metabolic function [221].

The CYP enzymes metabolism of carcinogens may result in active derivatives that start cancer. Phase II enzymes that degrade and release carcinogens consist of a variety of families. When DNA repair mechanisms fail to reverse the DNA damage caused by carcinogens, DNA adducts in oncogenes or tumor suppressor genes, mutations in these genes frequently result, which may cause cell death or cancer as shown in Figure 2.6 [214].

2.6 DETECTION OF CARCINOGENS

There are several techniques available for the sensitive detection of carcinogens in people. These include electrochemical conductance (ECC) [222], atomic absorbance spectrometry (AAS) [223], gas chromatography/mass spectrometry [224], fluorescence spectroscopy [225], enzyme

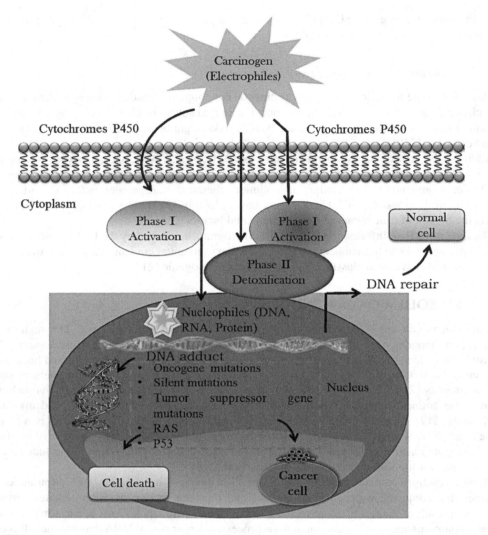

FIGURE 2.6 Metabolic pathways of carcinogen. Carcinogens introduced into cells are metabolized by phase I enzymes and detoxified by phase II enzymes. Phase I enzymes convert the carcinogens into DNA-binding compounds. The chromosomal DNA and the DNA-binding metabolites interact to generate DNA adducts, which can lead to mutations, cell death, or the emergence of cancer.

immunoassays [226] and the 32P-post labeling assay [225]. A few methods of carcinogen's detection are discussed below.

2.6.1 32P-POST LABELING ASSAY

For the detection of carcinogen-DNA adducts and other types of changed nucleotides in DNA, the 32P-post labeling technique is frequently used. It has been used to identify the DNA adducts created by a variety of genotoxic agents in bacterial, mammalian, and occasionally human tissues. In addition, to detecting apurinic sites in DNA, oxidative DNA damage, UV-induced photo dimers, and to a lesser extent, DNA damage brought by cytotoxic drugs, 32P-post labeling analysis has been applied to most classes of carcinogens ranging from bulky or aromatic compounds to small or aliphatic compounds. It has given the first concrete proof of some synthetic cancer-causing hormones, which have DNA-damaging abilities. It has demonstrated the capability of complex combinations like coal tar and tobacco smoke to cause DNA damage. It has been utilized in human biomonitoring investigations to identify DNA damage brought on by both occupational and non-occupational environmental exposures to carcinogens [227].

2.6.2 FLUORESCENCE SPECTROSCOPY

Due to its high sensitivity, fluorescence spectroscopy has been a key analytical tool in science and medicine for many years. As a result, it is ideal for analyzing traces of organic compounds. It makes sense that it would be used to examine carcinogen-DNA adducts [228, 229] that used fluorescence spectroscopy as "the sole thread that ran through the labyrinth" to isolate and characterize polycyclic aromatic hydrocarbons (PAHs), the first purified chemical carcinogens, from coal tar pitch [229].

2.6.3 PREVENTION OF CARCINOGEN EXPOSURE

Limiting carcinogenic emissions from a single vehicle, developing community mobility strategies, and altering an individual's typical behavior are all necessary preventive measures [213]. For instance, reducing the risk of skin cancer from sunshine involves international factors. The ozone layer should be preserved globally [230]. Adopting safety procedures and sharing accident information globally is necessary to reduce the danger of long-distance air pollution such as radiation from nuclear power plant accidents [231]. Reduced alcohol and cigarette consumption must continue as a priority. The expansion of human papillomavirus (HPV) vaccine coverage is another important goal. Reduced occupational exposure to carcinogens, worker's protection from carcinogen exposure, education on healthier diets and simple, inexpensive access to fruits and vegetables can all help to lower the risks of cancer [232].

2.7 CONCLUSION

A carcinogen is a substance, organism, or agent capable of causing cancer. According to the 15th report on carcinogens 2021, 256 substances are anticipated to cause cancer in humans. Mainly, there are three types of carcinogens, i.e., physical, chemical, and biological carcinogens, which occur naturally such as ultraviolet radiations, certain bacteria, and viruses, or chemically synthesized carcinogens, i.e., smoke, asbestos, and arsenic. Carcinogens can enter the body by the process of dermal contact, ingestion, inhalation, or injection. They continue to have a significant impact on the incidence, mortality, and social burdens of cancer worldwide. They alter a normal cell genetic makeup and result in cancer. They can bind to DNA and change structure to make DNA adducts. More research is needed to help better understanding of the non-genotoxic mechanisms, as they may not be enough to cause carcinogenesis and increased tumor risk. There are few techniques available for the detection of carcinogens. But there should be nano sensor-based methods that detect carcinogens in food and industry immediately on the basis of their mechanism, so that the risk of cancer can be minimized. Strategies should be made by the government to minimize carcinogenic emissions from vehicles and industries, avoid exposure to ultraviolet rays, ban tobacco products, and eliminate carcinogens from industries.

REFERENCES

1. Shonkwiler, R.W. and J. Herod, *Cancer: A Disease of the DNA*. In *Mathematical Biology*. 2009, Springer. pp. 399–416.
2. Woo, Y.R., et al., *The human microbiota and skin cancer. International Journal of Molecular Science*, 2022. **23**(3): p. 1813.
3. Rao, H.-L., et al., *Increased intratumoral neutrophil in colorectal carcinomas correlates closely with malignant phenotype and predicts patients' adverse prognosis. PloS One*, 2012. **7**(1): p. e30806.
4. Luch, A., *Nature and nurture – lessons from chemical carcinogenesis. Nature Reviews Cancer*, 2005. **5**(2): pp. 113–25.
5. Rastogi, S., et al., *Skin tumorigenic potential of aflatoxin B1 in mice. Food Chemical Toxicology*, 2006. **44**(5): pp. 670–7.
6. Anand, P., et al., *Cancer is a preventable disease that requires major lifestyle changes. Pharmaceutical Research*, 2008. **25**(9): pp. 2097–116.
7. Madia, F., et al., *Carcinogenicity assessment: Addressing the challenges of cancer and chemicals in the environment. Environment International*, 2019. **128**: pp. 417–29.
8. Suarez-Torres, J.D., J.P. Alzate, and M.E.J.J.o.A.T. Orjuela-Ramirez, *The NTP Report on Carcinogens: A valuable resource for public health, a challenge for regulatory science. Journal of Applied Toxicology*, 2020. **40**(1): pp. 169–75.
9. Krewski, D., et al., *Concordance between sites of tumor development in humans and in experimental animals for 111 agents that are carcinogenic to humans. Journal of Toxicology and Environmental Health, Part B Critical Reviews*, 2019. **22**(7–8): pp. 203–36.
10. Smith, M.T., et al., *The key characteristics of carcinogens: Relationship to the hallmarks of cancer, relevant biomarkers, and assays to measure them. Cancer Epidemiology Biomarkers and Preventation*, 2020. **29**(10): pp. 1887–903.
11. Smith, T.J., G.D. Stoner, and C.S. Yang, *Activation of 4-(methylnitrosamino)-1-(3-pyridyl)-1-butanone (NNK) in human lung microsomes by cytochromes P450, lipoxygenase, and hydroperoxides. Cancer Research*, 1995. **55**(23): pp. 5566–73.
12. Guyton, K.Z., et al., *Key characteristics approach to carcinogenic hazard identification. Chemical Research in Toxicology*, 2018. **31**(12): pp. 1290–2.
13. Jomova, K. and M. Valko, *Advances in metal-induced oxidative stress and human disease. Toxicology*, 2011. **283**(2–3): pp. 65–87.
14. Temkin, A.M., et al., *Application of the key characteristics of carcinogens to per and polyfluoroalkyl substances. International Journal of Environmental Research and Public Health*, 2020. **17**(5): p. 1668.
15. Schins, R.P. and A.M. Knaapen, *Genotoxicity of poorly soluble particles. Inhalation Toxicology*, 2007. **19**(Suppl 1): pp. 189–98.
16. Xie, X.L., et al., *Long-term treatment with L-isoleucine or L-leucine in AIN-93G diet has promoting effects on rat bladder carcinogenesis. Food Chemical Toxicology*, 2012. **50**(11): pp. 3934–40.
17. Chung, K.T. and G.S. Gadupudi, *Possible roles of excess tryptophan metabolites in cancer. Environmental and Molecular Mutagenesis*, 2011. **52**(2): pp. 81–104.
18. Tirino, V., et al., *Cancer stem cells in solid tumors: An overview and new approaches for their isolation and characterization. Faseb Journal*, 2013. **27**(1): pp. 13–24.
19. He, J., Y. Liu, and D.M. Lubman, *Targeting glioblastoma stem cells: Cell surface markers. Current Medicinal Chemistry*, 2012. **19**(35): pp. 6050–5.
20. Lee, W.J., et al., *Investigating the different mechanisms of genotoxic and non-genotoxic carcinogens by a gene set analysis. PLoS One*, 2014. **9**(1): p. e86700.
21. Preussmann, R., *The problem of thresholds in chemical carcinogenesis some views on theoretical and practical aspects. Journal of Cancer Research and Clinical Oncology*, 1980. **97**(1): pp. 1–14.
22. Faguet, G.B.J.I.j.o.c., *A brief history of cancer: Age-old milestones underlying our current knowledge database. Internation Journal of Cancer*, 2015. **136**(9): pp. 2022–36.
23. Sreedharan, S., et al., *Snuff-induced malignancy of the nasal vestibule: A case report. American Journal of Otolaryngology*, 2007. **28**(5): pp. 353–6.
24. Brown, J.R. and J.L. Thornton, *Percivall Pott (1714-1788) and chimney sweepers' cancer of the scrotum. British Jorunal of Industrial Medicine*, 1957. **14**(1): pp. 68–70.

25. Jethwa, A.R. and S.S. Khariwala, *Tobacco-related carcinogenesis in head and neck cancer. Cancer and Metastasis Reviews*, 2017. **36**(3): pp. 411–23.

26. Nabavizadeh, B., G.M. Amend, and B.N. Breyer, *Workers died of dyes: The discovery of occupational bladder cancers. Urology*, 2021. **154**: pp. 4–7.

27. Blackadar, C.B., *Historical review of the causes of cancer. World Journal of Clinical Oncology*, 2016. **7**(1): pp. 54–86.

28. Kuroki, T. and K.J.I.J.o.C. Wakabayashi, *100 Years of Cancer Research in Japan*. 2013, Wiley Online Library: Hoboken. pp. 1235–9.

29. Cox, E., D. Cruickshank, and J. Smith, *The crystal structure of benzene at -3°. Proceedings of the Royal Society*, 1958. **247**: pp. 1–21.

30. Bartrip, P.W., *History of asbestos related disease. Postgraduate Medical Journal*, 2004. **80**(940): pp. 72–6.

31. Baan, R.A. and Y. Grosse, *Man-made mineral (vitreous) fibres: Evaluations of cancer hazards by the IARC Monographs Programme. Mutation Research*, 2004. **553**(1–2): pp. 43–58.

32. Randi, G., et al., *The European Cancer Information System: Exploring linkages between indoor radon concentrations and data on cancer burden*. 2022. **3**: p. 607

33. Pflaum, T., et al., *Carcinogenic compounds in alcoholic beverages: An update. Archives of Toxicology*, 2016. **90**(10): pp. 2349–67.

34. Silverman, D.T., *Diesel exhaust causes lung cancer: Now what? Occupational and Environmental Medicine*, 2017. **74**(4): pp. 233–4.

35. Wong, I.C., Y.K. Ng, and V.W. Lui, *Cancers of the lung, head and neck on the rise: Perspectives on the genotoxicity of air pollution. Chinese Journal of Cancer*, 2014. **33**(10): pp. 476–80.

36. Lellis, B., et al., *Effects of textile dyes on health and the environment and bioremediation potential of living organisms. Biotechnology Research and Innovation*, 2019. **3**(2): pp. 275–90.

37. Lunn, R.M., et al., *Cancer hazard evaluations for contemporary needs: Highlights from new NTP evaluations and methodological advancements. Journal of National Cancer Institute*, 2022. **114**(11): pp. 1441–8.

38. Barrett, J.R., *Liver cancer and aflatoxin: New information from the Kenyan outbreak. Environmental Health Perspectives*. 2005. **113**(12): pp. A837–A838.

39. Carpenter, D.O. and S.J.J.o.A.H. Bushkin-Bedient, *Exposure to chemicals and radiation during childhood and risk for cancer later in life. Journal of Adolescent Health*. 2013. **52**(5): pp. S21–S29.

40. Centers for Disease Control, *Publications and reports of the surgeon general*. In *How Tobacco Smoke Causes Disease: The Biology and Behavioral Basis for Smoking-Attributable Disease: A Report of the Surgeon General*. 2010, Centers for Disease Control and Prevention (US): Atlanta (GA).

41. Heudorf, U., V. Mersch-Sundermann, and J. Angerer, *Phthalates: Toxicology and exposure. International Journal of Hygiene and Environmental Health*, 2007. **210**(5): pp. 623–34.

42. Kang, D.S., et al., *Application of the adverse outcome pathway framework to risk assessment for predicting carcinogenicity of chemicals. Journal of Cancer Preventaion*, 2018. **23**(3): pp. 126–33.

43. Ciliberti, A., C. Maltoni, and G.J.A.o.t.N.Y.A.o.S. Perino, *Long-term carcinogenicity bioassays on propylene administered by inhalation to Sprague-Dawley rats and Swiss mice. Annals of the New York Academy of Sciences*, 1988. **534**: pp. 235–45.

44. Infante, P.F., et al., *Fibrous glass and cancer. American Journal of Industrial Medicine*, 1994. **26**(4): pp. 559–84.

45. Baan, R.A., Y.J.M.R.F. Grosse, and M.M.o. Mutagenesis, *Man-made mineral (vitreous) fibres: evaluations of cancer hazards by the IARC Monographs Programme. Mutation Research*, 2004. **553**(1–2): pp. 43–58.

46. Shannon, H.S., et al., *Mortality experience of Ontario glass fibre workers--extended follow-up. Annals of Occupational Hygiene*, 1987. **31**(4b): pp. 657–62.

47. Enterline, P.E., et al., *Mortality update of a cohort of U.S. man-made mineral fibre workers. Annals of Occupational Hygiene*, 1987. **31**(4b): pp. 625–56.

48. Marsh, G.M., et al., *Mortality among a cohort of US man-made mineral fiber workers: 1985 follow-up. Journal of Occupational Medicine*, 1990. **32**(7): pp. 594–604.

49. Doll, R., *Symposium on MMMF, Copenhagen, October 1986: Overview and conclusions. Annals of Occupational Hygiene*, 1987. **31**(4b): pp. 805–19.

50. Heath, J.C., *The production of malignant tumours by cobalt in the rat. British Journal of Cancer*, 1956. **10**(4): pp. 668–73.

51. Hueper, W.C., *Experimental studies in metal cancerigenesis. IV. Cancer produced by parenterally introduced metallic nickel. Journal of National Cancer Institute*, 1955. **16**(1): pp. 55–73.

52. Pope, C.A., 3rd, et al., *Lung cancer, cardiopulmonary mortality, and long-term exposure to fine particulate air pollution. Jama*, 2002. **287**(9): pp. 1132–41.

53. Wartenberg, D., *Residential magnetic fields and childhood leukemia: A meta-analysis. Americal Journal of Public Health*, 1998. **88**(12): pp. 1787–94.

54. *Non-ionizing radiation, Part 1: Static and extremely low-frequency (ELF) electric and magnetic fields. IARC Monographs Eval Carcinogenic Risks to Humans*, 2002. **80**: pp. 1–395.

55. Appel, J.D., et al., *Asbestos fibers mediate transformation of monkey cells by exogenous plasmid DNA. Proceedings of the National Academy of Sciences USA*, 1988. **85**(20): pp. 7670–4.

56. Grassmé, H., V. Jendrossek, and E. Gulbins, *Molecular mechanisms of bacteria induced apoptosis. Apoptosis*, 2001. **6**(6): pp. 441–5.

57. Liu, X., et al., *Induction of apoptotic program in cell-free extracts: Requirement for dATP and cytochrome c. Cell*, 1996. **86**(1): pp. 147–57.

58. Susin, S.A., et al., *Molecular characterization of mitochondrial apoptosis-inducing factor. Nature*, 1999. **397**(6718): pp. 441–6.

59. Zou, H., et al., *Apaf-1, a human protein homologous to C. elegans CED-4, participates in cytochrome c-dependent activation of caspase-3. Cell*, 1997. **90**(3): pp. 405–13.

60. Joza, N., et al., *Essential role of the mitochondrial apoptosis-inducing factor in programmed cell death. Nature*, 2001. **410**(6828): pp. 549–54.

61. Newton, K. and A. Strasser, *Cell death control in lymphocytes. Advances in Immunology*, 2000. **76**: pp. 179–226.

62. Kimbrough, T.G. and S.I. Miller, *Contribution of Salmonella typhimurium type III secretion components to needle complex formation. Proceedings of the National Academy of Sciences USA*, 2000. **97**(20): pp. 11008–13.

63. Zychlinsky, A., M.C. Prevost, and P.J. Sansonetti, *Shigella flexneri induces apoptosis in infected macrophages. Nature*, 1992. **358**(6382): pp. 167–9.

64. Zychlinsky, A., et al., *IpaB mediates macrophage apoptosis induced by Shigella flexneri. Molecular Microbiology*, 1994. **11**(4): pp. 619–27.

65. Hilbi, H., et al., *Shigella-induced apoptosis is dependent on caspase-1 which binds to IpaB. Journal of Biological Chemistry*, 1998. **273**(49): pp. 32895–900.

66. Chen, Y., et al., *A bacterial invasin induces macrophage apoptosis by binding directly to ICE. Embo Journal*, 1996. **15**(15): pp. 3853–60.

67. Esen, M., et al., *Mechanisms of Staphylococcus aureus induced apoptosis of human endothelial cells. Apoptosis*, 2001. **6**(6): pp. 431–9.

68. Bleves, S. and G.R. Cornelis, *How to survive in the host: The Yersinia lesson. Microbes and Infection*, 2000. **2**(12): pp. 1451–60.

69. Monack, D.M., et al., *Yersinia-induced apoptosis in vivo aids in the establishment of a systemic infection of mice. Journal of Experimental Medicine*, 1998. **188**(11): pp. 2127–37.

70. Miller, E.C. and J.A.J.C. Miller, *Mechanisms of chemical carcinogenesis. Cancer*, 1981. **47**(S5): pp. 1055–64.

71. Vineis, P., A. Schatzkin, and J.D. Potter, *Models of carcinogenesis: An overview. Carcinogenesis*, 2010. **31**(10): pp. 1703–9.

72. Smith, A.H., et al., *Lung, bladder, and kidney cancer mortality 40 years after arsenic exposure reduction. Journal of National Cancer Institute*, 2018. **110**(3): pp. 241–9.

73. Abdul, K.S., et al., *Arsenic and human health effects: A review. Enviromental Toxicoogyl Pharmacology*, 2015. **40**(3): pp. 828–46.

74. Sawada, N., *Association between arsenic intake and cancer-from the viewpoint of epidemiological study. Nihon Eiseigaku Zasshi*, 2018. **73**(3): pp. 265–8.

75. Zhou, Q. and S. Xi, *A review on arsenic carcinogenesis: Epidemiology, metabolism, genotoxicity and epigenetic changes. Regulatory Toxicology Pharmacology*, 2018. **99**: pp. 78–88.

76. Lee, C.H., W.T. Liao, and H.S. Yu, *Aberrant immune responses in arsenical skin cancers. Kaohsiung Journal of Medical Science*, 2011. **27**(9): pp. 396–401.

77. Nurminen, M. and A. Tossavainen, *Is there an association between pleural plaques and lung cancer without asbestosis? Scandinavian Journal Work, Environment and Health*, 1994. **20**(1): pp. 62–4.

78. Maltoni, C., C. Pinto, and A. Mobiglia, *Mesotheliomas due to asbestos used in railroads in Italy. Annuals og the New York Academy of Sciences*, 1991. **643**: pp. 347–67.

79. *Report on cancer risks associated with the ingestion of asbestos. DHHS Committee to Coordinate Environmental and Related Programs. Environmental Health Perspect*, 1987. **72**: pp. 253–65.

80. Van Hemelrijck, M.J., et al., *Secondhand smoking, 4-aminobiphenyl, and bladder cancer: Two meta-analyses. Cancer Epidemiology Biomarkers and Preventation*, 2009. **18**(4): pp. 1312–20.

81. Bhattacharya, A., et al., *The inverse relationship between bladder and liver in 4-aminobiphenyl-induced DNA damage. Oncotarget*, 2015. **6**(2): pp. 836–45.

82. Cohen, S.M., et al., *4-aminobiphenyl and DNA reactivity: case study within the context of the 2006 IPCS Human Relevance Framework for analysis of a cancer mode of action for humans. Critical Reviews Toxicology*, 2006. **36**(10): pp. 803–19.

83. Kadlubar, F.F., *DNA adducts of carcinogenic aromatic amines. IARC Scientific Publications*, 1994. **1994**(125): pp. 199–216.

84. Bahadar, H., S. Mostafalou, and M. Abdollahi, *Current understandings and perspectives on non-cancer health effects of benzene: A global concern. Toxicology and Applied Pharmacology*, 2014. **276**(2): pp. 83–94.

85. Mungi, C., D. Lai, and X.L. Du, *Spatial analysis of industrial benzene emissions and cancer incidence rates in Texas. International Journal of Environmental Research and Public Health*, 2019. **16**(15): p. 2627

86. Warden, H., et al., *Associations between occupational exposure to benzene, toluene and xylene and risk of lung cancer in Montréal. Occupational and Environmental Medicine*, 2018. **75**(10): pp. 696–702.

87. Belingheri, M., et al., *Benzene and leukemia: From scientific evidence to regulations. A historical example. Medicina Lavoro*, 2019. **110**(3): pp. 234–40.

88. Rana, I., et al., *Benzene exposure and non-Hodgkin lymphoma: A systematic review and meta-analysis of human studies. Lancet Planet Health*, 2021. **5**(9): pp. e633–e643.

89. Panahi, Y., et al., *Complications and carcinogenic effects of mustard gas – a systematic review and meta-analysis in Iran. Asian Pacific Journal of Cancer Prevention*, 2015. **16**(17): pp. 7567–73.

90. Ghanei, M. and A.A. Harandi, *Lung carcinogenicity of sulfur mustard. Clinical Lung Cancer*, 2010. **11**(1): pp. 13–7.

91. Khateri, S., et al., *Incidence of lung, eye, and skin lesions as late complications in 34,000 Iranians with wartime exposure to mustard agent. Journal of Occupational and Environmental Medicine*, 2003. **45**(11): pp. 1136–43.

92. Dacre, J.C. and M. Goldman, *Toxicology and pharmacology of the chemical warfare agent sulfur mustard. Pharmacology Reviews*, 1996. **48**(2): pp. 289–326.

93. Emad, A. and G.R. Rezaian, *Immunoglobulins and cellular constituents of the BAL fluid of patients with sulfur mustard gas-induced pulmonary fibrosis. Chest*, 1999. **115**(5): pp. 1346–51.

94. Das, M., et al., *Inhibition of polycyclic aromatic hydrocarbon-DNA adduct formation in epidermis and lungs of SENCAR mice by naturally occurring plant phenols. Cancer Research*, 1987. **47**(3): pp. 767–73.

95. Hecht, S.S., *Tobacco smoke carcinogens and lung cancer. Journal of National Cancer Institute*, 1999. **91**(14): pp. 1194–210.

96. National Cancer Policy Forum, Board on Health Care Services, and Institute of Medicine. In *Reducing Tobacco-Related Cancer Incidence and Mortality: Workshop Summary*. 2013, National Academies Press (US): Washington (DC).

97. Jassem, E., et al., *Smoking and lung cancer. Pneumonologia i Alergologia Polska*, 2009. **77**(5): pp. 469–73.

98. de Groot, P. and R.F. Munden, *Lung cancer epidemiology, risk factors, and prevention. Radiologic Clinics of North America*, 2012. **50**(5): pp. 863–76.

99. Loeb, L.A., et al., *Smoking and lung cancer: An overview. Cancer Research*, 1984. **44**(12 Pt 1): pp. 5940–58.

100. Underner, M., et al., *Cannabis smoking and lung cancer. Revue des Maladies Respiratories*, 2014. **31**(6): pp. 488–98.

101. Tang, M.S., et al., *Electronic-cigarette smoke induces lung adenocarcinoma and bladder urothelial hyperplasia in mice. Proceedings of the National Acadedy of Sciences USA*, 2019. **116**(43): p. 21727–31.

102. Trédaniel, J., et al., *Exposure to environmental tobacco smoke and risk of lung cancer: the epidemiological evidence. European Respiratory Journal*, 1994. **7**(10): pp. 1877–88.

103. Middleton, G., et al., *Publisher Correction: The National Lung Matrix Trial of personalized therapy in lung cancer. Nature*, 2020. **585**(7826): p. E21.

104. Sasco, A.J., M.B. Secretan, and K. Straif, *Tobacco smoking and cancer: a brief review of recent epidemiological evidence. Lung Cancer*, 2004. **45**(Suppl 2): pp. S3–S9.

105. Karagueuzian, H.S., et al., *Cigarette smoke radioactivity and lung cancer risk. Nicotine and Tobacco Research*, 2012. **14**(1): pp. 79–90.

106. Steliga, M.A. and C.M. Dresler, *Epidemiology of lung cancer: Smoking, secondhand smoke, and genetics. Surgical Oncology Clinics of North America*, 2011. **20**(4): pp. 605–18.

107. Proctor, R.N., *The history of the discovery of the cigarette-lung cancer link: evidentiary traditions, corporate denial, global toll. Tobacco Control*, 2012. **21**(2): pp. 87–91.

108. North, C.M. and D.C. Christiani, *Women and lung cancer: What is new? Seminars in Thoracic and Cardiovascular Surgery*, 2013. **25**(2): pp. 87–94.

109. Hang, B., J.H. Mao, and A.M. Snijders, *Genetic susceptibility to thirdhand-smoke-induced lung cancer development. Nicotine and Tobacco Research*, 2019. **21**(9): pp. 1294–6.

110. Gómez Raposo, C., J. De Castro Carpeño, and M. González Barón, *Causes of lung cancer: Smoking, environmental tobacco smoke exposure, occupational and environmental exposures and genetic predisposition. Medicina Clinica (Barc)*, 2007. **128**(10): pp. 390–6.

111. *Smoking and laryngeal cancer. Medical Journal of Australia*, 1976. **2**(8): p. 284.

112. Jurkiewicz, D., K. Dzaman, and P. Rapiejko, *Laryngeal cancer risk factors. Polski Merkuriusz Lekarski*, 2006. **21**(121): pp. 94–8.

113. Ramroth, H., A. Dietz, and H. Becher, *Environmental tobacco smoke and laryngeal cancer: Results from a population-based case-control study. European Archives of Otorhinolaryngology*, 2008. **265**(11): pp. 1367–71.

114. Gregory, R.L., *Appearance and reality (1): A number of ideas. Perception*, 1990. **19**(4): pp. 419–23.

115. Mutlu, P., et al., *Association between XRCC3 Thr241Met polymorphism and laryngeal cancer susceptibility in Turkish population. European Archives of Otorhinolaryngology*, 2015. **272**(12): pp. 3779–84.

116. Cattaruzza, M.S., P. Maisonneuve, and P. Boyle, *Epidemiology of laryngeal cancer. Europena Journal of Cancer Part B Oral Oncology*, 1996. **32b**(5): pp. 293–305.

117. Shivappa, N., et al., *Inflammatory potential of diet and risk of laryngeal cancer in a case-control study from Italy. Cancer Causes Control*, 2016. **27**(8): pp. 1027–34.

118. Ramsey, T., et al., *Laryngeal cancer: Global socioeconomic trends in disease burden and smoking habits. Laryngoscope*, 2018. **128**(9): pp. 2039–53.

119. Bridger, G.P. and P. Reay-Young, *Laryngeal cancer and smoking. Medical Journal of Australia*, 1976. **2**(8): pp. 293–4.

120. Szyfter, K., *Molecular and cellular changes following exposure to tobacco smoke causing laryngeal cancer. An outline of the problem. Przegl Lek*, 2004. **61**(10): pp. 1197–9.

121. Zhang, Q.W., et al., *Variations in disease burden of laryngeal cancer attributable to alcohol use and smoking in 204 countries or territories, 1990-2019. BMC Cancer*, 2021. **21**(1): p. 1082.

122. Kumar, M., et al., *Oral cancer: Etiology and risk factors: A review. Journal of Cancer Research and Therapy*, 2016. **12**(2): pp. 458–63.

123. Ghantous, Y. and I. Abu Elnaaj, *Global incidence and risk factors of oral cancer. Harefuah*, 2017. **156**(10): pp. 645–9.

124. Nagler, R., A. Weizman, and A. Gavish, *Cigarette smoke, saliva, the translocator protein 18 kDa (TSPO), and oral cancer. Oral Diseases*, 2019. **25**(8): pp. 1843–9.

125. Ford, P.J. and A.M. Rich, *Tobacco use and oral health. Addiction*, 2021. **116**(12): pp. 3531–40.

126. Kademani, D., *Oral cancer. Mayo Clinical Proceeedings*, 2007. **82**(7): pp. 878–87.

127. Chen, Q., et al., *Relationship between selenium and the risk for oral cancer: A case-control study. Zhonghua Liu Xing Bing Xue Za Zhi*, 2019. **40**(7): pp. 810–4.

128. Byakodi, R., et al., *Oral cancer in India: An epidemiologic and clinical review. Journal of Community Health*, 2012. **37**(2): pp. 316–9.

129. Alqutaibi, A.Y., et al., *Early detection of oral cancer and potentially malignant disorders: Experiences, practices, and beliefs of prosthodontists practicing in Saudi Arabia. Journal of Prosthetic Dentistry,* 2021. **126**(4): pp. 569–74.

130. Mohanty, V., et al., *Molecular alterations in oral cancer between tobacco chewers and smokers using serum proteomics. Cancer Biomark,* 2021. **31**(4): pp. 361–73.

131. Nagler, R.M. and A.Z. Reznick, *Cigarette smoke effects on salivary antioxidants and oral cancer – novel concepts. Israel Medical Association Journal,* 2004. **6**(11): pp. 691–4.

132. Riechelmann, H., *Occupational exposure and cancer of the oral cavity and pharynx. Laryngorhinootologie,* 2002. **81**(8): pp. 573–9.

133. Rassekh, C.H., *Tobacco cancer of the oral cavity and pharynx. West Virginia Medical Journal,* 2001. **97**(1): pp. 8–12.

134. Damphousse, K.E., D.S. Mowls, and L.A. Beebe, *An ecological analysis of tobacco use and oral cavity and pharynx cancers in U.S. males. Journal of the Okla State Medical Association,* 2015. **108**(11): pp. 488–91.

135. Simarak, S., et al., *Cancer of the oral cavity, pharynx/larynx and lung in North Thailand: Case-control study and analysis of cigar smoke. British Journal of Cancer,* 1977. **36**(1): pp. 130–40.

136. La Vecchia, C., et al., *Epidemiology and prevention of oral cancer. Oral Oncology,* 1997. **33**(5): pp. 302–12.

137. Ellington, T.D., et al., *Trends in incidence of cancers of the oral cavity and pharynx – United States 2007-2016. MMWR Morbidity and Mortality Weekly Report,* 2020. **69**(15): pp. 433–8.

138. Dong, J. and A.P. Thrift, *Alcohol, smoking and risk of oesophago-gastric cancer. Best Practice and Research Clin Gastroenterology,* 2017. **31**(5): pp. 509–517.

139. Short, M.W., K.G. Burgers, and V.T. Fry, *Esophageal cancer. American Family Physician,* 2017. **95**(1): pp. 22–28.

140. Scherübl, H., *Smoking tobacco and cancer risk. Deutsch Medizinische Wochenschrift,* 2021. **146**(6): pp. 412–7.

141. Korc, M., et al., *Tobacco and alcohol as risk factors for pancreatic cancer. Best Practice and Research Clinical Gastroenterology,* 2017. **31**(5): pp. 529–36.

142. Capasso, M., et al., *Epidemiology and risk factors of pancreatic cancer. Acta Biomedica,* 2018. **89**(9-s): pp. 141–6.

143. Antoni, S., et al., *Bladder cancer incidence and mortality: A global overview and recent trends. European Urology,* 2017. **71**(1): pp. 96–108.

144. Cumberbatch, M.G.K., et al., *Epidemiology of bladder cancer: A systematic review and contemporary update of risk factors in 2018. European Urology,* 2018. **74**(6): pp. 784–95.

145. Rozanec, J.J. and F.P. Secin, *Epidemiology, etiology and prevention of bladder cancer. Archivos Espanoles de Urologia,* 2020. **73**(10): pp. 872–8.

146. Nesi, G., et al., *Environment and urinary bladder cancer. A historical perspective. Polish Journal of Pathology,* 2019. **70**(1): pp. 21–25.

147. Hektoen, H.H., et al., *Lifestyle associated factors and risk of urinary bladder cancer: A prospective cohort study from Norway. Cancer Medicine,* 2020. **9**(12): pp. 4420–32.

148. Tahbaz, R., M. Schmid, and A.S. Merseburger, *Prevention of kidney cancer incidence and recurrence: Lifestyle, medication and nutrition. Current Opinion in Urology,* 2018. **28**(1): pp. 62–79.

149. Capitanio, U., et al., *Epidemiology of renal cell carcinoma. European Urology,* 2019. **75**(1): pp. 74–84.

150. Su, B., et al., *The relation of passive smoking with cervical cancer: A systematic review and meta-analysis. Medicine (Baltimore),* 2018. **97**(46): p. e13061.

151. Kim, J.Y., et al., *Secondhand smoke exposure, diabetes, and high BMI are risk factors for uterine cervical cancer: A cross-sectional study from the Korea national health and nutrition examination survey (2010-2018). BMC Cancer,* 2021. **21**(1): p. 880.

152. Pate Capps, N., A. Stewart, and C. Burns, *The interplay between secondhand cigarette smoke, genetics, and cervical cancer: A review of the literature. Biological Research for Nursing,* 2009. **10**(4): pp. 392–9.

153. Hansen, B.T., S. Campbell, and M. Nygård, *Regional differences in cervical cancer incidence and associated risk behaviors among Norwegian women: A population-based study. BMC Cancer,* 2021. **21**(1): p. 935.

154. Praud, D., et al., *Cigarette smoking and gastric cancer in the Stomach Cancer Pooling (StoP) Project. European Journal of Cancer Prevention,* 2018. **27**(2): pp. 124–33.

155. Botteri, E., et al., *Smoking and colorectal cancer risk, overall and by molecular subtypes: A meta-analysis. Amermican Journal of Gastroenterology*, 2020. **115**(12): pp. 1940–9.
156. Chen, X., et al., *Smoking, genetic predisposition, and colorectal cancer risk. Clinical and Translational Gastroenterology*, 2021. **12**(3): p. e00317.
157. Wang, Y.Q., et al., *Analysis of liver cancer screening results and influencing factors of urban residents in Zhejiang Province from 2013 to 2018. Zhonghua Yu Fang Yi Xue Za Zhi*, 2021. **55**(3): pp. 346–52.
158. Abdul, K.S.M., et al., *Arsenic and human health effects: A review. Envionmental Toxicoloy Pharmacology*, 2015. **40**(3): pp. 828–46.
159. Belani, C.P., et al., *Women and lung cancer: Epidemiology, tumor biology, and emerging trends in clinical research. Lung Cancer*, 2007. **55**(1): pp. 15–23.
160. Devesa, S.S., et al., *International lung cancer trends by histologic type: Male:female differences diminishing and adenocarcinoma rates rising. International Journal of Cancer*, 2005. **117**(2): pp. 294–9.
161. Patel, J.D., P.B. Bach, and M.G. Kris, *Lung cancer in US women: A contemporary epidemic. Jama*, 2004. **291**(14): pp. 1763–8.
162. Lubin, J.H. and W.J. Blot, *Assessment of lung cancer risk factors by histologic category. Journal of National Cancer Institute*, 1984. **73**(2): pp. 383–9.
163. Bain, C., et al., *Lung cancer rates in men and women with comparable histories of smoking. Journal of National Cancer Institute*, 2004. **96**(11): pp. 826–34.
164. Warren, G.W. and K.M. Cummings, *Tobacco and lung cancer: risks, trends, and outcomes in patients with cancer. American Society of Clinical Oncology Educational Book*, 2013: pp. 359–64.
165. Kuper, H., P. Boffetta, and H.O. Adami, *Tobacco use and cancer causation: association by tumour type. Journal of Internal Medicine*, 2002. **252**(3): pp. 206–24.
166. Volanis, D., et al., *Environmental factors and genetic susceptibility promote urinary bladder cancer. Toxicology Letters*, 2010. **193**(2): pp. 131–7.
167. Gallaway, M.S., et al., *Surveillance for cancers associated with tobacco Use – United States, 2010-2014. MMWR Surveillance Summaries*, 2018. **67**(12): pp. 1–42.
168. Poon, R.T., et al., *Different risk factors and prognosis for early and late intrahepatic recurrence after resection of hepatocellular carcinoma. Cancer*, 2000. **89**(3): pp. 500–7.
169. Zeegers, M.P., et al., *The association between smoking, beverage consumption, diet and bladder cancer: A systematic literature review. World Journal of Urolology*, 2004. **21**(6): pp. 392–401.
170. Chapman, S., et al., *Cigarette smoke extract induces oral squamous cell carcinoma cell invasion in a receptor for advanced glycation end-products-dependent manner. European Journal of Oral Sciences*, 2018. **126**(1): pp. 33–40.
171. Hasnis, E., et al., *Synergistic effect of cigarette smoke and saliva on lymphocytes – the mediatory role of volatile aldehydes and redox active iron and the possible implications for oral cancer. International Journal of Biochemistry and Cell Biology*, 2004. **36**(5): pp. 826–39.
172. Sadri, G. and H. Mahjub, *Tobacco smoking and oral cancer: A meta-analysis. Journal of Research in Health Sciences*, 2007. **7**(1): pp. 18–23.
173. Chaturvedi, P., et al., *Tobacco related oral cancer. BMJ*, 2019. **365**: p. l2142.
174. Johnson, N.W., P. Jayasekara, and A.A. Amarasinghe, *Squamous cell carcinoma and precursor lesions of the oral cavity: Epidemiology and aetiology. Periodontol 2000*, 2011. **57**(1): pp. 19–37.
175. Jiang, X., et al., *Tobacco and oral squamous cell carcinoma: A review of carcinogenic pathways. Tobacco Induced Diseases*, 2019. **17**: p. 29.
176. Huang, H.-W., et al., *Arsenic-induced carcinogenesis and immune dysregulation. International Journal of Envionmental Research and Public Health*, 2019. **16**(15): p. 2746.
177. Zhou, Q., and S.J.R.T. Xi, *A review on arsenic carcinogenesis: Epidemiology, metabolism, genotoxicity and epigenetic changes. Regulatory Toxicology Pharmacology* 2018. **99**: pp. 78–88.
178. Faita, F., et al., *Arsenic-induced genotoxicity and genetic susceptibility to arsenic-related pathologies. International Journal of Envionmental Research and Public Health*, 2013. **10**(4): pp. 1527–46.
179. Dutheil, F., et al., *Prostate cancer and asbestos: A systematic review and meta-analysis. Permanente Journal*, 2020. **24**(19): p. PMC7039423.
180. Morinaga, K., et al., *Asbestos-related lung cancer and mesothelioma in Japan. Industrial Health*, 2001. **39**(2): pp. 65–74.
181. Slomovitz, B., et al., *Asbestos and ovarian cancer: Examining the historical evidence. International Journal of Gynecological Cancer*, 2021. **31**(1): pp. 122–28.

182. Sera, Y. and K.-Y.J.T.T.J.o.E.M. Kang, *Asbestos and cancer in the Sennan district of Osaka*. *Tohoku Journal of Experimental Medicins*, 1981. **133**(3): pp. 313–20.

183. Robles, H., *Aminobiphenyl, 4*. In Reference Module in Biomedical Sciences 2014. Elsevier: Amsterdam.

184. Wang, L., et al., *Stem cell and benzene-induced malignancy and hematotoxicity*. *Chemical Research in Toxicology*, 2012. **25**(7): pp. 1303–15.

185. Warden, H., et al., *Associations between occupational exposure to benzene, toluene and xylene and risk of lung cancer in Montréal*. *Occupational and Environmental Medicine*, 2018. **75**(10): pp. 696–702.

186. Rana, I., et al., *Benzene exposure and non-Hodgkin lymphoma: a systematic review and meta-analysis of human studies*. *The Lancet*, 2021. **5**(9): p. e633–43.

187. Mungi, C., et al., *Spatial analysis of industrial benzene emissions and cancer incidence rates in Texas*. *International Journal of Environmental Research and Public Health*, 2019. **16**(15): p. 2627.

188. Snyder, R., G. Witz, and B.D. Goldstein, *The toxicology of benzene*. *Environmental Health Perspect*, 1993. **100**: pp. 293–306.

189. Ghanei, M. and A.A.. Harandi, *Lung carcinogenicity of sulfur mustard*. *Clinical Lung Cancer*, 2010. **11**(1): pp. 13–7.

190. Dillman, J.F., et al., *Genomic analysis of rodent pulmonary tissue following bis-(2-chloroethyl) sulfide exposure*. *Chemical Research in Toxicology*, 2005. **18**(1): pp. 28–34.

191. Lecona, E. and O. Fernandez-Capetillo, *Targeting ATR in cancer*. *Nature Reviews Cancer*, 2018. **18**(9): pp. 586–95.

192. Mukaida, K., et al., *Mustard gas exposure and mortality among retired workers at a poisonous gas factory in Japan: A 57-year follow-up cohort study*. *Occupational and Environmental Medicine*, 2017. **74**(5): pp. 321–7.

193. Manning, K.P., et al., *Cancer of the larynx and other occupational hazards of mustard gas workers*. *Clinical Otolaryngology Allied Science*, 1981. **6**(3): pp. 165–70.

194. Doi, M., et al., *Effect of mustard gas exposure on incidence of lung cancer: A longitudinal study*. *American Journal of Epidemiology*, 2011. **173**(6): pp. 659–66.

195. Purchase, I., et al., *Lifetime carcinogenicity study of 1-and 2-naphthylamine in dogs*. *Br J Cancer*, 1981. **44**(6): pp. 892–901.

196. Humans, I.W.G.o.t.E.o.C.R.t., *2-naphthylamine*. In *Chemical Agents and Related Occupations*. 2012, International Agency for Research on Cancer.

197. Masuda, Y. and D. Hoffmann, *Determination of 1-naphthylamine and 2-naphthylamine in cigarette smoke*. Analytical Chemistry, 1969. **41**(4): p. 650-652.

198. Cameron, K.S., V. Buchner, and P.B. Tchounwou, *Exploring the molecular mechanisms of nickel-induced genotoxicity and carcinogenicity: A literature review*. *Reviews on Environmental Health*, 2011. **26**(2): pp. 81–92.

199. Sciannameo, V., et al., *Cancer mortality and exposure to nickel and chromium compounds in a cohort of Italian electroplaters*. *American Journal of Industrial Medicine*, 2019. **62**(2): pp. 99–110.

200. Zhao, J., et al., *Occupational toxicology of nickel and nickel compounds*. *Journal of Environmental Pathology, Toxicology and Oncology*, 2009. **28**(3): pp. 177–208.

201. Pavela, M., J. Uitti, and E. Pukkala, *Cancer incidence among copper smelting and nickel refining workers in Finland*. *Am J Ind Med*, 2017. **60**(1): pp. 87–95.

202. Schaumlöffel, D., *Nickel species: Analysis and toxic effects*. *Journal of Trace Elements in Medicine and Bioliogy*, 2012. **26**(1): pp. 1–6.

203. Norseth, T., *The carcinogenicity of chromium*. *Environmental Health Perspective*, 1981. **40**: pp. 121–30.

204. Fang, Z., et al., *Genotoxicity of tri- and hexavalent chromium compounds in vivo and their modes of action on DNA damage in vitro*. *PLoS One*, 2014. **9**(8): pp. e103194.

205. Yatera, K., et al., *Cancer risks of hexavalent chromium in the respiratory tract*. *Journal of Uoeh*, 2018. **40**(2): pp. 157–72.

206. Costa, M. and C.B. Klein, *Toxicity and carcinogenicity of chromium compounds in humans*. *Critical Reviews in Toxicology*, 2006. **36**(2): pp. 155–63.

207. Wang, Y., et al., *Carcinogenicity of chromium and chemoprevention: A brief update*. *Onco Targets Therapy*, 2017. **10**: pp. 4065–79.

208. Choudhary, G.J.C., *Human health perspectives on environmental exposure to benzidine: A review.* Chemosphere, 1996. **32**(2): pp. 267–91.
209. Rao, C.V., *Benzidine.* In *Encyclopedia of Toxicology (Third Edition),* P. Wexler, Editor. 2014. Academic Press: Oxford. pp. 419–22.
210. Boffetta, P. and F. Nyberg, *Contribution of environmental factors to cancer risk.* British Medical Bulletin, 2003. **68**: pp. 71–94.
211. Prüss-Üstün, A., et al., *Preventing disease through healthy environments: A global assessment of the burden of disease from environmental risks.* 2016. World Health Organization.
212. Schottenfeld, D., et al., *Current perspective on the global and United States cancer burden attributable to lifestyle and environmental risk factors.* Annual Review of Public Health, 2013. **34**: pp. 97–117.
213. Gatto, N.M., *Environmental carcinogens and cancer risk.* Cancers (Basel), 2021. **13**(4): p. 622.
214. Oyama, T., et al., *Lung cancer and CYP1A1 orGSTM1 polymorphisms.* Environmental Health and Preventive Medicine, 2003. **7**(6): pp. 230–4.
215. Guengerich, F.P., *Cytochrome p450 and chemical toxicology.* Chemical Research in Toxicology, 2008. **21**(1): pp. 70–83.
216. Moorthy, B., C. Chu, and D.J. Carlin, *Polycyclic aromatic hydrocarbons: From metabolism to lung cancer.* Toxicological Sciences, 2015. **145**(1): pp. 5–15.
217. Windmill, K.F., et al., *The role of xenobiotic metabolizing enzymes in arylamine toxicity and carcinogenesis: Functional and localization studies.* Mutation Research, 1997. **376**(1–2): pp. 153–60.
218. Lai, C. and P.G. Shields, *The role of interindividual variation in human carcinogenesis.* Journal of Nutrition, 1999. **129**(2S Suppl): p. 552s–555s.
219. Saengtienchai, A., et al., *Identification of interspecific differences in phase II reactions: Determination of metabolites in the urine of 16 mammalian species exposed to environmental pyrene.* Environmental Toxicology Chemistry, 2014. **33**(9): pp. 2062–9.
220. Vineis, P. and M. Porta, *Causal thinking, biomarkers, and mechanisms of carcinogenesis.* Journal of Clinical Epidemiology, 1996. **49**(9): pp. 951–6.
221. Bouchardy, C., et al., *Metabolic genetic polymorphisms and susceptibility to lung cancer.* Lung Cancer, 2001. **32**(2): pp. 109–12.
222. Floyd, R.A., et al., *Hydroxyl free radical adduct of deoxyguanosine: Sensitive detection and mechanisms of formation.* Free Radical Research Communications, 1986. **1**(3): pp. 163–72.
223. Weston, A.J.M.R.F. and M.M.o. Mutagenesis, *Physical methods for the detection of carcinogen-DNA adducts in humans.* Mutation Research, 1993. **288**(1): pp. 19–29.
224. Shuker, D.E., et al., *Urinary markers for measuring exposure to endogenous and exogenous alkylating agents and precursors.* Environmental Health Perspective, 1993. **99**: pp. 33–7.
225. Weston, A., et al., *Fluorescence detection of lesions in DNA.* Basic Life Sciences, 1990. **53**: pp. 63–81.
226. Sutherland, B.M. and A.D. Woodhead, *DNA Damage and Repair in Human Tissues.* Vol. 53. 2012: Springer Science & Business Media: Berlin.
227. Phillips, D.H., *Detection of DNA modifications by the 32P-postlabelling assay.* Mutatation Research, 1997. **378**(1–2): pp. 1–12.
228. Mayneord, W. and E.J.B.J. Roe, *Fluorescence spectrum of 1:2-benzpyrene.* Biochemical Journal, 1936. **30**(4): p. 707.
229. Kennaway, E., *The identification of a carcinogenic compound in coal-tar.* Brish Medical Journal, 1955. **2**(4942): pp. 749–52.
230. Turtiainen, T. and L. Salonen, *Prevention measures against radiation exposure to radon in well waters: Analysis of the present situation in Finland.* Journal of Water Health, 2010. **8**(3): pp. 500–12.
231. Keiding, L.M., *General preventive measures against carcinogenic exposure in the external environment.* Pharmacology Toxicology, 1993. **72**(Suppl 1): pp. 136–8.
232. Clementino, M., X. Shi, and Z. Zhang, *Prevention of polyphenols against carcinogenesis induced by environmental carcinogens.* Journal of Environmental Pathology Toxicology and Oncology, 2017. **36**(1): pp. 87–98.

3 Causes of Death from Cancer

*Hafiz Muhammad Irfan, Muhammad Ihtisham Umar,
Usman Sabir, Muhammad Yasir Ali, and
Ummaima Shahzad*

3.1 INTRODUCTION

Worldwide, cancer kills 244.6 million people every year; 137.4 million men and 107.1 million women are affected. While, ischemic heart disease kills 203.7 million people yearly, and 137.9 million people yearly die from stroke [1]. Leukemias (37%), then malignancies of the brain and central nervous system (16%), and lymphomas (14%), are the most prevalent among individuals younger than 13 years old. Breast cancer (13%) is the extremely prevalent tumor among 15–49-year-olds, followed by cancers of the liver (12%) and lung (9%) [2]. In the age group 50–60 years, the pulmonary tumor is the most prevalent malignant disease (19%), followed by the liver (12%) and breast (10%) cancers. In persons aged 60 or older, the most prevalent malignancies are lung (20%), stomach (8%), colorectal (9%), and hepatic (10%) [3].

The vast knowledge regarding the causes of cancer at the molecular level has exploded over recent years. The metastasis and cellular abnormalities at the genetic level result in cancer with poor or unfavorable prognosis and the molecular pathways that describe the malignant phenotype of distinct cancer have been described in different research [4]. Metastasis is the critical stage in the development of the fatal phenotype of cancer. Most solid tumor malignancies result in patient death because they spread away from the original site and metastasize [5].

The five stages of metastasis are invasion, neovascularization, bloodstream, extravasation, and colonization. Environmental cues like old age and circadian instabilities, sealant signals from extracellular matrix (ECM) components like collagen and fibronectin, ECM mechanical stressors like compression and tension, cell–cell interplay, soluble signals including growth factors and cytokines, and the intertumoral microbiota all contribute to the activation of metastasis and invasion [6]. Epithelial-to-mesenchymal transition (EMT) can happen through either solitary cell migration or mass movement. Many stages happen between the first epithelial cell and the invasive mesenchymal cell [7]. Circulating cancer cells can be lone wolves or large tumors. If a circulating tumor cell (CTC) stops at a secondary site or gets stuck in a blood vessel, it will extravasate and recolonize the nearby regions. Some cells hibernate as a protective mechanism against new conditions [5].

Based on their inherited genetic makeup, cells are attacked by several external factors that might cause gene damage, such as radiation, viruses, and other micro-organisms, chemical carcinogens, and free radicals as byproducts of physiological cell functions and build up with aging [8]. For example, TNF-α promotes tumor growth, produces angiogenesis, plays a crucial role in setting off the inflammatory cascade, controls the production of chemokines, and plays a major role in invasion and cachexia as well as thrombosis and bone metastasis [9]. Matrix metalloproteinases (MMPs) involve the dissolution of the extracellular matrix by an enzyme that is increased in most

DOI: 10.1201/9781003363958-4

malignancies and facilitates tumor cell infiltration and metastasis. The frequent sites of cancer metastasis are the lung, breast, colon, prostate, and ovary [10]. Several genes, such as collagen type I alpha 1 (COL1A1) and pituitary tumor-transforming 1 (PTTG1), are increased, whereas other genes, such as myosin heavy polypeptide 11, and smooth muscle (MYH1), a significant component of the contractile apparatus, are down-regulated. Nuclear receptors sub-family 4, group-A, member-1 (NR4A1) – a gene involved in the transcription factor and apoptosis inducer – is also suppressed [11]. The characteristics that cancer develops in various clinical syndromes may be fatal for the patient [12]. These disorders can be generally connected to organ failure and systemic cytokine overproduction [13].

3.2 CAUSES OF DEATH IN THE CANCER PATIENTS

Cancers of the liver, pancreatic, esophagus, lung, and brain were associated with the highest relative index-cancer mortality (Figure 3.1). Patients with malignancies of the colorectum, bladder, kidney, endometrial, breast, prostate, and testis had the highest incidence of non-cancer causes of mortality; where greater than 40% of deaths were due to heart disease [14]. Cachexia is the leading cause of death in cancer patients [9]. Progressive weight loss, anorexia, anemia, and fatigue can be traced back to an imbalance in proinflammatory cytokines, which are released because of an inflammatory cascade initiated by the host defense and tumor. These cytokines have multiple targets, including myocytes, hepatocytes, adipocytes, bone marrow, neurons, and endothelial cells [15]. In addition to endothelial cell damage and activation of the clotting cascade, endothelial cell damage promotes the cancer cells to infiltrate locally, and metastasis is related to the thromboembolic phenomenon [16].

Pain, fractures, and compressed spinal cord are all results of metastases in the skeleton and the stimulation of osteoblasts and osteoclasts by cancer cells, which starts a vicious cycle of bone degradation and accelerated tumorigenesis [17]. Similarly, in the last 6 weeks of life, the leading cause of death is gastroesophageal blockage and severe dyspnea, which affect 10% to 60% of cancer

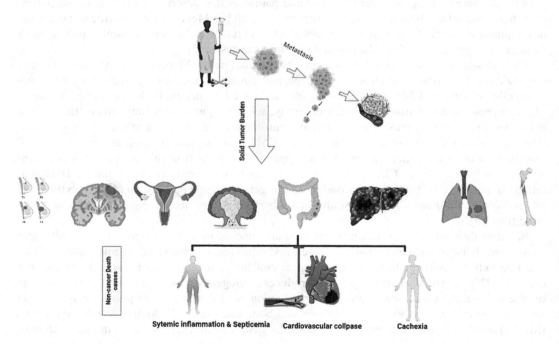

FIGURE 3.1 Schematic presentation of cancer and non-cancer causes of deaths and respective organs.

patients [18]. The other most prevalent non-cancerous causes of mortality are septicemia, infectious illnesses, and parasitic infections, and nearly all fatalities (93.8%) happened within 3 years of diagnosis. All deaths occurred due to cardiovascular and cerebrovascular illness as the secondary non-cancer cause [19]. Additionally, chemotherapy can cause more than 25% of deaths in patients with cancers. The major causative factors are pulmonary, lung, cardiac, and renal fibrosis [20]. The detail of the most prevalent fetal cancers and causes of death is as follows.

3.2.1 HEPATIC CANCER

Liver and bile duct malignancies have the fastest-growing mortality rates among men and women. Hepatocellular carcinoma, intrahepatic cholangiocarcinoma, fibrolamellar carcinoma, and hepatoblastoma are all types of primary liver cancer [21]. It is generally believed that the ends of the bile duct tree are the sites of the liver progenitor and stem cells. In response to stress, hepatocytes have the potential to dedifferentiate into hepatocyte-derived progenitor-like cells via a process known as reversible ductal metaplasia. It is theorized that hepatocytes originate from progenitor/oval cells, hepato-blasts, and cholangiocytes [22]. Liver cancer and the immune system have been connected through several pathways. To begin, the inflammatory signaling pathways in hepatocytes (through JAK-STAT, nuclear factor κB, etc.) can be activated when immune cells produce cytokines such as TNFα and interleukin (IL)-6 [23]. Stem cell characteristics, such as NOTCH, are enriched in tumors pertaining to the proliferation class, as are signaling pathways involved in propagation, such as insulin-like growth factor-I and the mechanistic target of rapamycin (mTOR) [24]. Mutations in CTNNB1, an S3 gene expression signature, and the traditional Wnt signaling pathway are hallmarks of the non-proliferation subtype [25].

3.2.2 LUNG CANCER

Lung infection, emphysema, pneumonia, airway obstruction, bleeding, embolism, excision, and lung damage are all major causes of death in lung cancer apart from tumor burden [26]. Neutrophils and monocytes are important effector cells in chronic obstructive pulmonary disease (COPD) because they produce cytokines, reactive oxygen species, extracellular matrix proteins, lipoxygenases, leukotrienes, and MMPs [27]. Increased CD8+ T lymphocytes in the airways and lung parenchyma may result in permanent abnormalities in the epithelium [28]. Participation of the CXCR4/CXCL12 (SDF-1) axis in the etiology of lung cancer is conceivable [29]. The enzymes COX-2 and PGE 2 may be involved in the development of both COPD and lung cancer via their effects on cell growth, cell death, and angiogenesis, hence enhancing the inflammatory response and carcinogenesis [30]. Overactivation of PI3K, glycogen synthase kinase-3, and PKC-zeta contributes to COPD and tumor formation [31].

In addition, abnormal overexpression of epidermal growth factor receptor (EGFR) is one of the earliest abnormalities in both high-risk smokers and COPD patients who develop squamous cell lung carcinoma (SCLC) [32]. Similarly, epithelial cells in bronchi and malignant cells of SCLC both overexpress protein aldo-keto reductase family 1 member B10 (AKR1B10) in COPD patients [33]. Significant associations exist between lung cancer and mutations in the genes encoding the major metabolizing enzymes of xenobiotics found in human lung tissues, such as cytochrome P450 (CYP) enzymes, microsomal epoxide hydrolases (EPHX), flavin monooxygenases, and myeloperoxidases (MPO) [34, 35]. Furthermore, SNP mutations in a region of chromosome 15's long arm (15q25.1) containing the nicotinic acetylcholine receptor alpha (nAChR) subunits 3 (CHRNA3) and 5 (CHRNA5), as well as the 4 nAChR subunit (CHRNB4), cannot be overruled [36]. Some p53 SNPs have been linked to an increased risk of developing COPD, and cigarette smoking is known to greatly increase the risk of lung cancer overall and the risk of lung cancer in people who already have a p53 mutation in their genes [37]. In the same way, it is said that the p16 INK4a tumor suppressor gene and the O-6-methylguanine-DNA methyltransferase (MGMT) promoters in the DNA samples of sputum of all SCLC patients are methylated in an abnormal way [38].

3.2.3 BREAST CANCER

In 95% of breast tumor patients, the estrogen receptor (ER), progesterone receptor (PR), and human epidermal growth factor receptor 2 (HER2) are overexpressed. Regardless of the stage of disease, size of the tumor, ER status, or age at the time of diagnosis, breast cancer affects mortality in individuals with various phenotypes [39]. In all age categories, women with positive lymph nodes at the time of diagnosis had an elevated risk of death over the 10 years of follow-up [40]. Due to the aggressive nature of the tumors, the prognosis for disease in young women at an early stage may be poorer. Deaths caused by problems with the circulatory system are probably caused by more than one thing [41, 42].

3.2.4 BONE CANCER

Abnormal features like hypercalcemia, bone discomfort, fractures, and nerve compression result from bone metastases [43]. Furthermore, in breast cancer, osteolytic metastases are the most prevalent, although considerable numbers of patients also develop mixed and osteoblastic metastases [44]. Common osteolytic factors include interleukins 8 and 11, parathyroid hormone related protein, and the vascular endothelial growth factor [45]. Osteoblastic metastases may be triggered by tumor-secreted endothelin–1 (ET-1), although there are several other possible osteoblastic agents. As bone-forming osteoblasts are the primary regulators of bone-degrading osteoclasts, stimulation of osteoblasts might paradoxically boost osteoclast function [46]. Thus, the co-expression of the osteolytic and osteoblastic proteins can result in the development of mixed metastases or an increase in osteolysis [47].

Bone tumor cells secrete osteolytic factors including PTHrP and osteoblastic factors like ET-1 [48]. Certain osteolytic agents induce osteoblast production of RANK ligand, activating its receptor on the surface of osteoclasts. Furthermore, osteoblasts secrete growth factors that can encourage tumor cells, which are then liberated by osteoclast activity from the bone matrix [49]. High local concentrations of components drive the development of tumor and bone cells, hence perpetuating a vicious cycle. Hypoxia may act as an extra stimulus for the vicious cycle by activating many genes for tumor and bone-related proteins [50]. In addition, the skeleton is the most frequent location of metastasis in men with end-stage prostate cancer [51].

3.2.5 TUMORS OF THE GASTROINTESTINAL TRACT

Colorectal cancer (CRC) is the third most occurring tumor worldwide. It is expected to cause about 52,580 deaths in 2022. Metastasis development can be lethal, generating mass effects and interfering with body homeostasis [52]. Esophageal cancer is highly lethal, and esophagectomy combined with lymph node dissection is the gold standard for treating locally advanced malignancies. Pulmonary comorbidities such as pneumonia colonic/jejunal interposition, blood transfusion, and heart failure are the main cause of death [53].

Pancreatic cancer is also the main cause of cancer-related mortality and one of the deadliest malignant neoplasms worldwide [54]. Developed nations have the greatest incidence and fatality rates of pancreatic cancer. The 5-year predicted survival rate for the pancreatic tumor is nearly 5% [55]. Diabetes is linked with an increased probability of pancreatic cancer. Both types of diabetes quadruple the risk of developing pancreatic malignancy [56]. Similarly, chronic pancreatitis resulting from severe alcohol consumption, or an underlying genetic condition is connected with an increased risk of tumor development [57]. Heart illnesses, cerebrovascular diseases, and septicemia are the common reasons for non-cancer mortality [58].

3.2.6 Ovarian Carcinoma

Despite being the most lethal form of gynecological cancer, the mechanisms by which the genes contribute to epithelial ovarian cancer are not well understood [59]. Typically, ovarian cancer manifests after 3–4 months of stomach pain, which may be misdiagnosed as irritable bowel disease. The disorder may reach the pelvis and include several lymph nodes [60]. Most deaths occur from cardiovascular disease, stroke, and COPD. For both Lynch syndrome (linked to endometrial and colorectal tumors) and hereditary nonpolyposis coli, it has been determined that genes associated with base mismatch repair play a major part in carcinogenesis [61]. Nearly a decade ago, a new categorization was presented that distinguished type I and type II ovarian tumors. Some type I cancers (endometrioid, mucinous, and clear cell types) possessed microsatellite instability and mutations in PTEN, BRAF, and KRAS. Type-II malignancies include high-grade serous and carcinosarcoma, which have BRCA1, BRCA2, and p53, mutations often [62]. Several hundred ovarian cancer tumors were subjected to an integrated genomic study, which showed mutations in NF1, BRCA2, and CDK12. Notably, approximately 50% of high-grade serous cancers lack homologous recombination repair of DNA damage, and NOTCH and FOXM1 signaling are associated with the progress of serous tumors [63].

3.2.7 Leukemias

Chronic lymphocytic leukemia (CLL) is the most prevalent type of leukemia in the West [64]. Acute myocardial infarction, peripheral vascular disease, and congestive heart failure are all examples of common co-morbidities. Patients with these conditions are also likely to have a cerebrovascular disease, chronic lung disease, diabetes, hemiplegia, kidney disease, malignant metastatic tumors, cirrhosis, and AIDS [65]. Diabetes without end-organ damage is the leading cause of mortality (99.5%). Other reasons for death include lymphoma and COPD [66].

3.2.8 Tumors in the Nervous System

The advancement of clinical tumors in the nervous system is the top cause of mortality (77.0%) especially in pediatrics, followed by infection [67]. Glioblastoma is a highly prevalent primary brain cancer in adult patients and is nearly always fatal, despite therapeutic improvements [68]. Specific neurologic consequences of tumor advancement, such as refractory seizures, intra-tumoral bleeding, and cerebral edema, were found as rare clinical events resulting in death in addition to clinical tumor advancement [69]. Seizures are the major complication of gliomas, especially in the last weeks of life, and they frequently have a negative effect on the quality of life. Pneumonia, ventricular meningitis, and pulmonary and cardiac arrhythmias are additional causes of death [70].

Once nerve endings release neuro-related substances like neurotrophins and neuropeptides, the nervous system promotes tumor metastasis [71]. Proteolytic enzymes like MMPs aid in this process by destroying the surrounding normal tissues. Neurological factors and neurotransmitters regulate MMP overexpression [72]. Elevated levels of brain-derived neurotrophic factor (BDNF) and related receptor tropomyosin-related kinase B (TrkB) prevent anoikis in epithelial cells. Both overexpression of TrkB and BDNF activation in the human cancer cell line of the endometrium may lead to changes in the expression of EMT cellular mediators [73].

Neuropeptides like substance P and bradykinin have been discovered to increase vascular permeability, hence encouraging tumor sarcoma cell extravasation and colonization [74]. Vascular endothelial growth factor (VEGF) plays a crucial role in the angiogenesis of tumors, which ultimately leads to metastasis, where Neuropeptide Y (NPY) increases its expression [75]. Stromal cells create neural-related substances and express the β-adrenergic receptor, which results in the production and the survival of tumor cells at the primary location and secondary organ [76]. Perineural invasion mediates cancer spread by triggering the production of NGF and GDNF via distinct signaling pathways. The ingrown nerve endings of tumors emit neurotransmitters, such as norepinephrine and substance P initiating the spread of metastases [77, 78].

3.3 MORTALITY-PROVOKING IMMUNOSUPPRESSION AND METASTASIS IN CANCER

Owing to the highly complex molecular attributes of cancer pathogenesis, one cannot nominate a specific factor accountable for the aggressiveness of cancers. However, the crosstalk between the cells of the tumor, the immune system, and tissue stroma gradually transforms the immune system in favor of the proliferating cancer cells. The resultant decline in immune attack also supports the metastasis of these rapidly diving cells from the site of initiation to the distant tissues. The infiltration of vital organs like the brain, liver, lungs, and kidneys drastically limit the therapeutic options with a poor prognosis of chemotherapy and a decline in the patient's survival. In the following section, we will focus on the mechanisms used by the cancer cells to attenuate immune attacks and provoke metastasis.

3.3.1 IMMUNOSUPPRESSION

At early disease stages, immune cells play a vital role in inhibiting the growth and proliferation of cancer cells, thus limiting these aberrant cells to their site of initiation. The myeloid cells such as the tumor-associated macrophages (TAMs) and dendritic cells (DCs) identify cancer antigens and unleash a cytotoxic attack on the cancer cells. Moreover, they also present these antigens to the cytotoxic CD8+ T cells (Tc) and the natural killer cells (NKs) to initiate a more specific antitumor immunity. NKs are armed with cytotoxic granules such as perforins and granzymes in a much more similar way as the Tc. The cytotoxic Tc are directly activated by antigens that are mounted on the major histocompatibility complex -I (MHC-I) self-marker proteins expressed by the host cells. The aberrant expression or complete downregulation of these self-antigens is common in viral infected and tumor cells. The tumor cells downregulate the self-antigens to protect themselves from the cytotoxic Tc attack. However, the NKs have an in-built potential to detect and demolish such deviant cells because of the specialized killer immunoglobulin-like (KIR) receptors that these cells are equipped with. Depending upon the expression of CD16 and the intensity of CD56 expression, NKs are grouped as $CD56^{bright}$ $CD16^-$ regulatory NKs and $CD56^{dim}$ $CD16^+$ cytotoxic NKs. The $CD56^{bright}$ NKs are believed to exhibit less cytotoxic potential because of a lower expression of KIR. Moreover, these cells exhibit a relatively lower expression of perforins and granzyme B but a higher expression of granzyme K as compared to the $CD56^{dim}$ NKs [79]. It is also a fact that the tumor stroma is more infiltrated by the $CD56^{bright}$ cells as compared to the $CD56^{dim}$ NKs, however, these NKs remain within the stromal tissue and do not interact directly with the cancer cells [80]. Within the stromal tissue, these regulatory NKs release cytokines and chemokines to boost Tc-mediated cytotoxicity by potentiating the recruitment and maturation of DCs. Primarily, these regulatory NKs are not acting directly as effector cytotoxic cells within the tumor microenvironment (TME) but play a crucial regulatory role in governing an immune response against cancer cells. However, the $CD56^{bright}$ cells within the TME express KIR and get differentiated into the effector $CD56^{dim}$ cells by the cytokines released from the stromal fibroblasts [81]. With a few exceptions of tumors where the collagen IV and laminin content is higher in TME [82], the cytokines and chemokine signature of the TME profoundly recruit NKs in the TME.

The effector immune cells, such as the macrophages, neutrophils, Tc, and NKs, selectively identify and target a comparatively much lesser population of the diseased cells from the normal tissues. However, the activation of Tc and NKs-mediated cytotoxicity is greatly affected by the myeloid cells. These are the myeloid cells that shape the immune signatures of the TME from a highly hostile pro-inflammatory state to an immunosuppressive and cancer-supportive state. For instance, TAMs infiltrate into the tumors and selectively attack the tumor cells in the earlier stages of the disease [83]. The infiltration of tumors by the CD68+ TAMs has been reported to increase survival in gastric [84], endometrial [85] and colon cancers [86]. Likewise, the infiltration of classic dendritic cells (cDCs) in lung cancers promote T cell-mediated cytotoxicity against the cancer cells [87, 88]. Particularly, the CD103hi cDCs have been found positively associated with survival in breast, lung, and head or neck cancers [89]. In addition to the cDCs, the neutrophils also promote the cytotoxic properties of

TABLE 3.1
Role of Myeloid Cells in Inhibiting Cancer Cell Proliferation and Metastasis

Immune Cells	Anticancer Effects of Myeloid Cells
Mononuclear cells and tumor associated macrophages (TAMs)	TAMs may have divergent functions with some antitumor activity as well [83]. High infiltration of CD68+ TAMs is associated with improved survival in colon [86]; Gastric [84] and Endometrial cancer [85]. M1 like phenotype of TAMs engulf tumor cells, release angiostatic mediators and promote T cell cytotoxicity against the cancer cells [91–93]. Subcapsular macrophages suppress the melanoma in mice by limiting the spread of tumor vesicles in the lymph drainage of the tumors [94].
Dendritic Cells	High infiltration of cDCs in lung cancers are found beneficial because of an enhanced T cell mediated cytotoxicity [87, 88]. Activated cDCs and T cells are found clustered within the tertiary structures of lymphoids in lung cancers [95]. A high CD103hi/CD103lo ratio in murine models have been found associated with increased T cell activation [89]. A higher infiltration of CD103hi cDCs in tumor stroma is found to enhance survival in many human cancers, including breast, head or neck, and lung cancers [89]. Tumors use many ways to suppress the anti-tumor activity of DCs [96]. For instance, (a) In murine ovarian cancer models, the tumor cells induce an upregulation of XBP1 proteins in cDCs that results into an enhanced endoplasmic reticulum stress in cDCs with an accumulation of oxidized lipids. This transformation of cDC biology attenuates the capability of these cells to present antigens to T cells [97]. (b) Activation of β-catenin signaling in cancer cells inhibits DC mediated immunity [98]. (c) Release of cyclooxygenases from tumor cells inhibits DC activity [99] and TAMs release IL-10 to inhibit DC functions [100].
Polymorphonuclear cells such as the neutrophils and myeloid derived suppressor cells (MDSCs)	Tumor infiltrating neutrophils inhibit seeding in the premetastatic lung [101]. Neutrophils exhibit cytotoxic effect against cancer cells in mouse models [102, 103]. Neutrophils that are retrieved from the patients with early stage lung cancer activate T cell cytotoxicity [104]. Intratumor neutrophil infiltrates showed modest positive impact on the patient condition [90].
Eosinophils	Infiltration of eosinophils in TME and their degranulation is associated with increased prognosis in (a) oral squamous cell carcinoma, (b) prostate cancer, and (c) colon cancer [105, 106] and cytotoxic effect by releasing cytotoxic proteins [105]. They inhibited progression of metastatic melanoma in mouse model [107] and help in normalizing vasculature and activate T cell cytotoxicity against cancer cells [108].
Mast cells	The density of tumor infiltrating inflammatory cells in colorectal cancers declines with the stage of cancer. However, within the infiltrates of the cancer tissue, mast cells were not found much as compared to other inflammatory cells, showing that these do not tend to infiltrate the tumor microenvironment. This proves that the mast cells are dispensable for tumor growth [109]. Developing better murine models (Cre-recombinase models) have revealed that mast cells are dispensable for tumor growth [110].

Tc and a higher infiltration of these cells has been associated with better prognosis [90]. The role of myeloid cells in inhibiting the survival and proliferation of cancer cells in the earlier stages of the disease is well established. Some of the reported studies are presented in Table 3.1 that confirm their protective role against the initiation and spread of cancers.

The crosstalk between the tumor and stromal cells gradually transforms the cellular micro-environment to favor these cancer cells by controlling the immune checkpoints. Tumor-associated neutrophils, monocytes myeloid-derived suppressive cells, and the regulatory T lymphocytes play a major role in such an immunosuppressive shift of the cellular microenvironment to support the cancer cell's survival. The different mechanisms involved in the immune evasion of cancer cells are enlisted in Table 3.2. Moreover, crosstalk between the tumor and immune cells, and some co-existing factors also facilitate such tumbling of TME immune surveillance. For instance, the hypoxia that is induced within the TME by the rapidly proliferating cells promotes angiogenesis to enhance the survival of the cancer cells. Further, the hypoxia-induced upregulation of HIF-1α has been associated with a decline in the sensitivity of lung cancers [111] and ovarian cancers [112] to radiotherapy and paclitaxel-induced cytotoxicity, respectively. HIF-1α also upregulates the expression of CD47 on cancer cells, which is related to immune evasion and cancer proliferation [113].

TABLE 3.2
Mechanism of Promoting Cancer Cell Survival and Metastasis by Immune Cells

Immune Cells	Cancer Promoting Effects
Mononuclear cells	TAMs infiltrate in cancers and the high densities of TAM like cells are linked with poor prognosis in a number of cancers, such as the breast, kidney, pancreatic, ovarian, oral, endometrial, lungs, and Hodgkin lymphoma [83, 150, 151].
	TAMs support the proliferation and the survival of cancer cells by releasing the following:
	1. Proliferative cytokines and growth factors such as EGF, IL6, TNF) [152, 153].
	2. Extracellular matrix degrading proteins that enhance invasion and intravasation (MMPs, cysteine, cathepsins) [154, 156].
	3. Proangiogenic agents (VEGFA, IL8, semaphorin 4D) [153, 157, 158].
	Release of immunosuppressive markers or their expression on the cell surface (arginase 1, TGFβ, IL10, programmed cell death ligand 1, i.e., PDL1) [153, 159, 160].
	M2 like lineage of TAMs in tumors promote tumor proliferation, invasion, angiogenesis and facilitate cancer cell survival by inhibiting immune attack in TME [159].
	M2 infiltration is negatively associated with prognosis and survival [161].
	TAMs release several miRNAs that play a significant role in cancer cell proliferation, angiogenesis. (Reviewed in [162].) These TAMs include perivascular CD163[hi] TAMs and CD163[lo] TAMs in the necrotic tissue of tumors.
	TAMs release IL-10 to attenuate T cell cytotoxicity by inhibiting DC functions [100].
	High densities of monocytes are associated with advanced disease stage and poor prognosis in many different cancers, such as adenocarcinoma, breast and the colorectal carcinoma [161, 163].
	M-CSF/M-CSFR signaling is involved in the recruitment of TAMs in TME with subsequent promotion in tumor growth. Genetic ablation of M-CSF reduces TAM density and delays tumor progression [164, 165].
	Elevated levels of CCL2, M-CSF are found to be associated with poor prognosis in many human cancers, such as the breast [166, 167], pancreatic [168], colorectal [169], hepatocellular [170], and the endometrial cancers [171].
Dendritic cells	High infiltration of CD123+ pDCs is associated with decreased total and relapse free survival in the breast tumor patients [172] and melanoma [173].

TABLE 3.2 (Continued)
Mechanism of Promoting Cancer Cell Survival and Metastasis by Immune Cells

Immune Cells	Cancer Promoting Effects
Polymorphonuclear cells such as the neutrophils and myeloid derived suppressor cells (MDSCs)	High densities of neutrophils, monocytes, and MDSCs is associated with advanced disease stage and poor prognosis in many different cancers, such as adenocarcinoma, breast, and the colorectal carcinoma [161, 163].
	Higher blood levels of monocytes, neutrophils, monocytes [174, 175] and MDSCs [176] are associated with poor prognosis in cancer patients.
	Granulocytic cells use ROS to inhibit immunity against cancer cells [152].
	Neutrophils promote tumor growth as follows:
	1. Limiting cancer cell senescence [177].
	2. Promoting angiogenesis [178].
	3. Triggering thrombosis via neutrophil extracellular traps [179].
	4. Inducing genotoxic damage [180].
	5. Recruiting tumor promoting cells in TME [181].
Mast cells	B lymphocytes and humoral immune machinery induces FCγR on mast cells and other myeloid cells. These receptors help these cells to promote inflammation that results into carcinogenesis.
	By releasing tryptophane 5 hydroxylase 1 (TPH1), these cells exhaust tryptophane that results into immunosuppression and promotion of tumor [182].
	Mast cells foster tumor growth by inhibiting anticancer immunity via the following:
	a. Activating tumor promoting T_{reg} [183-185].
	b. Activating tumor promoting neutrophils [185, 186].
	Tumor infiltration by mast cells resulted into poor prognosis in patients with colorectal cancers [187].
Common myeloid cell markers	CD11b (also called integrin αM) and Gr1 (a surface antigen that is comprised of both Ly6C and Ly6G epitopes) are expressed on the surface of monocytes, granulocytes as well as MDSCs. These cells inhibit antitumor cytotoxicity of T cells upto varying degrees [188, 189].
	Different mechanisms that the myeloid cells use to inhibit T cell immunity include secretion &/or surface expression of immunosuppressive cytokines/markers that include the following:
	1. Arginase 1 [190].
	2. NO [191].
	3. PDL1 [160].
	4. COX2 [192].
	5. TGFβ [193].
	Myeloid cells produce ROS and peroxynitrite that can
	1. Interfere with MHC-T receptor interaction [194].
	2. Attenuate T cell migration [195].
	Activate Treg cells via CD40-CD40L signaling to induce tolerance against tumor antigens [196].
B lymphocytes	B lymphocytes and humoral immune machinery induce FCγR on mast cells and other myeloid cells. These receptors help these cells to promote inflammation that results in carcinogenesis [197].

3.3.2 METASTASIS

The escape of cancer cells from the immune checkpoints allows them to detach from the site of origin to migrate from distant locations, a phenomenon that is accountable for more than 90% of deaths in cancer patients [114]. The extent of metastasis greatly varies in different types of cancers, which indicates a probable existence of co-relation between the gene expression and metastatic potential. For instance, the extent of metastasis has been found extremely rare in basal cell carcinomas. However, an immensely aggressive and early metastasis in pancreatic cancers makes them extremely difficult to treat. Likewise, the metastasizing to lungs has been found much more common in bone sarcomas [115]. Initially, the cancer cells get detached from their neighboring cells and interact with the extracellular matrix to invade. This initial phase of metastasis is therefore termed the local invasion [116]. In some cancers, the cells invade locally however they seldom tend to advance further to metastasis. For instance, the extent of local invasion is highly noticeable in dermal carcinomas and brain tumors. However, both of these tumors seldom exhibit metastasis [117]. To invade in the surrounding extracellular matrix, these cells get transformed from having epithelial characteristics to containing more mesenchymal attributes via a complex mechanism, defined as the epithelial-to-mesenchymal transition (EMT). Once invaded into the extracellular matrix, the cancer cells enter the nearby blood vessels via the process of intravasation, spread to the distant tissues, and extravasate to the locations where they find a relatively better chance to survive. On the new locations, these cells retransform to regain the epithelial attributes via a reverse mesenchymal to epithelial transition (MET) [118, 119].

The stromal cells of the tumor microenvironment ensure a pivotal role in triggering alterations in gene expression during EMT. The major stromal cells that instigate EMT include the cancer-associated fibroblasts [120], T lymphocytes (CD8[+] cytotoxic T cells, CD4[+] T helper cells, and regulatory T cells) [121, 122], the tumor-associated macrophages [123] and the myeloid-derived suppressor cells [124]. In the epithelium, the cancer cells are attached to the neighboring cells through E-cadherin (epithelial cadherin) molecules. These tumor cells release colony-stimulating factors (CSF) to attract macrophages and stromal cells. The attracted macrophages further release epidermal growth factor (EGF) to induce CSF expression in cancer cells, thus enhancing the attracted population of macrophages and stromal cells through positive feedback. Various cytokines including transforming growth factor β (TGF β) [120], vascular endothelial growth factor (VEGF) [125], hepatocyte growth factor (HGF) [126, 127], EGF [128], tumor necrosis factor (TNF) [129], interleukin 6 (IL-6) [128] and chemokine C-C motif ligand 18 (CCL18) [130] are released from the stromal cells as well as from the cancer cells that act in a paracrine or autocrine fashion to induce a set of transcription factors in the cancer cells. These factors include SNAIL1/2 [131], ZEB1/2, TWIST1 [132], FOXA1/2 [133], FOXC2 [134], FOXD3 [135], FOXF1 [136], FOXO3A [137], FOXQ1 [138], ZNF703 [139], and PRX1 [140]. Once induced, these transcription factors downregulate the epithelial cell adhesion molecules particularly the E-cadherins, occludins, claudins [141], and cytokeratin [142]. Cathepsin B released from the macrophages degrades E-cadherins on the cancer cell surface, thus detaching these modified cells from epithelium. EGF, TNF-α and other mediators from these macrophages downregulate the synthesis of E-cadherin and upregulate N-cadherins [136], fibronectin [136], α_5 integrin [143], vimentin [133, 140], laminin [140], collagen [144], and matrix metalloproteinases (MMPs), such as MMP1, MMP2, MMP9, and MMP15 [145]. These MMPs degrade the basement membrane to detach the cancer cells from the epithelium. Further, HGF released from the macrophages stimulates the cancer cells to develop lamellipodia for their movement toward the HGF-releasing cells. The N-cadherins help these cells get attached to the endothelial cells and invade the bloodstream where platelets mask these cells to evade from the immune system [146]. In addition, integrins, such as α_5 and $\alpha_6\beta_4$, also govern EMT and metastasis by cell survival induction, regulating cell attachment/detachment characteristics, and inducing invasion and migration [147]. It is important to mention here that the expression of $\alpha_6\beta_4$ integrins was previously reported to be downregulated in EMT [148], the recent studies have suggested its up-regulation in hepatocellular carcinoma where it promotes EMT via slug upregulation [149].

3.4 CONCLUSION

Metastasis is the crucial stage in the development of the lethal cancer trait that is accountable for more than 90% of deaths in cancer patients. Immune cells like mononuclear cells, dendritic cells, mast cells, and lymphocytes try to stifle the survival of cancer cells early on but eventually assist them in proliferating in later stages. Similarly, cells in stroma communicate with tumor cells by secreting cytokines like transforming growth factor, interleukins, and vascular endothelial growth factor, which then induces a cluster of transcription factors. Patients with cancer may also die due to the symptoms they experience from various clinical syndromes. Organ failure and systemic inflammation have been linked to these diseases. The highest relative index-cancer mortality is seen in liver, pancreatic, colorectal, pulmonary, breast, and central nervous system tumors. Heart disease, including thromboembolism, is the leading cause of death among non-cancerous causes and occupy 40% of death.

REFERENCES

1. Kim, H.-I., H. Lim, and A. Moon, *Sex differences in cancer: Epidemiology, genetics and therapy.* Biomol. Ther., 2018. **26**(4): p. 335.
2. Zheng, R., et al., *Report of cancer epidemiology in China, 2015. Zhonghua Zhong Liu Za Zhi [Chin. J. Oncol.]*, 2019. **41**(1): pp. 19–28.
3. Mattiuzzi, C. and G. Lippi, *Current cancer epidemiology. J. Epidemiol. Glob. Health*, 2019. **9**(4): p. 217.
4. Frank, S.A., *Dynamics of cancer*. 2018. Princeton University Press: Princeton.
5. Fares, J., et al., *Molecular principles of metastasis: A hallmark of cancer revisited. Signal Transduct. Target. Ther.*, 2020. **5**(1): pp. 1–17.
6. Jin, X., et al., *A metastasis map of human cancer cell lines. Nature*, 2020. **588**(7837): pp. 331–6.
7. Bergers, G. and S.-M. Fendt, *The metabolism of cancer cells during metastasis. Nat. Rev. Cancer*, 2021. **21**(3): pp. 162–80.
8. Lewandowska, A.M., et al., *Environmental risk factors for cancer-review paper. Ann. Agric. Environ. Med.*, 2018. **26**(1): pp. 1–7.
9. Argilés, J.M., F.J. López-Soriano, and S. Busquets, *Mediators of cachexia in cancer patients. Nutrition*, 2019. **66**: pp. 11–15.
10. Klaunig, J.E., *Oxidative stress and cancer. Current Pharm. Des.*, 2018. **24**(40): pp. 4771–8.
11. Martínez-Jiménez, F., et al., *A compendium of mutational cancer driver genes. Nat. Rev. Cancer*, 2020. **20**(10): pp. 555–72.
12. Lyden, D., et al., *Metastasis. Cancer Cell*, 2022. **40**(8): pp. 787–91.
13. Suhail, Y., et al., *Systems biology of cancer metastasis. Cell Syst.*, 2019. **9**(2): pp. 109–27.
14. Zaorsky, N.G., et al., *Causes of death among cancer patients. Ann. Oncol.*, 2017. **28**(2): pp. 400–7.
15. Argilés, J.M., et al., *Inter-tissue communication in cancer cachexia. Nat. Rev. Endocrinol.*, 2019. **15**(1): pp. 9–20.
16. Schmaier, A.A., P. Ambesh, and U. Campia, *Venous thromboembolism and cancer. Current Cardiol. Rep.*, 2018. **20**(10): pp. 1–10.
17. Ferguson, J.L. and S.P. Turner, *Bone cancer: Diagnosis and treatment principles. Am. Fam. Physician*, 2018. **98**(4): pp. 205–13.
18. Loberg, R.D., et al., *The lethal phenotype of cancer: the molecular basis of death due to malignancy. CA: Cancer J. Clin.*, 2007. **57**(4): pp. 225–41.
19. Friedenreich, C.M., et al., *Physical activity and mortality in cancer survivors: a systematic review and meta-analysis. JNCI Cancer Spectr.*, 2020. **4**(1): p. pkz080.
20. Chu, E. and A. Sartorelli, *Cancer chemotherapy. In Lange's Basic and Clinical Pharmacology.* 2018, McGraw-Hill: New York. pp. 948–76.

21. Craig, A.J., et al., *Tumour evolution in hepatocellular carcinoma. Nat. Rev. Gastroenterol. Hepatol.*, 2020. **17**(3): pp. 139–52.

22. Yin, Z., et al., *Heterogeneity of cancer-associated fibroblasts and roles in the progression, prognosis, and therapy of hepatocellular carcinoma. J. Hematol. Oncol.*, 2019. **12**(1): p. 1–9.

23. van der Heide, D., R. Weiskirchen, and R. Bansal, *Therapeutic targeting of hepatic macrophages for the treatment of liver diseases. Front. Immunol.*, 2019. **10**: p. 2852.

24. Hibdon, E.S., et al., *Notch and mTOR signaling pathways promote human gastric cancer cell proliferation. Neoplasia*, 2019. **21**(7): pp. 702–12.

25. Sia, D., et al., *Liver cancer cell of origin, molecular class, and effects on patient prognosis. Gastroenterol.*, 2017. **152**(4): pp. 745–61.

26. Nichols, L., R. Saunders, and F.D. Knollmann, *Causes of death of patients with lung cancer. Arch. Pathol. Lab. Med.*, 2012. **136**(12): pp. 1552–57.

27. Parris, B.A., et al., *Chronic obstructive pulmonary disease (COPD) and lung cancer: common pathways for pathogenesis. J. Thorac. Dis.*, 2019. **11**(Suppl 17): p. S2155.

28. Horton, B.L., et al., *Lack of CD8+ T cell effector differentiation during priming mediates checkpoint blockade resistance in non–small cell lung cancer. Sci. Immunol.*, 2021. **6**(64): p. eabi8800.

29. Kamihara, Y., et al., *Tumor-to-tumor metastasis of diffuse large B cell lymphoma to gastric adenocarcinoma via CXCL12 (SDF-1)/CXCR4 axis: a case report. BMC Gastroenterol.*, 2021. **21**(1): p. 1–5.

30. Cadassou, O., et al., *Enhanced migration of breast and lung cancer cells deficient for cN-II and CD73 via COX-2/PGE2/AKT axis regulation. Cell. Oncol.*, 2021. **44**(1): pp. 151–65.

31. Bade, B.C. and C.S.D. Cruz, *Lung cancer 2020: epidemiology, etiology, and prevention. Clin. Chest Med.*, 2020. **41**(1): pp. 1–24.

32. Friedlaender, A., et al., *Next generation sequencing and genetic alterations in squamous cell lung carcinoma: where are we today? Front. Oncol.*, 2019. **9**: p. 166.

33. Kanno, M., et al., *Serum aldo–keto reductase family 1 member B10 predicts advanced liver fibrosis and fatal complications of nonalcoholic steatohepatitis. J. Gastroenterol.*, 2019. **54**(6): pp. 549–57.

34. Ramesh, V., T. Brabletz, and P. Ceppi, *Targeting EMT in cancer with repurposed metabolic inhibitors. Trends in Cancer*, 2020. **6**(11): pp. 942–50.

35. Mohammed, F., A. Baydaa Abed Hussein, and T. Ahmed, *Evaluation of methylation panel in the promoter region of p16INK4a, RASSF1A, and MGMT as a biomarker in sputum for lung cancer. Arch. Razi Inst.*, 2022. **77**(3): pp. 1075–81.

36. Jones, S.K., et al., *A systematic review of genetic variation within nicotinic acetylcholine receptor genes and cigarette smoking cessation. Drug Alcohol Depend.*, 2022: p. 109596.

37. Hou, W., et al., *Cigarette smoke induced lung barrier dysfunction, EMT, and tissue remodeling: a possible link between COPD and lung cancer. BioMed Res. Int.*, 2019. **2019**.

38. Adcock, I.M., G. Caramori, and P.J. Barnes, *Chronic obstructive pulmonary disease and lung cancer: New molecular insights. Respiration*, 2011. **81**(4): pp. 265–84.

39. Gholamalizadeh, M., et al., *Association between FTO gene polymorphisms and breast cancer: The role of estrogen. Expert Rev. Endocrinol. Metab.*, 2020. **15**(2): pp. 115–21.

40. Chen, A., et al., *Intermittent hypoxia induces a metastatic phenotype in breast cancer. Oncogene*, 2018. **37**(31): pp. 4214–25.

41. Colzani, E., et al., *Prognosis of patients with breast cancer: Causes of death and effects of time since diagnosis, age, and tumor characteristics. J. Clin. Oncol.*, 2011. **29**(30): pp. 4014–21.

42. Massarweh, S.A., et al., *Molecular characterization and mortality from breast cancer in men. J. Clin. Oncol.*, 2018. **36**(14): p. 1396.

43. Zekry, K.M., et al., *Reconstruction of intercalary bone defect after resection of malignant bone tumor. J. Orthop. Surg.*, 2019. **27**(1): p. 2309499019832970.

44. Alter, B.P., et al., *Cancer in the National Cancer Institute inherited bone marrow failure syndrome cohort after fifteen years of follow-up. Haematologica*, 2018. **103**(1): p. 30.

45. Tulotta, C. and P. Ottewell, *The role of IL-1B in breast cancer bone metastasis. Endocr. Relat Cancer*, 2018. **25**(7): pp. R421–R434.

46. Lu, N. and C.J. Malemud, *Extracellular signal-regulated kinase: a regulator of cell growth, inflammation, chondrocyte and bone cell receptor-mediated gene expression. Int. J. Mol. Sci.*, 2019. **20**(15): p. 3792.

47. Roca, H., et al., *Apoptosis-induced CXCL5 accelerates inflammation and growth of prostate tumor metastases in bone.* J. Clin. Invest., 2018. **128**(1): pp. 248–66.

48. Wong, S.K., et al., *Prostate cancer and bone metastases: The underlying mechanisms.* Int. J. Mol. Sci., 2019. **20**(10): p. 2587.

49. Jakob, T., et al., *Bisphosphonates or RANK-ligand-inhibitors for men with prostate cancer and bone metastases: A network meta-analysis.* Cochrane Database Syst. Rev., 2020(12): p. Cd013020.

50. Hiraga, T., *Hypoxic microenvironment and metastatic bone disease.* Int. J. Mol. Sci., 2018. **19**(11): p. 3523.

51. Guise, T.A., et al., *Molecular mechanisms of breast cancer metastases to bone.* Clin. Breast Cancer, 2005. **5**: pp. S46–S53.

52. Riihimäki, M., et al., *Patterns of metastasis in colon and rectal cancer.* Sci. Rep., 2016. **6**(1): pp. 1–9.

53. Kakuta, T., et al., *Prognostic factors and causes of death in patients cured of esophageal cancer.* Ann. Surg. Oncol., 2014. **21**(5): p. 1749–55.

54. Mizrahi, J.D., et al., *Pancreatic cancer.* The Lancet, 2020. **395**(10242): pp. 2008–20.

55. McGuigan, A., et al., *Pancreatic cancer: a review of clinical diagnosis, epidemiology, treatment and outcomes.* World J. Gastroentero., 2018. **24**(43): p. 4846.

56. Rawla, P., T. Sunkara, and V. Gaduputi, *Epidemiology of pancreatic cancer: global trends, etiology and risk factors.* World J. Oncol., 2019. **10**(1): p. 10.

57. Ilic, M. and I. Ilic, *Epidemiology of pancreatic cancer.* World J. Gastroenterolo., 2016. **22**(44): p. 9694.

58. Carioli, G., et al., *European cancer mortality predictions for the year 2021 with focus on pancreatic and female lung cancer.* Ann. Oncol., 2021. **32**(4): pp. 478–487.

59. Lee, J.M., L. Minasian, and E.C. Kohn, *New strategies in ovarian cancer treatment.* Cancer, 2019. **125**: pp. 4623–29.

60. Lheureux, S., et al., *Epithelial ovarian cancer.* The Lancet, 2019. **393**(10177): pp. 1240–53.

61. Orr, B. and R.P. Edwards, *Diagnosis and treatment of ovarian cancer.* Hematol. Oncol. Clin. North Am., 2018. **32**(6): pp. 943–64.

62. Chandra, A., et al., *Ovarian cancer: Current status and strategies for improving therapeutic outcomes.* Cancer Med., 2019. **8**(16): pp. 7018–31.

63. Jayson, G.C., et al., *Ovarian cancer.* The Lancet, 2014. **384**(9951): pp. 1376–88.

64. Burger, J.A., *Treatment of chronic lymphocytic leukemia.* N. Eng. J. Med., 2020. **383**(5): pp. 460–73.

65. Parikh, S.A., *Chronic lymphocytic leukemia treatment algorithm 2018.* Blood Cancer J., 2018. **8**(10): pp. 1–10.

66. Villavicencio, A., et al., *Comorbidities at diagnosis, survival, and cause of death in patients with chronic lymphocytic leukemia: A population-based study.* Int. J. Env. Res. Public Health, 2021. **18**(2): p. 701.

67. Udaka, Y.T. and R.J. Packer, *Pediatric brain tumors.* Neurol. Clin., 2018. **36**(3): pp. 533–56.

68. Barnholtz-Sloan, J.S., Q.T. Ostrom, and D. Cote, *Epidemiology of brain tumors.* Neurol. Clin., 2018. **36**(3): pp. 395–419.

69. Farmanfarma, K.K., et al., *Brain cancer in the world: an epidemiological review.* World Cancer Res. J., 2019. **6**(5): p. e1356.

70. Barbaro, M., et al., *Causes of death and end-of-life care in patients with intracranial high-grade gliomas: a retrospective observational study.* Neurology, 2022. **98**(3): pp. e260–6.

71. Cacho-Díaz, B., et al., *Tumor microenvironment differences between primary tumor and brain metastases.* J. Trans. Med., 2020. **18**(1): pp. 1–12.

72. Ahir, B.K., H.H. Engelhard, and S.S. Lakka, *Tumor development and angiogenesis in adult brain tumor: glioblastoma.* Mol. Neurobiol., 2020. **57**(5): pp. 2461–78.

73. Meng, L., et al., *Targeting the BDNF/TrkB pathway for the treatment of tumors.* Oncol. Lett., 2019. **17**(2): pp. 2031–9.

74. Królicki, L., et al. *225Ac-and 213Bi-substance P analogues for glioma therapy.* In *Seminars in Nuclear Medicine.* 2020. Elsevier: Amsterdam.

75. Song, E., et al., *VEGF-C-driven lymphatic drainage enables immunosurveillance of brain tumours.* Nature, 2020. **577**(7792): pp. 689–94.

76. Mravec, B., L. Horvathova, and L. Hunakova, *Neurobiology of cancer: the role of β-adrenergic receptor signaling in various tumor environments.* Int. J. Mol. Sci., 2020. **21**(21): p. 7958.

77. Ray, R., et al., *Regulation of cisplatin resistance in lung cancer cells by nicotine, BDNF, and a β-adrenergic receptor blocker. Int. J. Mol. Sci.*, 2022. **23**(21): p. 12829.

78. Kuol, N., et al., *Role of the nervous system in cancer metastasis. J. Exp. Clin. Cancer Res.*, 2018. **37**(1): pp. 1–12.

79. Bengsch, B., et al., *Deep immune profiling by mass cytometry links human T and NK cell differentiation and cytotoxic molecule expression patterns. J. Immunol. Methods*, 2018. **453**: pp. 3–10.

80. Carrega, P., et al., *Natural killer cells infiltrating human nonsmall-cell lung cancer are enriched in CD56 bright CD16(-) cells and display an impaired capability to kill tumor cells. Cancer*, 2008. **112**(4): pp. 863–75.

81. Chan, A., et al., *CD56bright human NK cells differentiate into CD56dim cells: role of contact with peripheral fibroblasts. J. Immunol.*, 2007. **179**(1): pp. 89–94.

82. Hagenaars, M., et al., *Characteristics of tumor infiltration by adoptively transferred and endogenous natural-killer cells in a syngeneic rat model: Implications for the mechanism behind anti-tumor responses. Int. J. Cancer*, 1998. **78**(6): pp. 783–9.

83. Ruffell, B. and L.M. Coussens, *Macrophages and therapeutic resistance in cancer. Cancer Cell*, 2015. **27**(4): pp. 462–72.

84. Ohno, S., *The degree of macrophage infiltration into the cancer cell nest is a significant predictor of survival in gastric cancer patients. Anticancer Res.*, 2003. **23**(6D): pp. 5015–22.

85. Ohno, S., *Correlation of histological localization of tumor-associated macrophages with clinicopathological features in endometrial cancer. Anticancer Res.*, 2004. **24**(5C): pp. 3335–42.

86. Forssell, J., *High macrophage infiltration along the tumor front correlates with improved survival in colon cancer. Clin. Cancer Res.*, 2007. **13**(5): pp. 1472–9.

87. Ladányi, A., *Density of DC-LAMP+ mature dendritic cells in combination with activated T lymphocytes infiltrating primary cutaneous melanoma is a strong independent prognostic factor. Cancer Immunol. Immunother.*, 2007. **56**(9): pp. 1459–69.

88. Goc, J., *Dendritic cells in tumor-associated tertiary lymphoid structures signal a Th1 cytotoxic immune contexture and license the positive prognostic value of infiltrating CD8+ T cells. Cancer Res.*, 2014. **74**(3): pp. 705–15.

89. Broz, M.L., *Dissecting the tumor myeloid compartment reveals rare activating antigen-presenting cells critical for T cell immunity. Cancer Cell*, 2014. **26**. pp. 638–52.

90. Bindea, G., *Spatiotemporal dynamics of intratumoral immune cells reveal the immune landscape in human cancer. Immunity*, 2013. **39**: pp. 782–95.

91. Hibbs, J.B., *Macrophage cytotoxicity: Role for L-arginine deiminase and imino nitrogen oxidation to nitrite. Science*, 1987. **235**(4787): pp. 473–6.

92. Nathan, C.F., *Extracellular cytolysis by activated macrophages and granulocytes. II. Hydrogen peroxide as a mediator of cytotoxicity. J. Exp. Med.*, 1979. **149**: pp. 100–13.

93. Urban, J.L., *Tumor necrosis factor: a potent effector molecule for tumor cell killing by activated macrophages. Proc. Natl. Acad. Sci. USA*, 1986. **83**(14): pp. 5233–7.

94. Pucci, F., *SCS macrophages suppress melanoma by restricting tumor-derived vesicle–B cell interactions. Science*, 2016. **352**: pp. 242–6.

95. Dieu-Nosjean, M.C., *Long-term survival for patients with non-small-cell lung cancer with intratumoral lymphoid structures. J. Clin. Oncol.*, 2008. **26**(27): pp. 4410–7.

96. Gabrilovich, D., *Mechanisms and functional significance of tumour-induced dendritic-cell defects. Nat. Rev. Immunol.*, 2004. **4**(12): pp. 941–52.

97. Cubillos-Ruiz, J.R., *ER stress sensor XBP1 controls anti-tumor immunity by disrupting dendritic cell homeostasis. Cell*, 2015. **161**(7): pp. 1527–38.

98. Spranger, S., *Melanoma-intrinsic β-catenin signalling prevents anti-tumour immunity. Nature*, 2015. **523**(7559): pp. 231–5.

99. Zelenay, S., *Cyclooxygenase-dependent tumor growth through evasion of immunity. Cell*, 2015. **162**: pp. 1257–70.

100. Ruffell, B., *Macrophage IL-10 blocks CD8+ T cell-dependent responses to chemotherapy by suppressing IL-12 expression in intratumoral dendritic cells. Cancer Cell*, 2014. **26**(5): pp. 623–37.

101. Granot, Z., *Tumor entrained neutrophils inhibit seeding in the premetastatic lung. Cancer Cell*, 2011. **20**: pp. 300–14.

102. Finisguerra, V., *MET is required for the recruitment of anti-tumoural neutrophils. Nature*, 2015. **522**: pp. 349–53.

103. Fridlender, Z.G., *Polarization of tumor-associated neutrophil phenotype by TGF-β: "N1" versus "N2" TAN. Cancer Cell*, 2009. **16**: pp. 183–94.

104. Eruslanov, E.B., *Tumor-associated neutrophils stimulate T cell responses in early-stage human lung cancer. J. Clin. Invest.*, 2014. **124**: pp. 5466–5480.

105. Davis, B.P. and M.E. Rothenberg, *Eosinophils and cancer. Cancer Immunol. Res.*, 2014. **2**: pp. 1–8.

106. Nielsen, H.J., *Independent prognostic value of eosinophil and mast cell infiltration in colorectal cancer tissue. J. Pathol.*, 1999. **189**: pp. 487–95.

107. Tepper, R.I., *An eosinophil-dependent mechanism for the antitumor effect of interleukin-4. Science*, 1992. **257**: pp. 548–51.

108. Carretero, R., *Eosinophils orchestrate cancer rejection by normalizing tumor vessels and enhancing infiltration of CD8+ T cells. Nat. Immunol.*, 2015. **16**(6): pp. 609–17.

109. Väyrynen, J.P., *Detailed analysis of inflammatory cell infiltration in colorectal cancer. Br. J. Cancer*, 2013. **109**(7): pp. 1839–47.

110. Schönhuber, N., *A next-generation dual-recombinase system for time- and host-specific targeting of pancreatic cancer. Nat. Med.*, 2014. **20**(11): pp. 1340–47.

111. Wan, J., et al., *The effects of HIF-1alpha on gene expression profiles of NCI-H446 human small cell lung cancer cells. J. Exp. Clin. Cancer Res.*, 2009. **28**(1): p. 150.

112. Huang, L., et al., *Hypoxia induced paclitaxel resistance in human ovarian cancers via hypoxia-inducible factor 1alpha. J. Cancer. Res. Clin. Oncol.*, 2010. **136**(3): pp. 447–56.

113. Liu, X., et al., *Is CD47 an innate immune checkpoint for tumor evasion? J. Hematol. Oncol.*, 2017. **10**(1): p. 12.

114. Seyfried, T.N. and L.C. Huysentruyt, *On the origin of cancer metastasis. Crit. Rev. Oncog.*, 2013. **18**(1–2): pp. 43–73.

115. Garcia Franco, C.E., et al., *Long-term results after resection for bone sarcoma pulmonary metastases. Eur. J. Cardiothorac. Surg.*, 2010. **37**(5): pp. 1205–8.

116. Pachmayr, E., C. Treese, and U. Stein, *Underlying Mechanisms for Distant Metastasis – Molecular Biology. Visc. Med.*, 2017. **33**(1): pp. 11–20.

117. Piva de Freitas, P., et al., *Metastatic basal cell carcinoma: a rare manifestation of a common disease. Case Rep. Med.*, 2017. **2017**: p. 8929745–8929745.

118. Scheel, C. and R.A. Weinberg, *Cancer stem cells and epithelial–mesenchymal transition: concepts and molecular links. Semin. Cancer Biol.*, 2012. **22**(5): pp. 396–403.

119. Hamilton, G. and B. Rath, *Mesenchymal-epithelial transition and circulating tumor cells in small cell lung cancer. In Isolation and Molecular Characterization of Circulating Tumor Cells*, M.J.M. Magbanua and J.W. Park, Editors. 2017, Springer International Publishing: Cham. pp. 229–45.

120. Yu, Y., et al., *Cancer-associated fibroblasts induce epithelial-mesenchymal transition of breast cancer cells through paracrine TGF-beta signalling. Br. J. Cancer*, 2014. **110**(3): pp. 724–32.

121. Kmieciak, M., et al., *HER-2/neu antigen loss and relapse of mammary carcinoma are actively induced by T cell-mediated anti-tumor immune responses. Eur. J. Immunol.*, 2007. **37**(3): pp. 675–85.

122. Romeo, E., et al., *The vicious cross-talk between tumor cells with an EMT phenotype and cells of the immune system. Cells*, 2019. **8**(5): p. 460.

123. Fan, Q.M., et al., *Tumor-associated macrophages promote cancer stem cell-like properties via transforming growth factor-beta1-induced epithelial-mesenchymal transition in hepatocellular carcinoma. Cancer Lett.*, 2014. **352**(2): pp. 160–8.

124. Toh, B., et al., *Mesenchymal transition and dissemination of cancer cells is driven by myeloid-derived suppressor cells infiltrating the primary tumor. PLoS Biol.*, 2011. **9**(9): p. e1001162.

125. Gonzalez-Moreno, O., et al., *VEGF elicits epithelial-mesenchymal transition (EMT) in prostate intraepithelial neoplasia (PIN)-like cells via an autocrine loop. Exp. Cell. Res.*, 2010. **316**(4): pp. 554–67.

126. Elliott, B.E., et al., *The role of hepatocyte growth factor (scatter factor) in epithelial-mesenchymal transition and breast cancer. Can. J. Physiol. Pharmacol.*, 2002. **80**(2): pp. 91–102.

127. Sagi, Z. and T. Hieronymus, *The impact of the epithelial-mesenchymal transition regulator hepatocyte growth factor receptor/MET on skin immunity by modulating langerhans cell migration. Front Immunol.*, 2018. **9**: p. 517–517.

128. Shintani, Y., et al., *IL-6 Secreted from cancer-associated fibroblasts mediates chemoresistance in NSCLC by increasing epithelial-mesenchymal transition signaling. J. Thorac. Oncol.*, 2016. **11**(9): pp. 1482–92.

129. Bates, R.C. and A.M. Mercurio, *Tumor necrosis factor-alpha stimulates the epithelial-to-mesenchymal transition of human colonic organoids. Mol. Biol. Cell*, 2003. **14**(5): pp. 1790–1800.

130. Wang, H., et al., *Chemokine (CC motif) ligand 18 upregulates Slug expression to promote stem-cell like features by activating the mammalian target of rapamycin pathway in oral squamous cell carcinoma. Cancer Sci.*, 2017. **108**(8): pp. 1584–93.

131. Wang, Y., et al., *The role of snail in EMT and tumorigenesis. Curr. Cancer Drug Targets*, 2013. **13**(9): pp. 963–72.

132. Peinado, H., D. Olmeda, and A. Cano, *Snail, Zeb and bHLH factors in tumour progression: an alliance against the epithelial phenotype? Nat Rev Cancer*, 2007. **7**(6): pp. 415–28.

133. Song, Y., M.K. Washington, and H.C. Crawford, *Loss of FOXA1/2 is essential for the epithelial-to-mesenchymal transition in pancreatic cancer. Cancer Res.*, 2010. **70**(5): pp. 2115–25.

134. Mani, S.A., et al., *Mesenchyme Forkhead 1 (FOXC2) plays a key role in metastasis and is associated with aggressive basal-like breast cancers. Proc. Natl. Acad. Sci. USA*, 2007. **104**(24): pp. 10069–74.

135. Cheung, M., et al., *The transcriptional control of trunk neural crest induction, survival, and delamination. Dev. Cell*, 2005. **8**(2): pp. 179–92.

136. Nilsson, J., et al., *Nuclear Janus-activated kinase 2/nuclear factor 1-C2 suppresses tumorigenesis and epithelial-to-mesenchymal transition by repressing forkhead box F1. Cancer Res.*, 2010. **70**(5): pp. 2020–29.

137. Belguise, K., S. Guo, and G.E. Sonenshein, *Activation of FOXO3a by the green tea polyphenol epigallocatechin-3-gallate induces estrogen receptor alpha expression reversing invasive phenotype of breast cancer cells. Cancer Res.*, 2007. **67**(12): pp. 5763–70.

138. Qiao, Y., et al., *FOXQ1 regulates epithelial-mesenchymal transition in human cancers. Cancer Res.*, 2011. **71**(8): pp. 3076–86.

139. Slorach, E.M., J. Chou, and Z. Werb, *Zeppo1 is a novel metastasis promoter that represses E-cadherin expression and regulates p120-catenin isoform expression and localization. Genes Dev.*, 2011. **25**(5): pp. 471–84.

140. Ocana, O.H., et al., *Metastatic colonization requires the repression of the epithelial-mesenchymal transition inducer Prrx1. Cancer Cell*, 2012. **22**(6): pp. 709–24.

141. Ikenouchi, J., et al., *Regulation of tight junctions during the epithelium-mesenchyme transition: Direct repression of the gene expression of claudins/occludin by snail. J. Cell Sci.*, 2003. **116**(Pt 10): pp. 1959–67.

142. Hemangini, H.V., et al., *Cytokeratin and vimentin expression in breast cancer. Int. J. Biol. Markers*, 2009. **24**(1): pp. 38–46.

143. White, L.R., et al., *The characterization of alpha5-integrin expression on tubular epithelium during renal injury. Am. J. Physio.l Renal Physiol.*, 2007. **292**(2): pp. F567–76.

144. Zhu, X., et al., *Epithelial derived CTGF promotes breast tumor progression via inducing EMT and collagen I fibers deposition. Oncotarget*, 2015. **6**(28): pp. 25320–38.

145. Radisky, E.S. and D.C. Radisky, *Matrix metalloproteinase-induced epithelial-mesenchymal transition in breast cancer. J. Mammary Gland Biol. Neoplasia*, 2010. **15**(2): p. 201–12.

146. Li, N., *Platelets in cancer metastasis: To help the "villain" to do evil. Int. J. Cancer*, 2016. **138**(9): pp. 2078–87.

147. Ganguly, K.K., et al., *Integrins and metastasis. Cell. Adh. Migr.*, 2013. **7**(3): pp. 251–261.

148. Yang, X., et al., *Regulation of beta 4-integrin expression by epigenetic modifications in the mammary gland and during the epithelial-to-mesenchymal transition. J. Cell Sci.*, 2009. **122**(Pt 14): pp. 2473–80.

149. Li, X.-L., et al., *Integrin β4 promotes cell invasion and epithelial-mesenchymal transition through the modulation of Slug expression in hepatocellular carcinoma. Sci. Rep.*, 2017. **7**(1): p. 40464.

150. Zhang, Q.W., *Prognostic significance of tumor-associated macrophages in solid tumor: A meta-analysis of the literature. PLoS ONE*, 2012. **7**(12): p. e50946.

151. Steidl, C., *Tumor-associated macrophages and survival in classic Hodgkin's lymphoma. N. Engl. J. Med.*, 2010. **362**(10): pp. 875–85.

152. Gabrilovich, D.I., *Coordinated regulation of myeloid cells by tumours. Nat. Rev. Immunol.*, 2012. **12**(4): pp. 253–68.

153. Noy, R. and J.W. Pollard, *Tumor-associated macrophages: From mechanisms to therapy. Immunity*, 2014. **41**(1): pp. 49–61.

154. Harney, A.S., *Real-time imaging reveals local, transient vascular permeability, and tumor cell intravasation stimulated by TIE2hi macrophage-derived VEGFA. Cancer Discov.*, 2015. **5**(9): pp. 932–43.

155. Mohamed, M.M. and B.F. Sloane, *Cysteine cathepsins: multifunctional enzymes in cancer. Nat. Rev. Cancer*, 2006. **6**(10): pp. 764–75.

156. Kessenbrock, K., *Matrix metalloproteinases: regulators of the tumor microenvironment. Cell*, 2010. **141**(1): pp. 52–67.

157. Lewis, J.S., *Expression of vascular endothelial growth factor by macrophages is up-regulated in poorly vascularized areas of breast carcinomas. J. Pathol.*, 2000. **192**(2): pp. 150–8.

158. Sierra, J.R., *Tumor angiogenesis and progression are enhanced by Sema4D produced by tumor-associated macrophages. J. Exp. Med.*, 2008. **205**(7): pp. 1673–85.

159. Biswas, S.K. and A. Mantovani, *Macrophage plasticity and interaction with lymphocyte subsets: cancer as a paradigm. Nat. Immunol.*, 2010. **11**(10): pp. 889–96.

160. Kuang, D.M., *Activated monocytes in peritumoral stroma of hepatocellular carcinoma foster immune privilege and disease progression through PD-L1. J. Exp. Med.*, 2009. **206**(6): pp. 1327–37.

161. Gentles, A.J., *The prognostic landscape of genes and infiltrating immune cells across human cancers. Nat. Med.*, 2015. **21**(8): pp. 938–45.

162. Squadrito, M.L., *MicroRNA-mediated control of macrophages and its implications for cancer. Trends Immunol.*, 2013. **34**(7): pp. 350–9.

163. Parker, K.H., *Myeloid-derived suppressor cells: critical cells driving immune suppression in the tumor microenvironment. Adv. Cancer Res.*, 2015. **128**: pp. 95–139.

164. Lin, E.Y., *Colony-stimulating factor 1 promotes progression of mammary tumors to malignancy. J. Exp. Med.*, 2001. **193**(6): pp. 727–40.

165. Kubota, Y., *M-CSF inhibition selectively targets pathological angiogenesis and lymphangiogenesis. J. Exp. Med.*, 2009. **206**(5): pp. 1089–102.

166. Richardsen, E., *Macrophage-colony stimulating factor (CSF1) predicts breast cancer progression and mortality. Anticancer Res.*, 2015. **35**(2): pp. 865–74.

167. Ueno, T., *Significance of macrophage chemoattractant protein-1 in macrophage recruitment, angiogenesis, and survival in human breast cancer. Clin. Cancer Res.*, 2000. **6**(8): pp. 3282–9.

168. Groblewska, M., *Serum levels of granulocyte colony-stimulating factor (G-CSF) and macrophage colony-stimulating factor (M-CSF) in pancreatic cancer patients. Clin. Chem. Lab Med.*, 2007. **45**(1): pp. 30–4.

169. Mroczko, B., *Serum macrophage-colony stimulating factor levels in colorectal cancer patients correlate with lymph node metastasis and poor prognosis. Clin. Chim. Acta*, 2007. **380**(1–2): p. 208–12.

170. Zhu, X.D., *High expression of macrophage colony-stimulating factor in peritumoral liver tissue is associated with poor survival after curative resection of hepatocellular carcinoma. J. Clin. Oncol.*, 2008. **26**(16): pp. 2707–16.

171. Smith, H.O., *The role of colony-stimulating factor 1 and its receptor in the etiopathogenesis of endometrial adenocarcinoma. Clin. Cancer Res.*, 1995. **1**(3): pp. 313–25.

172. Treilleux, I., *Dendritic cell infiltration and prognosis of early stage breast cancer. Clin. Cancer Res.*, 2004. **10**(22): pp. 7466–74.

173. Jensen, T.O., *Intratumoral neutrophils and plasmacytoid dendritic cells indicate poor prognosis and are associated with pSTAT3 expression in AJCC stage I/II melanoma. Cancer*, 2012. **118**(9): pp. 2476–85.

174. Jiang, L., *Prognostic value of monocyte and neutrophils to lymphocytes ratio in patients with metastatic soft tissue sarcoma. Oncotarget*, 2015. **6**(11): pp. 9542–50.

175. Huang, S.H., *Prognostic value of pretreatment circulating neutrophils, monocytes, and lymphocytes in oropharyngeal cancer stratified by human papillomavirus status. Cancer*, 2015. **121**(4): pp. 545–55.

176. Gabitass, R.F., *Elevated myeloid-derived suppressor cells in pancreatic, esophageal and gastric cancer are an independent prognostic factor and are associated with significant elevation of the Th2 cytokine interleukin-13. Cancer Immunol. Immunother.*, 2011. **60**(10): pp. 1419–30.

177. Di Mitri, D., *Tumour-infiltrating Gr-1+ myeloid cells antagonize senescence in cancer. Nature*, 2014. **515**(7525): pp. 134–7.

178. Shojaei, F., *Bv8 regulates myeloid-cell-dependent tumour angiogenesis. Nature*, 2007. **450**(7171): pp. 825–31.

179. Demers, M., *Cancers predispose neutrophils to release extracellular DNA traps that contribute to cancer-associated thrombosis. Proc. Natl. Acad. Sci. USA*, 2012. **109**(32): pp. 13076–81.

180. Wilson, C.L., *NFκB1 is a suppressor of neutrophil-driven hepatocellular carcinoma. Nat. Commun.*, 2015. **6**(1): pp. 6818–32.

181. Ortiz, M.L., *Immature myeloid cells directly contribute to skin tumor development by recruiting IL-17-producing CD4+ T cells. J. Exp. Med.*, 2015. **212**(3): pp. 351–67.

182. Nowak, E.C., *Tryptophan hydroxylase-1 regulates immune tolerance and inflammation. J. Exp. Med.*, 2012. **209**(11): pp. 2127–35.

183. Blatner, N.R., *In colorectal cancer mast cells contribute to systemic regulatory T-cell dysfunction. Proc. Natl. Acad. Sci. USA*, 2010. **107**(14): p. 6430–35.

184. Gounaris, E., *Mast cells are an essential hematopoietic component for polyp development. Proc. Natl. Acad. Sci. USA*, 2007. **104**(50): pp. 19977–82.

185. Yang, Z., *Mast cells mobilize myeloid-derived suppressor cells and Treg cells in tumor microenvironment via IL-17 pathway in murine hepatocarcinoma model. PLoS ONE*, 2010. **5**(1): p. e8922.

186. Saleem, S.J., *Cutting edge: mast cells critically augment myeloid-derived suppressor cell activity. J. Immunol.*, 2012. **189** (2): pp. 511–5.

187. Malfettone, A., *High density of tryptase-positive mast cells in human colorectal cancer: a poor prognostic factor related to protease-activated receptor 2 expression. J. Cell. Mol. Med.*, 2013. **17**(8): pp. 1025–37.

188. Marvel, D. and D.I. Gabrilovich, *Myeloid-derived suppressor cells in the tumor microenvironment: Expect the unexpected. J. Clin. Invest.*, 2015. **125**(9): pp. 3356–64.

189. Lu, T., *Tumor-infiltrating myeloid cells induce tumor cell resistance to cytotoxic T cells in mice. J. Clin. Invest.*, 2011. **121**(10): pp. 4015–29.

190. Vasquez-Dunddel, D., *STAT3 regulates arginase-I in myeloid-derived suppressor cells from cancer patients. J. Clin. Invest.*, 2013. **123**(4): pp. 1580–9.

191. Mazzoni, A., *Myeloid suppressor lines inhibit T cell responses by an NO-dependent mechanism. J. Immunol.*, 2002. **168**(2): pp. 689–95.

192. Mao, Y., *Melanoma-educated CD14+ cells acquire a myeloid-derived suppressor cell phenotype through COX-2-dependent mechanisms. Cancer Res.*, 2013. **73** (13): pp. 3877–87.

193. Young, M.R., *Suppression of T cell proliferation by tumor-induced granulocyte-macrophage progenitor cells producing transforming growth factor-β and nitric oxide. J. Immunol.*, 1996. **156**(5): pp. 1916–22.

194. Nagaraj, S., *Altered recognition of antigen is a mechanism of CD8+ T cell tolerance in cancer. Nat. Med.*, 2007. **13**(7): pp. 828–35.

195. Molon, B., *Chemokine nitration prevents intratumoral infiltration of antigen-specific T cells. J. Exp. Med.*, 2011. **208**(10): pp. 1949–62.

196. Pan, P.Y., *Immune stimulatory receptor CD40 is required for T-cell suppression and T regulatory cell activation mediated by myeloid-derived suppressor cells in cancer. Cancer Res.*, 2010. **70**(1): pp. 99–108.

197. Andreu, P., *FcRγ activation regulates inflammation-associated squamous carcinogenesis. Cancer Cell*, 2010. **17**(2): pp. 121–34.

4 Passive Targeting

Malik Saadullah, Amna Sehar, Khurram Afzal,
Ijaz Ali, Shams ul Hassan, and Muhammad Yasir Ali

4.1 INTRODUCTION

Cancer is a multidimensional disorder and the leading cause of death globally, and the number of cancer-diagnosed patients is increasing day by day [1]. According to the evaluation from the World Health Organization, about 84 million people died from cancer from 2005 to 2015 [2]. In 2012, approximately 14.1 million patients were diagnosed with cancer, of which approximately 8.2 million cases were incurable. This figure is predicted to increase, with 19.3 million new cases of cancer by 2025 [3]. At present, the management of cancer is a more significant goal of research [4]. For the effectual treatment of cancer, it is crucial to advance our understanding of cancer pathophysiology. Traditional chemotherapeutic drugs are incredibly ineffective in their treatment profiles because of their weak solubility, dreary pharmacokinetic profiles, and confusing side effects. One approach that has attained considerable attention in recent years is passive targeting. Passive targeting is a novel drug delivery system in cancer-treating therapies that allude to providing unique therapeutic properties to the drugs that are otherwise not presented by these drugs in raw form. These unique parameters of the drug may be defined in terms of improved efficacy, feasibility in administration, minimizing harmful side effects, and reduced toxicity in comparison with conventional therapies (surgery, radiation, and chemotherapies). The term passive targeted drug delivery can be reciprocally used as "site-specific" drug delivery and "controlled" drug delivery [5]. However, the term targeted drug delivery is more relevant in the context, for example, drug delivery displayed by delayed-release systems, including enteric-coated systems or colon-specific systems, hold up the release of drugs until they reach a specific tissue site in the body [6].

Targeted therapies are aimed to block specific biological transduction pathways or cancer proteins that are involved in tumor growth and progression, i.e., molecular targets (receptors, growth factors, kinase cascades, or molecules related to apoptosis and angiogenesis) that are present in normal tissues, but are found overexpressed or mutated in cancer. The idea of these revolutionary therapies is either to block the signals that help malignant cells to grow and divide uncontrollably, produce the death of cancer cells using induction of apoptosis, stimulate the immune system, or target the delivery of chemotherapy agents specifically to cancer cells, minimizing the death of normal cells and avoiding the undesirable side effects [7, 8]

Drug delivery systems (DDS), which use synthetic polymers either by covalent conjugation or as part of a composite with micellar medicines, have emerged as a brand-new area of research for the creation of new medications in a variety of illnesses. Drugs delivered by micellar or stealth liposomes and protein-polymer conjugates both need the use of synthetic polymers. These polymer-based new drug entities are known as "polymer therapeutics" and they overlap with nanomedicine

DOI: 10.1201/9781003363958-5

that has become popular in recent years. The pathophysiological peculiarities of solid tumors, with standard low molecular weight treatments that cannot be addressed, are used to increase drug performance through polymer therapies or nanomedicines. Nanomedicines show improved tumor-selective targeting, improved therapeutic efficacy, and minimized side effects, in which prolonged circulation time plays a crucial role.

The most significant finding is that practically all human malignancies, except hypovascular tumors like pancreatic or prostate cancer, exhibit the EPR effect. As clinical examples for this, researchers have experienced that SMANCS/Lipiodol given via the hepatic artery accumulated selectively in hepatocellular carcinoma. A similar result in a clinical setting was also reported for doxil, a liposomal carrier system of doxorubicin. Another clinical example based on the EPR effect can be demonstrated in the traditional tumor imaging in the clinic that utilizes (gamma)-emitting gallium scintigraphy based on the selective accumulation of radioactive gallium (used as citrate) in the tumor [9].

4.2 ANATOMICAL AND PATHOPHYSIOLOGICAL CHANGES IN TUMOR VASCULATURE

Once a malignant tumor reaches a size of >2–3 mm^3, the transport of both nutrients and oxygen is diffusion-limited, and the creation of additional blood vessels is necessary to keep up with the continually rising demands of the malignant cells' quickly expanding malignancy. This is achieved by the malignant tissue releasing angiogenic factors to enhance the microvasculature within the tumor and support future growth [10]. Vascular structures in neoplastic tissues are extremely disordered, and dilated, have numerous holes, and have broad gap junctions between endothelium cells as a result of an imbalance of angiogenic factors and matrix metalloproteinases (MMPs) in these tissues. Basement membrane and microvascular cells are missing or damaged. Additionally, the smooth muscle layer that generally covers endothelial cells is commonly absent from tumor arteries. Whereas the leaky vasculature of cancerous tissue permits macromolecules with a thickness of less than 600 nm to extravasate into the neoplastic tissues, the normal vasculature is equipped with tight junctions that are impermeable to molecules sized >2–4 nm, retaining nanoparticles inside the circulation. These extravasated nanoparticles tend to stagnate inside the proliferative cells since tumors are lacking in a well-developed lymphatic system (Figure 4.1). This phenomenon of leaky vasculature as well as impaired lymphatic drainage has been referred to as the enhanced permeation and retention (EPR) effect [11, 12].

4.3 PASSIVE TARGETING STRATEGIES

The passive targeting technique involves drug-delivering strategies where the drug is delivered to a target site passively by manipulating the attributes of the target tissue. The passive targeting strategies rely upon the principle of the EPR, which is summarized by the selective accumulation of the drug at the target site due to the leaky vasculature and poor lymphatic drainage of tumor tissue. The passive targeting strategies have shown assuring results in the field of drug delivery. The choice of the targeting strategy should depend on the specific characteristics of the drug and the target tissue.

4.3.1 FORMULATION BASED STRATEGIES

4.3.1.1 Size and Shape-Based Targeting

Targeting based on size and shape is a tactic that makes use of the characteristics of the nanoparticle's size and shape to enable passive targeting. Due to the EPR effect, nanoparticles with a size range of 10–200 nm can extravasate through the fenestrations in the tumor vasculature and accumulate in the tumor tissue. Nanoparticles with larger sizes do not extravasate across the blood vessel,

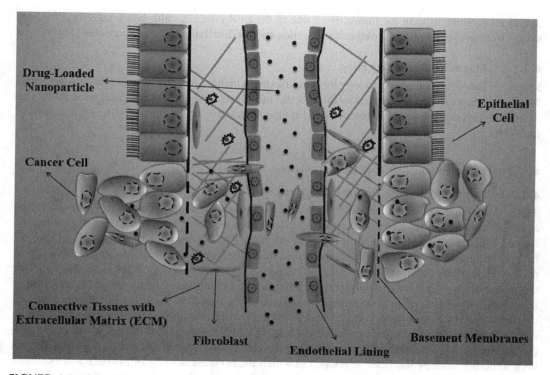

FIGURE 4.1 Schematic drawing of enhanced permeation and retension. Drug-loaded nanoparticles are extrasated into a tumor tissue from the pores of enhanced size between endothelial linings.

and small nanoparticles travel deep into the tumor site but remain there only transiently. In addition, the shape of the nanoparticles can also affect their targeting ability. For example, rod-shaped nanoparticles have been proven to have better tumor penetration and aggregation than spherical nanoparticles [13].

4.3.1.2 Surface Modification-Based Targeting

Surface modification-based targeting is a strategy that involves modifying the surface of nanoparticles with ligands that target specific receptors on the tumor cells. Ligands, such as antibodies, peptides, and aptamers, can be conjugated to the surface of nanoparticles to achieve targeted drug delivery. The ligands bind to the over-expressed receptors on the tumor cells, leading to the internalization of the nanoparticles and the release of the drug.

4.3.1.3 Charge-Based Targeting

Charge-based targeting is a strategy that utilizes the charge of nanoparticles to achieve passive targeting. The surface charge of nanoparticles plays a key role in finding their interactions with affected cells and tissues. Negatively charged nanoparticles have displayed better tumor accumulation because of the negative charge of the tumor tissue. In contrast, positively charged nanoparticles have been shown to accumulate in off-target tissues, such as the liver and spleen [14].

4.3.1.4 Stealth-Based Targeting

Stealth-based targeting is a technique that involves the coating of hydrophilic polymers such as polyethylene glycol (PEG) on the surface of nanoparticles to avoid recognition by the immune system. PEGylation prolonged the circulation time of nanoparticles in the bloodstream, leading to enhanced accumulation in the tumor tissue due to the EPR effect. Stealth-based targeting has been shown to improve the pharmacokinetic properties and biodistribution of drug particles [15].

4.3.1.5 Magnetic-Based Targeting

Magnetic-based targeting is a strategy that uses magnetic nanoparticles to achieve passive targeting. Magnetic nanoparticles are guided to the specific target site using an external magnetic field. This technique has been used to cure tumors located near the surface of the skin or in the gastrointestinal tract [16].

4.3.2 TUMOR ENVIRONMENT-BASED STRATEGIES

4.3.2.1 Targeting Specific Tumor Conditions

The passive targeting strategies utilize specific conditions in a body part (organ) bearing a tumor or in the tumor environment itself to facilitate drug release. These conditions involve (but are not limited to) particular pH, certain enzymes, or microflora in the organ or tumor site. For example, by preparing tablets drug delivery to the colon might be targeted with a specific coating that is destroyed in situ by colon pH and/or resident bacteria [17]. The limitation of this method is targeting the whole organ, not only the tumor itself, potentially opening the door to severe organ cytotoxicity. The curing way of passive targeting cancer cells is based on the use of metalloproteinases disclosed only in certain tumors. It was found that the growth of malignant melanoma was noted by overexpression of several matrix metalloproteinases (MMPs), especially MMP-2, which play a crucial role in the degradation of basal membranes as well as the extracellular matrix. Consequently, a drug targeting strategy has been developed in which the protease activity of MMP-2 was exploited to release the anticancer agent from a macromolecular carrier, i.e., circulating albumin [18]. For this purpose, a water-soluble maleimide derivative of doxorubicin incorporating a MMP-2 specific peptide sequence (Gly-Pro-Leu-Gly-Ile-Ala-Gly-Gln) was developed. This compound binds rapidly and selectively to the circulating albumin using the latter as a carrier. The albumin-bound form of this prodrug increased efficacy and was specifically cleaved by MMP-2 liberating a doxorubicin tetrapeptide (Ile-AlaGly-Gln-DOX) and subsequently doxorubicin [17].

4.3.2.2 Local Delivery to Tumor

Local delivery to tumors is a basic approach to targeting specific tissues that provide local administration of anticancer agents directly into the tumor site. This method has the obvious benefit of keeping the medicine out of systemic circulation. This strategy may be able to reduce the negative effects of drugs on healthy organs, as long as drugs used topically are kept in the tumor and do not circulate in the whole body. Some tumors, such as lung malignancies, are difficult to access for local drug delivery, although topical distribution for some tumors may be accomplished by injections or surgical procedures. To overcome these difficulties, for the treatment of lung cancer, numerous anticancer aerosols have been manufactured [19, 20]. These two passive targeting strategies for tumors are occasionally used in cancer therapy, despite the possibility of doing so.

4.4 ENHANCED PERMEABILITY AND RETENTION (EPR)

It is necessary to find a more comprehensive strategy for creating anticancer medications that are highly selective for cancerous tissue. To solve this problem, the phenomenon of "enhanced permeability and retention (EPR) effect" introduced by Maeda and Matsumura is now becoming the gold standard in cancer-targeting drug designing that is based on macromolecules, micellar, and lipidic particles, all of these utilize the EPR-effect as a guiding principle, and the EPR effect is observed in, almost all rapidly growing solid tumors. The EPR effect is a collaboration of two phenomena, i.e., enhanced permeation and enhanced retention [14].

4.4.1.1 Enhanced Permeation

In cancer, the cells grow quickly and improperly, therefore, for these fast-growing tissue's nutritional needs cannot be met by the usual vasculature. The result is angiogenesis (the creation of new blood vessels from existing ones). Because there are so many proliferating endothelial cells present, the newly created arteries have an uneven endothelium layer, an aberrant basement membrane, and insufficient pericytes (contractile cells surrounding the endothelial cells). The result is enlarged pores and leaky vasculature (10–1000 nm). As a result, materials of a tiny enough size can easily pass through the pores and into the tumor interstitium.

4.4.1.2 Enhanced Retention

Lymphatic systems are in control of drainage in healthy tissue. More chemicals than needed are transported by the lymphatic vessels once they leak into the interstitium. These lymphatic vessels are absent or broken in tumor tissue. As a result, materials that have entered extracellular fluid are not effectively eliminated and are instead maintained in tumor tissue, resulting in the release of their drug contents at local site (Figure 4.2) [21].

4.4.1.3 Mechanism of Passive Targeting Through the EPR Effect

When compared to normal tissues, tumors accumulate macromolecules preferentially. The tumor interstitium, an interstitial space between the capillary's basement membrane and cells, is where the buildup occurs. High tumoral vascular permeability, slow venous return from tumor tissues, and decreased lymphatic outflow are the root causes of these preferential accumulations [22]. Many drug carriers with diameters above renal filtration have the effect recognized (6 nm). Larger molecules stay at tumor sites for a longer time, but smaller molecules accumulate more quickly (Figure 4.1). Sizes 20–200 nm seem to be ideal for drug particle extravasation and accumulation in the interstitium. The EPR's impact on drug accumulation varies in strength, although it almost never exceeds 10% of the initial dose. The liver and spleen still contain the majority of the dosage [23, 24]. Compared to liposomes larger than 300 nm or smaller than 50 nm, tumor tissues exhibit a four-fold increase in the uptake of non-PEGylated liposomes of sizes between 100 nm and 200 nm [25].

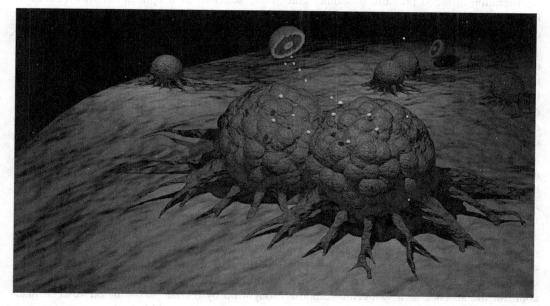

FIGURE 4.2 Drug release at tumor site due to enhanced permeation and retention (EPR) of liposome.

Preferential accumulation of drug particles in the tumor is also the result of a combination of prolonged circulation time and enhanced vascular permeability. As the maximum is attained after a few hours (often more than 24 hours), the increase in circulation time allows for more time for the slow vascular access process. That is why "long-circulating" drug particles are necessary for the EPR effect. Different approaches have been checked to increase the scope of the EPR effect and overcome the heterogeneity of the tumor vasculature that limits efficacy, including the administration of the pro-inflammatory bradykinin, inducing systemic hypertension with angiotensin II (increased blood flow in tumors), or vasodilatation with nitric oxide generators, such as nitroglycerine [26, 27].

4.4.1.4 Factors Affecting Enhanced Permeability and Retention

In the field of cancer therapies, researchers have long been aware of the EPR effect. It turns out that there is a lot more to the preferential accumulation of these nanoparticles in the tumor location than was originally thought. Angiogenesis, hemodynamic control, vascular permeability, lymphangiogenesis, and heterogeneity of the tumor microenvironment are some of the biological processes included in this process. These aforementioned factors have a great deal of subject-to-subject variation. The physicochemical nature of each material, for example, play a role in the accumulation of the nanoparticles. Although the blood arteries surrounding the tumor are sufficient to deliver the necessary amount of oxygen for cell growth, a quickly expanding tumor requires an increased blood supply. To supply the nutritional needs of the tumor cells, new blood vessels grow [28].

4.4.1.4.1 *Structural Abnormalities of the Neoplastic Vessels and Blood Pressure*

Structural as well as architectural abnormalities refer to structural changes in blood vessels that occur in tumors. Increased vessel diameter, atypical vessel form, and enhanced vessel wall permeability are a few examples of these modifications. These deviations may lead to increased blood flow and chemical and fluid leakage from the arteries, which may permit medications or other substances to gather in the tumor tissue. This irregular fluid and solute transport dynamics across tumor vasculature caused by these aberrant neoplastic vessels can be used to further enhance the EPR effect.

Alteration in blood pressure is another crucial characteristic of neoplastic arteries. Interstitial fluid pressure is frequently high in tumors, which can result in a reduction in blood flow and oxygen delivery to the tumor tissue. Because of this, there may be tumor areas that are poorly perfused and difficult to treat. High interstitial fluid pressure, on the other hand, may facilitate the leakage of molecules from blood vessels, which, according to some research, may also contribute to the accumulation of pharmaceuticals in the tumor tissue. Overall, the aberrant blood pressure and architectural features of neoplastic arteries contribute to the passive targeting buildup of medications and other therapeutic substances in tumors. Drugs with weak solubility or limited capacity to permeate normal tissues may benefit from this method of delivery [29]. It was demonstrated that elevating the mean arterial blood pressure by infusion of angiotensin II resulted in an ~5.7-fold selective increase in blood flow in tumor tissue, without an associated increase in normal tissue [30]. It is also verified that angiotensin II-induced hypertension augments the EPR effect. Raising the systolic blood pressure in tumor-bearing rats by angiotensin II infusion resulted in a two–six-fold selective increase in tumor blood flow volume, depending on the blood pressure attained. In addition to the increased blood flow, the authors of that study observed a preferential accumulation of drugs with a molecular mass of ~80 kDa within the tumor tissue. Moreover, drug accumulation in normal organs, such as kidney and bone marrow, was reduced to 60–80%. Tight endothelial gap junctions and normal vasogenic response to angiotensin in healthy tissues permit less transvascular transfer of macromolecules. Also, it is established that angiotensin II-induced hypertension increases. In contrast, the absence of a vasogenic response brought on by the neoplastic blood vessels' inadequate vascular smooth muscle layer causes an increase in intratumoral blood flow in response to a generalized increase in blood pressure. Macromolecular or nanomedicines accumulate in cancerous tissues as a result of increased blood flow and leaky vasculature. Patients with multiple solid tumors who received systemic macromolecular medications in a hypertensive state caused by angiotensin II showed similar outcomes. Although the hypertension was only present for around 20 minutes, utilizing macromolecular agents in a hypertensive condition led to a >five-fold higher concentration of anticancer medications in the tumor, whereas low-molecular-weight anticancer treatments had dose-limiting toxicity [31].

4.4.1.4.2 Vasogenic Mediators

Vasogenic mediators are crucial for controlling blood pressure and blood circulation in the body. Both endogenous and exogenous mediators that may induce vasodilation or constriction of blood arteries in response to injury or inflammation can be present. In an effort to enhance the EPR and improve drug targeting to the neoplastic tissue, several mediators have been studied.

Bradykinin: Bradykinin is a peptide secreted by injured tissue that stimulates vascular permeability as well as vasodilation. In the peritoneal and pleural fluids of both humans and animals with cancer, bradykinin is found in high concentrations. The suppression of kallikrein (a subgroup of serine protease enzyme) provided additional evidence of bradykinin's critical function in the extravasation of plasma components into the peritoneal or pleural cavities. As a result, a major mediator influencing the EPR effect in tumor sites is bradykinin, a fundamental regulator of vascular permeability. Bradykinin is also known to activate NO production through the activation of endothelial NO synthase (eNOS) NO production contributes to the angiogenic properties of VEGF in human endothelial cells, also referred to as vascular permeability factor (VPF) [32]. Bradykinin is degraded by several peptidases, particularly angiotensin-converting enzyme (ACE). More importantly, ACE inhibitors increase the release of macromolecular drugs to tumors, even under normotensive conditions ACE inhibitors may work selectively at tumor sites in normotensive patients with neoplasia to potentiate the EPR effect [33].

Nitric oxide (NO): Nitric oxide is generated from L-arginine and oxygen by three isoforms of NOs. Inducible NOs, the most potent isoform, is produced in macrophages and neutrophils, which are known to extensively infiltrate tumor tissues. NO is a well-known mediator of vasodilation, angiogenesis, and extravasation. It has been shown that increased vascular permeability in solid tumors is caused by NO and is prevented by NO synthase inhibitors and NO scavengers. NO is anticipated to be a key factor influencing tumor vascular permeability, boosting the EPR impact in solid tumors. In addition to having a direct impact on EPR, superoxide anion, which is primarily produced by leukocytes, and NO quickly react to form peroxynitrite. A possible additional factor in the EPR effect is the activation of proMMPs into MMPs by the generated peroxynitrite. The site-specific delivery of SMANCS-Lipiodol was improved when the NO-releasing drug isosorbide dinitrate was pumped into the local tumor feeding artery and angiotensin II were concurrently administered systemically, confirming the idea that NO promotes the EPR [34, 35].

Peroxynitrite and MMPs: Neoplastic tissues produce NO, which reacts with the inflammatory cells' produced superoxide anion to produce peroxynitrite. Peroxynitrite causes a reaction in proMMPs that activates them into MMPs. By destroying the extracellular matrix and promoting angiogenesis, MMPs are known to promote cancer spread and the development of solid tumors. MMPs have also been shown to increase the vascular permeability of solid tumors in mice, and MMP inhibitors have been shown to oppose this effect. Over the past 20 years, a number of MMP inhibitors have been created, but none of them have found clinical use. The first potential explanation for this failure is that some tumor cells are still alive and might start growing again when the drug treatment is stopped. The second factor could be that MMPs are essential proteases for cellular metabolism and that MMP inhibitors can be harmful in high dosages. This has caused the development of several anti-MMP medications to be stopped [34].

Vascular endothelial growth factor (VEGF): With the exception of the lung, it has been demonstrated that formerly known as VPF, levels are 2 to 30 times higher in neoplastic tissues than in healthy tissues. In addition to being an endothelial cell mitogen, VEGF is essential for the development of vascular permeability. It has been demonstrated that intradermal injection of VEGF, considerably increases the extravasation of Evans blue dye in a dose-dependent manner, underscoring its significance in boosting the EPR effect [35, 36].

PGs: PGE2 in particular is a key modulator of vascular permeability mediated by PGs. Cyclooxygenase (COX) isozymes, such as COX-2, which is noticeably enhanced in tumors, are responsible for producing PGE2. The fact that COX inhibitors such as indomethacin and salicylic acid limit vascular permeability in sarcoma 180 and other solid tumors offers strong support for the contribution of PGs to promoting vascular permeability. Beraprost sodium, a PGI2 analog, has a half-life in vivo that is substantially longer (>1 h) than PGI2, which only lasts for a few seconds. It has been shown that PGI2 analogs can increase the EPR effect by two to three times, making them an effective method of macromolecule distribution [37, 38].

4.5 DELIVERY VEHICLES

Drugs, imaging agents, or other therapeutic payloads may be delivered to the tumor site by means of vehicles while limiting their distribution to healthy regions. To achieve high medication concentrations in the tumor tissue, and aims to attain high therapeutic value, selective carriers are used in this note. Numerous drug delivery and drug targeting systems, such as synthetic polymers, microcapsules, liposomes, and micelles are currently developed or under development. Their use aims to minimize drug degradation upon administration, prevent undesirable side effects, and increase drug bioavailability and the fraction of the drug accumulated in the pathological area. To better achieve these goals, drug carriers can be made slowly degradable, stimuli-reactive (for example, pH- or temperature sensitive), and targeted (for example, by conjugating them with ligands specific towards certain characteristic components/receptors of the area of interest). In addition, drug carriers are expected to stay in the blood (prolonged time intervals) in order to maintain the required therapeutic level of pharmaceuticals in the blood over an extended period [39] to allow for their slow accumulation in pathological sites with affected and leaky vasculature (tumors, inflammations, and infarcted areas) via the enhanced permeability and retention (EPR) effect, and facilitate targeted delivery of specific ligand-modified drugs and drug carriers into poorly accessible areas [40].

Pharmaceutical drug carriers, especially those for parenteral administration, are expected to be easy and reasonably cheap to prepare, biodegradable, have a small particle size, possess high loading capacity, demonstrate prolonged circulation, and, ideally, accumulate specifically or non-specifically in required pathological sites in the body [41].

4.5.1 POLYMERIC NANOPARTICLES

A new class of delivery agents called polymeric nanoparticles can passively accumulate in the tumor microenvironment. To increase their specificity for cancer cells, these nanoparticles can be surface-modified with targeting ligands and used to encapsulate a variety of medicines. Polymeric nanoparticles may potentially be programmed to release drugs at the tumor site in response to environmental factors like temperature or pH. Because of their stability in the GIT, preservation of encapsulated actives, and ease of control over their physicochemical and drug release features, polymeric NCs are one of the most promising methods to improve oral administration [42]. In comparison to other NCs, polymeric NPs have a number of benefits for GIT delivery, especially because they are more stable and evenly distributed throughout the GIT. In comparison to other dose forms, this means that the medicine is absorbed more consistently and there is a lower chance of local irritation [43]. It is noteworthy that the percentage of dose actually crossing the GIT mucosa is increased but stays low (a few % of bioavailability), requiring higher doses, increasing potential toxic effects, and underlining the limitations of these approaches [42]. The generation of nanoparticles includes biodegradable and biocompatible natural or synthetic polymers that already have FDA approval. Synthetic polymers, such as polyglutamic acid and polyglycolic acid (PGA), polyethylene glycol (PEG), polycaprolactone (PCL), polylactic acid (PLA), polyaspartate (PAA), poly(D,L-lactide-co-glycolic) acid (PLGA), and N-(2-hydroxypropyl)-methacrylamide copolymer (HPMA), are frequently used since they are easily manufactured and degraded after use and produce a sustained release of the active compounds over time [44]. However, natural polymers, such as chitosan, alginate, dextran, heparin, albumin, gelatin, or collagen, are less used since, in spite of being nontoxic, abundant in nature, inexpensive, and easily biodegraded, they present relatively fast release profiles, and they are not naturally pure and homogeneous, requiring a purification step before their use [45]. Nevertheless, natural polymers are recently gaining interest as usable options, since the generation of nanocarriers with them is performed by mild methods (ionic gelation, coacervation, or complex complexation) [46].

Polymeric nanoparticles are currently in preclinical and clinical development, but despite their promising characteristics described above, in general, they have not reached FDA approval. Currently there is only one polymeric nanoparticle available in the market, Abraxane (ABI-007), an albumin-bound paclitaxel nanoparticle that was approved by the FDA in 2005 for the treatment of metastatic breast cancer. Later, it was approved for the first-line treatment of advanced non-small cell lung cancer (October, 2012) and for metastatic pancreatic cancer (September, 2013). Also, it is in phase III trials for the treatment of malignant melanoma [47, 48]. Moreover, there are some other nanoparticles-based formulations under clinical trials [49].

4.5.2 Liposomes

Liposomes are artificially prepared lipid bilayer vesicles of size range between 50 to 1000 nm [50]. They can be classified on different bases; size (small, large or gigantic), number of bilayers (uni, oligo, or multilamellar) and phospholipid (cation, anionic, or neutral). They can entrap hydrophilic drugs (in the central aqueous core) and hydrophobic drugs (in the lipid bilayer). Their surface can be modified by various strategies to get intentional purposes, e.g., long systemic circulation, increased tumor accumulation by active targeting, and enhanced cellular internalization [51, 52]. Liposomes are made up of distinctive lipid bilayered membrane of amphiphilic phospholipids that can also host hydrophobic cytotoxic agents in its (hydrophobic) membrane. However, due to the restricted space in the membrane and the drug's destabilizing influence on outer space, the drug loading capacity of poorly soluble medications is constrained; as a result, they are primarily thought of as carriers of water-soluble drugs, though with low loading limits [53]. These structures display additional beneficial qualities, such as biocompatibility and nearly biologically inert profiles in most patients, not generating antigenic or toxic reactions in a large percentage of cases, in addition to the amphiphilic drug loading characteristics. The so-called "complement activation-related pseudoallergy" (CARPA), a drug-induced acute immunological toxicity characterized by hypersensitivity reactions, can be brought on by the intravenous administration of liposomal medications [54, 55]. Liposomes have simple adjustable surfaces and long-lasting blood circulation, which can be improved by conjugating polyethylene glycol (PEG) to the liposome surface (stealth liposomes). Additionally, by combining various commercial lipid molecules, it is possible to change the physiochemical characteristics of liposomes, allowing for easy control of their size, surface charge, and utility without the need for additional conventional chemical steps or laborious modifications that are required for the preparation of other carriers, i.e., polymer conjugates [56, 57]. However, in addition to the above-mentioned low drug loading, they also have some other drawbacks, including issues with stability and industrial reproducibility, difficulties with sterilization, phospholipid oxidation, and the restricted control of drug release by conventional formulations, which have profiles of release in rapid bursts. This behavior can be improved by using techniques like drug release that is thermossensitive, pH-sensitive, and/or ultrasound-sensitive. Several promising clinical investigations are being conducted to improve the antitumoral efficacy of cytotoxic medicines and decrease their toxicity by combining them with liposomal formulations that have longer blood circulation times [58]. Recently, new strategies in liposomal research have gained interest, and some clinical trials based on the combination of different chemotherapeutic agents, and stimuli-responsive release approaches, have been started [59, 60]. This is the situation with the phase I, phase II, and phase III trials for the treatment of acute myeloid leukemia using liposomes carrying cytarabine and daunorubicin (CPX-351). The thermosensitive liposomes containing doxorubicin (ThermoDox) in phase III for the therapy of hepatocellular carcinoma and the phase II trials of liposomes encapsulating irinotecan HCl and floxuridine (CPX-1) as a therapeutic for aggressive colorectal cancer [18] and in phase I/II to recurrent chest wall breast cancer, locally recurrent breast cancer, primary and metastatic tumors of the liver, and metastatic colorectal cancer [61]. Despite the above-mentioned advantages of liposomal nanocarriers, only five liposome-based anticancer drugs have been approved by the FDA [62]. Doxorubicin HCl stealth liposome injection (Doxil) was, in 1995, the first liposomal carrier approved by the FDA and vincristine sulfate liposome injection (Marqibo, ONCO TCS) has been the last liposomal cytotoxic drug to be approved by the FDA in August 2012 [63].

Since it was repeatedly shown that like macromolecules, long-circulating liposomes are capable of accumulating in various pathological areas with affected vasculature via the EPR effect [64]. Long circulating polymer (PEG)-coated liposomes have been utilized frequently for passive accumulation medication delivery into malignancies (Figure 4.3). The adaptability of protective polymers, which enables a very small number of surface-grafted polymer molecules to produce an impermeable covering over the liposome surface, is a crucial property. While PEG continues to be the industry standard for liposome interfacial shielding for passively targeted preparations, efforts are still being made to find additional polymers that could be employed to create long-circulating liposomes [65]. Long-circulating liposomes prepared using poly[N-(2-hydroxypropyl) methacrylamide)], poly N-vinylpyrrolidones, L-amino acid-based biodegradable polymer-lipid conjugates, and polyvinyl alcohol [66]. The relative importance of protective polymer molecular size and liposome charge was examined, and the results suggested that opsonins of various molecular forms may be involved in the elimination of liposomes containing various charged lipids. Moreover, PEG was added to the

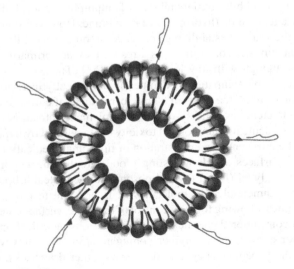

FIGURE 4.3 Surface-modified liposome.

liposome surface in a releasable manner to make it easier for cells to acquire the liposomes once they accumulate at the target region due to the EPR effect and the PEG coating detaches due to the presence of local pathological circumstances (decreased pH in tumors) [64]. New detachable PEG conjugates described in PEG were also attached to the liposome surface in a removable fashion to facilitate liposome capture by the cell after PEG liposomes accumulate in the target site via the EPR effect and the PEG coating is detached under the action of local pathological conditions (decreased pH in tumors). New detachable PEG conjugates are described in where the detachment process is based on the mild thiolysis of the dithiobenzylurethane linkage between PEG and an amino-containing substrate (such as PE). Low pH-degradable PEG-lipid conjugates based on the hydrazone linkage between PEG and lipid have also been described [67].

Doxorubicin in PEG-coated liposomes (Doxil1 and Caelyx1) is successfully used for the treatment of solid tumors in patients with breast carcinoma metastases, with subsequent survival improvement [68]. The same set of indications was targeted by the combination therapy involving liposomal doxorubicin and paclitaxel or Doxil/Caelyx and carboplatin [69]. Caelyx is currently also in phase II studies for patients with squamous cell cancer of the head, neck, and ovarian cancer. Clinical data showed the impressive effect of doxorubicin in PEG-liposomes against unresectable hepatocellular carcinoma cutaneous T-cell lymphoma, and sarcoma [70]. Nonetheless, it should be emphasized that recent research revealed that PEG-liposomes, once thought to be physiologically inert, could still cause some negative effects by activating the complement system [57, 71]. It is typically considered that the low pH and other conditions inside the endosome cause the liposomal barrier to become unstable. This interaction with the endosomal membrane then causes the latter to become secondarily unstable, causing drug release into the cytoplasm. To make liposomes pH sensitive, fusogenic lipids like unsaturated DOPE (dioleoyl-sn-glycero-3-phosphatidylethanolamine) are typically needed in the liposome formulation [72].

4.5.3 Polymeric Micelles

These are potential delivery systems that enable a regulated drug release for less soluble cytotoxic medicines. Polymeric micelles are made of amphiphilic block copolymers and have a hydrophobic core that can contain anticancer medications that are poorly soluble in water and a hydrophilic shell that allows the inclusion of hydrophilic medications and gives the micelle stability. The prolonged blood circulation caused by this formulation is one of the reasons that make these kinds of vehicles suitable for drug delivery [73]. Numerous anticancer drug solubility issues can be resolved by incorporating them into polymeric micelles, but their uniformity and smaller size (20–80 nm), which allows for a large number of anticancer drugs to fit inside, also lengthens the time that the drug spends circulating in the bloodstream and improves the permeability of the anticancer drugs, which enhances their transmission from the vascular system depth into the tumors [74, 75]. As several limitations of the current formulations, such as their poor stability in the circulatory system and the early drug leakage, which may induce side effects and a decline in effectiveness, are solved, polymeric micelles will become more clinically significant [76]. In spite of the promising characteristics of the polymeric micelles, there are only eight polymeric micelle-based formulations included [77]. Genexol-PM (paclitaxel encapsulated in mono methoxy-poly(ethylene glycol)-block-poly(D,L-lactide)), which is curently involved in 13 clinical trials, is the polymeric micelle with a more advanced state of development. It is undergoing phase II, III, and IV clinical trials for the treatment of advanced, recurrent, or metastatic breast cancer; phase II clinical trials for the treatment of severe non-small-cell lung cancer; advanced urothelial cancer; phase I/II clinical studies for the treatment of ovarian cancer; and phase I/II clinical trials for the treatment of advanced or metastatic pancreatic cancer; and it has received Korean Medication Management approval for the treatment of breast and lung cancer [78].

The other clinical trials currently under development with this structures are, the phase I trial with polymeric micelles composed of methoxy-poly(ethylene glycol)-block-poly(D,L-lactide) loaded with docetaxel (Nanoxel-PM) [79]. The phase I trial of NC 4016, a PEG–poly(glutamic acid) polymeric micelle of oxaliplatin the polymeric micelles composed of PEG and PAA that incorporate doxorubicin (NK911) (phase I/II 650 trials) [80] or paclitaxel (NK105) (phase II/III trials), the phase I/II trials of the pegylated polymeric micelles NC-6004 (Nanoplain: PEG + poly-glutamic acid) and NK012 (PEG + poly-glycolic acid) [81, 82] containing cisplatin or SN38, respectively, and the phase II/III trials of the P-glycoprotein-targeting pluronic micelle of doxorubicin (SP1049C) that was labeled as an orphan drug by the FDA in 2008 [83].

When loaded micelles consisting of PEG-b-poly(4-phenyl1-butanoate)-l-aspartamide conjugate, paclitaxel was demonstrated to accumulate in tumors substantially better than its commercial formulation Taxoll among medications administered by passively targeted micelles. This formulation led to a 25-fold improvement in drug accumulation in the C-26 tumor in mice and a corresponding rise in anticancer activity. It also resulted in an almost 100-fold increase in the AUC, a 15-fold decrease in the volume of distribution, and a considerable reduction in drug clearance. With varying degrees of efficacy, various alternative micellar preparations for passively targeting paclitaxel have also been studied [84, 85].

4.5.4 DENDRIMERS

They are three-dimensional synthetic macromolecules with many branches (10–100 nm). By fine-tuning the chemical synthesis of the dendrimer, the biocompatibility and pharmacokinetics of the carrier can be changed. This is possible because dendrimers can be chemically synthesized from a central core in a series of controlled polymeric reactions that allow for a high degree of control over their architecture. With uniform properties (monodisperse size and well-defined shape), biodegradability and biocompatibility, good water solubility, high drug loading capacity, and multiple functional groups in its surface that influence its toxicity and allow the conjugation of multiple molecules simultaneously, such as anticancer drugs, targeting moieties, and PEG to increase the water solubility, this novel and emerging carrier family bear promising properties for its use in the field of oncology and the circulation time of the drugs in blood [86]. Dendrimers have a special uniformity that allows them to penetrate cancer cell membranes and reduce carrier removal by macrophages. Despite these encouraging traits, dendrimers have the same production-cost-increasing multistep synthesis 676 as polymer therapies. The anticancer medication can be covalently conjugated to the dendrimer's surface or non-covalently encapsulated in the dendrimers core, allowing for the customization of the drug release patterns [87, 88]. The encapsulation of anticancer drugs in amphiphilic dendrimers with a hydrophobic core surrounded by hydrophilic branches permits only the utilization of these dendrimers in local treatments (intratumoral injections), because, although it solubilizes the hydrophobic drugs and leaves the drug unaltered, it produces toxicity and generates an uncontrolled drug release [89, 90]. In addition to improving the drugs' solubilization, chemical conjugation of anticancer prodrugs to the dendrimer's surface groups has other benefits over non-covalent encapsulation of the drugs, including the ability to attach multiple hydrophobic or hydrophilic anticancer drugs at the same time and controlled drug release depending on the linkers employed [91]. Dendrimers have been used as passive anticancer nanocarriers [92]. An early example of in vivo passive targeting is the conjugation of a sodium carboxyl-terminated G-3.5 polyamidoamine (PAMAM) dendrimer with cisplatin for the treatment of B16F10-induced melanomas, achieving an enhanced antitumor efficacy compared with the free drug [93].

4.6 DRAWBACKS OF PASSIVE TARGETING

Although passive targeting has considerable success in the treatment of cancer, there are several serious limitations that must be taken into account. These drawbacks emphasize the need for more specialized and focused methods of treating cancer, which can reduce side effects, improve drug delivery, and overcome tumor resistance.

As a result of passive targeting, it is anticipated that the majority of medication particles will gather at the tumor site. Hence, the level of tumor vascularization and angiogenesis has a significant impact on this passive targeting. Unfortunately, the EPR effect is not always present in all malignancies. Moreover, there may be differences in the permeability of arteries inside a tumor and between various tumor types. The same tumor can exhibit substantially distinct EPR effects when growing subcutaneously or orthotopically [94]. Thus, to provide anticancer treatment at the appropriate moment, extensive information on the characteristics of tumor vascularization and tumor type is needed. Also, a lot of solid tumors have high interstitial fluid pressure, which hinders the efficient uptake and uniform distribution of nanocarriers and/or drugs in the tumor tissues by limiting the movement of these substances across interstitial spaces upon extravasation [95].

Parallel modifications to the NP surface's physicochemical characteristics in an effort to make them stealth NPs may have significant downsides. For instance, raising the PEG concentration is known to have interesting effects on the surface polymer architecture and lower the surface charge of the nanocarriers. Parallel to this, there are several drawbacks to the polymers employed to give NPs' stealth qualities. The eventual fate of the polymer ingredients involved in NP is a crucial factor in clinical treatments. The metabolism and excretion of NPs and their components, as well as the clearance mechanism, have received less attention. After internalization in macrophages, as well as in liver, spleen, kidney, and lung cells, where a sizable portion of NPs may be identified, it cannot be ruled out that PEG influences cell functioning at the long-term follow-up after internalization [96]. It is necessary for pharmaceutical carriers to be internalized to the target tumor cell in order to deliver the encapsulated drug to the correct location inside the cell when biopharmaceutical agents, such as proteins, peptides, or nucleic acids, are not membrane permeable. This prevents the extracellular release of the drug from occurring in these cases. Consequently, a crucial step in drug delivery, which is still a scientific issue, is the improved intracellular delivery by employing PEGylated NPs without loss of pharmacological activity (i.e., the improved bioavailability of drug). Third-generation nanocarriers based on precise targeting have therefore been created in order to boost tumor localization as well as tumor cell internalization [94].

4.7 CONCLUSION

With the potential to increase the efficacy and lessen the toxicity of cancer treatments, passive targeting has emerged as a viable strategy for cancer therapy. However, a number of obstacles, including the diversity of malignancies and the intricate interactions between the therapeutic drug and the tumor microenvironment, have hindered its clinical translation.

Future research should concentrate on creating more advanced nanocarriers, integrating passive targeting with other therapeutic modalities, and customizing the therapy to the unique features of particular cancers in order to overcome these difficulties. Passive targeting has the potential to transform cancer therapy and enhance the quality of life for cancer patients with these initiatives.

A revolutionary method of treating cancer that is less intrusive and more targeted than conventional chemotherapy, passive targeting in cancer therapies has shown considerable promise in recent years. There is great potential for the future of passive targeting in cancer therapy, even though the area is relatively young.

The capacity of passive targeting is to specifically target cancer cells while sparing healthy cells is one of its most encouraging features. This can lessen the negative effects of cancer treatment while also enhancing patient outcomes. Additionally, passive targeting offers the potential for more precise delivery of therapeutic agents to the tumor site. This could result in higher efficacy and lower toxicity, making treatment more tolerable for patients.

It is expected that increasingly sophisticated technologies and tactics will evolve as passive targeting keeps on developing. To increase the precision and potency of passive targeting, these techniques can include the use of nanoparticles, biomaterials, and gene therapies.

REFERENCES

1. Stewart, B. and C. Wild, *World cancer report 2014. Lyon: International Agency for Research on Cancer; 2014. Google Scholar*, 2015.
2. Ogawara, K.-i., et al., *Nanoparticle-based passive drug targeting to tumors: considerations and implications for optimization. Biological and Pharmaceutical Bulletin*, 2013. **36**(5): pp. 698–702.
3. McDaniel, J.T., et al., *Social determinants of cancer incidence and mortality around the world: An ecological study. Global Health Promotion*, 2019. **26**(1): pp. 41–49.
4. Bazak, R., et al., *Passive targeting of nanoparticles to cancer: A comprehensive review of the literature. Molecular and Clinical Oncology*, 2014. **2**(6): pp. 904–908.
5. Khan, S.A. and H. Ali, *Novel drug delivery systems.* In *Essentials of Industrial Pharmacy.* 2022, Springer: Berlin. pp. 235–250.
6. Kang, H., et al., *Size-dependent EPR effect of polymeric nanoparticles on tumor targeting. Advanced Healthcare Materials*, 2020. **9**(1): p. 1901223.
7. Hanahan, D. and R.A. Weinberg, *Hallmarks of cancer: The next generation. Cell*, 2011. **144**(5): pp. 646–674.
8. Chabner, B.A. and T.G. Roberts Jr, *Chemotherapy and the war on cancer. Nature Reviews Cancer*, 2005. **5**(1): pp. 65–72.
9. Maeda, H., G. Bharate, and J. Daruwalla, *Polymeric drugs for efficient tumor-targeted drug delivery based on EPR-effect. European Journal of Pharmaceutics and Biopharmaceutics*, 2009. **71**(3): pp. 409–419.
10. LaRocque, J., D.J. Bharali, and S.A. Mousa, *Cancer detection and treatment: the role of nanomedicines. Molecular Biotechnology*, 2009. **42**: pp. 358–366.
11. Skinner, S.A., P.J. Tutton, and P.E. O'Brien, *Microvascular architecture of experimental colon tumors in the rat. Cancer Research*, 1990. **50**(8): pp. 2411–2417.
12. Talekar, M., et al., *Targeting of nanoparticles in cancer: drug delivery and diagnostics. Anti-Cancer Drugs*, 2011. **22**(10): pp. 949–962.
13. Albanese, A., P.S. Tang, and W.C. Chan, *The effect of nanoparticle size, shape, and surface chemistry on biological systems. Annual Review of Biomedical Engineering*, 2012. **14**: pp. 1–16.
14. M Rabanel, J., et al., *Drug-loaded nanocarriers: passive targeting and crossing of biological barriers. Current Medicinal Chemistry*, 2012. **19**(19): pp. 3070–3102.
15. Kommareddy, S. and M. Amiji, *Biodistribution and pharmacokinetic analysis of long-circulating thiolated gelatin nanoparticles following systemic administration in breast cancer-bearing mice. Journal of Pharmaceutical Sciences*, 2007. **96**(2): pp. 397–407.
16. Dobson, J., *Magnetic nanoparticles for drug delivery. Drug DevelopmentResearch*, 2006. **67**(1): pp. 55–60.
17. Minko, T., et al., *Molecular targeting of drug delivery systems to cancer. Current Drug Targets*, 2004. **5**(4): pp. 389–406.
18. Mansour, A.M., et al., *A new approach for the treatment of malignant melanoma: enhanced antitumor efficacy of an albumin-binding doxorubicin prodrug that is cleaved by matrix metalloproteinase 2. Cancer Research*, 2003. **63**(14): pp. 4062–4066.
19. Gautam, A. and N. Koshkina, *Paclitaxel (taxol) and taxoid derivates for lung cancer treatment: potential for aerosol delivery. Current Cancer Drug Targets*, 2003. **3**(4): pp. 287–296.
20. Khanna, C. and D.M. Vail, *Targeting the lung: preclinical and comparative evaluation of anticancer aerosols in dogs with naturally occurring cancers. Current Cancer Drug Targets*, 2003. **3**(4): pp. 265–273.
21. Attia, M.F., et al., *An overview of active and passive targeting strategies to improve the nanocarriers efficiency to tumour sites. Journal of Pharmacy and Pharmacology*, 2019. **71**(8): pp. 1185–1198.
22. Maeda, H., *Tumor-selective delivery of macromolecular drugs via the EPR effect: background and future prospects. Bioconjugate Chemistry*, 2010. **21**(5): pp. 797–802.
23. Gabizon, A., et al., *Long-circulating liposomes for drug delivery in cancer therapy: A review of biodistribution studies in tumor-bearing animals. Advanced Drug Delivery Reviews*, 1997. **24**(2–3): pp. 337–344.
24. Bae, Y.H. and K. Park, *Targeted drug delivery to tumors: myths, reality and possibility. Journal of Controlled Release*, 2011. **153**(3): p. 198.

25. Liu, D., A. Mori, and L. Huang, *Role of liposome size and RES blockade in controlling biodistribution and tumor uptake of GM1-containing liposomes. Biochimica et Biophysica Acta (BBA)-Biomembranes*, 1992. **1104**(1): pp. 95–101.

26. Maeda, H., *Nitroglycerin enhances vascular blood flow and drug delivery in hypoxic tumor tissues: Analogy between angina pectoris and solid tumors and enhancement of the EPR effect. Journal of Controlled Release: Official Journal of the Controlled Release Society*, 2010. **142**(3): pp. 296–298.

27. Fang, J., H. Nakamura, and H. Maeda, *The EPR effect: Unique features of tumor blood vessels for drug delivery, factors involved, and limitations and augmentation of the effect. Advanced Drug Delivery Reviews*, 2011. **63**(3): pp. 136–151.

28. Bates, D., et al., *Regulation of microvascular permeability by vascular endothelial growth factors. Journal of Anatomy*, 2002. **200**(5): pp. 523–534.

29. Kuruppu, D., et al., *Changes in the microvascular architecture of colorectal liver metastases following the administration of SMANCS/lipiodol. Journal of Surgical Research*, 2002. **103**(1): pp. 47–54.

30. Suzuki, M., et al., *A new approach to cancer chemotherapy: Selective enhancement of tumor blood flow with angiotensin II. Journal of the National Cancer Institute*, 1981. **67**(3): pp. 663–669.

31. Li, C., et al., *Augmentation of tumour delivery of macromolecular drugs with reduced bone marrow delivery by elevating blood pressure. British Journal of Cancer*, 1993. **67**(5): pp. 975–980.

32. Kou, R., D. Greif, and T. Michel, *Dephosphorylation of endothelial nitric-oxide synthase by vascular endothelial growth factor: Implications for the vascular responses to cyclosporin A. Journal of Biological Chemistry*, 2002. **277**(33): pp. 29669–29673.

33. Maeda, H., *Vascular permeability in cancer and infection as related to macromolecular drug delivery, with emphasis on the EPR effect for tumor-selective drug targeting. Proceedings of the Japan Academy, Series B*, 2012. **88**(3): pp. 53–71.

34. Iyer, A.K., et al., *Exploiting the enhanced permeability and retention effect for tumor targeting. Drug Discovery Today*, 2006. **11**(17–18): pp. 812–818.

35. Seki, T., J. Fang, and H. Maeda, *Tumor-targeted macromolecular drug delivery based on the enhanced permeability and retention effect in solid tumor. Pharmaceutical Perspectives of Cancer Therapeutics*, 2009: pp. 93–120.

36. Maeda, H., et al., *Vascular permeability enhancement in solid tumor: Various factors, mechanisms involved and its implications. International Immunopharmacology*, 2003. **3**(3): pp. 319–328.

37. Greish, K., *Enhanced permeability and retention of macromolecular drugs in solid tumors: A royal gate for targeted anticancer nanomedicines. Journal of Drug Targeting*, 2007. **15**(7–8): pp. 457–464.

38. Wu, J., T. Akaike, and H. Maeda, *Modulation of enhanced vascular permeability in tumors by a Bradykinin antagonist, a cyclooxygenase inhibitor, and a nitric oxide scavenger. Cancer Research*, 1998. **58**(1): pp. 159–165.

39. Torchilin, V.P., *Passive and active drug targeting: drug delivery to tumors as an example. Drug Delivery*, 2010: pp. 3–53.

40. Hobbs, S.K., et al., *Regulation of transport pathways in tumor vessels: role of tumor type and microenvironment. Proceedings of the National Academy of Sciences*, 1998. **95**(8): pp. 4607–4612.

41. Gref, R., et al., *Biodegradable long-circulating polymeric nanospheres. Science*, 1994. **263**(5153): pp. 1600–1603.

42. des Rieux, A., et al., *Nanoparticles as potential oral delivery systems of proteins and vaccines: a mechanistic approach. Journal of Controlled Release*, 2006. **116**(1): pp. 1–27.

43. Pan, Y., et al., *Bioadhesive polysaccharide in protein delivery system: chitosan nanoparticles improve the intestinal absorption of insulin in vivo. International Journal of Pharmaceutics*, 2002. **249**(1–2): pp. 139–147.

44. Wang, X., et al., *Advances of cancer therapy by nanotechnology. Cancer Research and Treatment: Official Journal of Korean Cancer Association*, 2009. **41**(1): pp. 1–11.

45. Liu, Z., et al., *Polysaccharides-based nanoparticles as drug delivery systems. Advanced Drug Delivery Reviews*, 2008. **60**(15): pp. 1650–1662.

46. Herrero, E.P., M.J. Alonso, and N. Csaba, *Polymer-based oral peptide nanomedicines. Therapeutic Delivery*, 2012. **3**(5): pp. 657–668.

47. Miele, E., et al., *Albumin-bound formulation of paclitaxel (Abraxane® ABI-007) in the treatment of breast cancer. International Journal of Nanomedicine*, 2009: pp. 99–105.

48. Kottschade, L.A., et al., *A phase II trial of nab-paclitaxel (ABI-007) and carboplatin in patients with unresectable stage IV melanoma: A North Central Cancer Treatment Group Study, N057E1. Cancer*, 2011. **117**(8): pp. 1704–1710.

49. Duncan, R. and R. Gaspar, *Nanomedicine(s) under the microscope. Molecular Pharmacology*, 2011. **8**: pp. 2101–41.

50. Bharali, D.J., et al., *Nanoparticles and cancer therapy: A concise review with emphasis on dendrimers. International Journal of Nanomedicine*, 2009: pp. 1–7.

51. Deshpande, P.P., S. Biswas, and V.P. Torchilin, *Current trends in the use of liposomes for tumor targeting. Nanomedicine*, 2013. **8**(9): pp. 1509–1528.

52. Patil, Y.P. and S. Jadhav, *Novel methods for liposome preparation. Chemistry and Physics of Lipids*, 2014. **177**: pp. 8–18.

53. Malam, Y., M. Loizidou, and A.M. Seifalian, *Liposomes and nanoparticles: nanosized vehicles for drug delivery in cancer. Trends in Pharmacological Sciences*, 2009. **30**(11): pp. 592–599.

54. Szebeni, J., et al., *Liposome-induced pulmonary hypertension: properties and mechanism of a complement-mediated pseudoallergic reaction. American Journal of Physiology-Heart and Circulatory Physiology*, 2000. **279**(3): pp. H1319–H1328.

55. Szebeni, J., *Complement activation-related pseudoallergy caused by liposomes, micellar carriers of intravenous drugs, and radiocontrast agents. Critical Reviews™ in Therapeutic Drug Carrier Systems*, 2001. **18**(6): pp. 567–606.

56. Zalipsky, S., et al., *Antitumor activity of new liposomal prodrug of mitomycin C in multidrug resistant solid tumor: insights of the mechanism of action. Journal of Drug Targeting*, 2007. **15**(7–8): pp. 518–530.

57. Moghimi, S.M. and J. Szebeni, *Stealth liposomes and long circulating nanoparticles: Critical issues in pharmacokinetics, opsonization and protein-binding properties. Progress in Lipid Research*, 2003. **42**(6): pp. 463–478.

58. Kono, K., et al., *Highly temperature-sensitive liposomes based on a thermosensitive block copolymer for tumor-specific chemotherapy. Biomaterials*, 2010. **31**(27): pp. 7096–7105.

59. Dicko, A., L.D. Mayer, and P.G. Tardi, *Use of nanoscale delivery systems to maintain synergistic drug ratios in vivo. Expert Opinion on Drug Delivery*, 2010. **7**(12): pp. 1329–1341.

60. Kleinstreuer, C. and Z. Xu, *Computational microfluidics applied to drug delivery in pulmonary and arterial systems. Microfluidics: Fundamentals, Devices, and Applications,* Weinheim: Wiley, 2018.

61. Fan, Y. and Q. Zhang, *Development of liposomal formulations: From concept to clinical investigations. Asian Journal of Pharmaceutical Sciences*, 2013. **8**(2): pp. 81–87.

62. Northfelt, D.W., et al., *Pegylated-liposomal doxorubicin versus doxorubicin, bleomycin, and vincristine in the treatment of AIDS-related Kaposi's sarcoma: results of a randomized phase III clinical trial. Journal of Clinical Oncology*, 1998. **16**(7): pp. 2445–2451.

63. Silverman, J.A. and S.R. Deitcher, *Marqibo®(vincristine sulfate liposome injection) improves the pharmacokinetics and pharmacodynamics of vincristine. Cancer Chemotherapy and Pharmacology*, 2013. **71**(3): pp. 555–564.

64. Maeda, H., *The enhanced permeability and retention (EPR) effect in tumor vascularture: the key role of tumor-selective macromolecular drug targeting. Advan Enzyme Regul*, 2001. **41**: pp. 1898–207.

65. Torchilin, V.P. and V.S. Trubetskoy, *Which polymers can make nanoparticulate drug carriers long-circulating? Advanced Drug Delivery Reviews*, 1995. **16**(2–3): pp. 141–155.

66. Takeuchi, H., et al., *Evaluation of circulation profiles of liposomes coated with hydrophilic polymers having different molecular weights in rats. Journal of Controlled Release*, 2001. **75**(1–2): pp. 83–91.

67. Kale, A.A. and V.P. Torchilin, *Design, synthesis, and characterization of pH-sensitive PEG– PE conjugates for stimuli-sensitive pharmaceutical nanocarriers: the effect of substitutes at the hydrazone linkage on the pH stability of PEG–PE conjugates. Bioconjugate Chemistry*, 2007. **18**(2): pp. 363–370.

68. O'Shaughnessy, J.A., *Pegylated liposomal doxorubicin in the treatment of breast cancer. Clinical Breast Cancer*, 2003. **4**(5): pp. 318–328.

69. Goncalves, A., et al., *Phase I study of pegylated liposomal doxorubicin (Caelyx) in combination with carboplatin in patients with advanced solid tumors. Anticancer Research*, 2003. **23**(4): pp. 3543–3548.

70. Wollina, U., et al., *Multicenter study of pegylated liposomal doxorubicin in patients with cutaneous T-cell lymphoma. Cancer: Interdisciplinary International Journal of the American Cancer Society*, 2003. **98**(5): pp. 993–1001.

71. Moein Moghimi, S., et al., *Activation of the human complement system by cholesterol-rich and pegylated liposomes—modulation of cholesterol-rich liposome-mediated complement activation by elevated serum ldl and hdl levels. Journal of Liposome Research*, 2006. **16**(3): pp. 167–174.

72. Shalaev, E.Y. and P.L. Steponkus, *Phase diagram of 1, 2-dioleoylphosphatidylethanolamine (DOPE): Water system at subzero temperatures and at low water contents. Biochimica et Biophysica Acta (BBA)-Biomembranes*, 1999. **1419**(2): pp. 229–247.

73. Torchilin, V.P., *Micellar nanocarriers: pharmaceutical perspectives. Pharmaceutical Research*, 2007. **24**: pp. 1–16.

74. Kwon, G.S. and K. Kataoka, *Block copolymer micelles as long-circulating drug vehicles. Advanced Drug Delivery Reviews*, 1995. **16**(2–3): pp. 295–309.

75. Cabral, H., et al., *Accumulation of sub-100 nm polymeric micelles in poorly permeable tumours depends on size. Nature Nanotechnology*, 2011. **6**(12): pp. 815–823.

76. Lu, Y. and K. Park, *Polymeric micelles and alternative nanonized delivery vehicles for poorly soluble drugs. International Journal of Pharmaceutics*, 2013. **453**(1): pp. 198–214.

77. Gong, J., et al., *Polymeric micelles drug delivery system in oncology. Journal of Controlled Release*, 2012. **159**(3): pp. 312–323.

78. Kim, D.-W., et al., *Multicenter phase II trial of Genexol-PM, a novel Cremophor-free, polymeric micelle formulation of paclitaxel, with cisplatin in patients with advanced non-small-cell lung cancer. Annals of Oncology*, 2007. **18**(12): pp. 2009–2014.

79. Lee, S.-W., et al., *Development of docetaxel-loaded intravenous formulation, Nanoxel-PM™ using polymer-based delivery system. Journal of Controlled Release*, 2011. **155**(2): pp. 262–271.

80. Matsumura, Y., et al., *Phase I clinical trial and pharmacokinetic evaluation of NK911, a micelle-encapsulated doxorubicin. British Journal of Cancer*, 2004. **91**(10): pp. 1775–1781.

81. Plummer, R., et al., *A phase I clinical study of cisplatin-incorporated polymeric micelles (NC-6004) in patients with solid tumours. British Journal of Cancer*, 2011. **104**(4): pp. 593–598.

82. Hamaguchi, T., et al., *Phase I study of NK012, a novel SN-38–incorporating micellar nanoparticle, in adult patients with solid tumors. Clinical Cancer Research*, 2010. **16**(20): pp. 5058–5066.

83. Valle, J.W., et al., *A phase 2 study of SP1049C, doxorubicin in P-glycoprotein-targeting pluronics, in patients with advanced adenocarcinoma of the esophagus and gastroesophageal junction. Investigational New Drugs*, 2011. **29**: pp. 1029–1037.

84. Hamaguchi, T., et al., *NK105, a paclitaxel-incorporating micellar nanoparticle formulation, can extend in vivo antitumour activity and reduce the neurotoxicity of paclitaxel. British Journal of Cancer*, 2005. **92**(7): pp. 1240–1246.

85. Kim, T.-Y., et al., *Phase I and pharmacokinetic study of Genexol-PM, a cremophor-free, polymeric micelle-formulated paclitaxel, in patients with advanced malignancies. Clinical Cancer Research*, 2004. **10**(11): pp. 3708–3716.

86. Nanjwade, B.K., et al., *Dendrimers: Emerging polymers for drug-delivery systems. European Journal of Pharmaceutical Sciences*, 2009. **38**(3): pp. 185–196.

87. Lee, C.C., et al., *Designing dendrimers for biological applications. Nature Biotechnology*, 2005. **23**(12): pp. 1517–1526.

88. Svenson, S., *Dendrimers as versatile platform in drug delivery applications. European Journal of Pharmaceutics and Biopharmaceutics*, 2009. **71**(3): pp. 445–462.

89. Kojima, C., et al., *Synthesis of polyamidoamine dendrimers having poly (ethylene glycol) grafts and their ability to encapsulate anticancer drugs. Bioconjugate Chemistry*, 2000. **11**(6): pp. 910–917.

90. Dhanikula, R.S. and P. Hildgen, *Influence of molecular architecture of polyether-co-polyester dendrimers on the encapsulation and release of methotrexate. Biomaterials*, 2007. **28**(20): pp. 3140–3152.

91. Gurdag, S., et al., *Activity of dendrimer– methotrexate conjugates on methotrexate-sensitive and -resistant cell lines. Bioconjugate Chemistry*, 2006. **17**(2): pp. 275–283.

92. Morgan, M.T., et al., *Dendritic molecular capsules for hydrophobic compounds. Journal of the American Chemical Society*, 2003. **125**(50): pp. 15485–15489.

93. Malik, N., E.G. Evagorou, and R. Duncan, *Dendrimer-platinate: a novel approach to cancer chemotherapy*. Anti-Cancer Drugs, 1999. **10**(8): pp. 767–776.

94. Huynh, N.T., et al., *The rise and rise of stealth nanocarriers for cancer therapy: passive versus active targeting*. Nanomedicine, 2010. **5**(9): pp. 1415–1433.

95. Heldin, C.-H., et al., *High interstitial fluid pressure—an obstacle in cancer therapy*. Nature Reviews Cancer, 2004. **4**(10): pp. 806–813.

96. Shan, X., et al., *In vitro macrophage uptake and in vivo biodistribution of long-circulation nanoparticles with poly (ethylene-glycol)-modified PLA (BAB type) triblock copolymer*. Colloids and Surfaces B: Biointerfaces, 2009. **72**(2): pp. 303–311.

5 Cancer Active Targeting Strategies

Tanzeela Awan, Ghazala Ambreen, Uzma Saher,
Saira Afzal, Muhammad Yasir Ali, and Asia Naz Awan

5.1 INTRODUCTION

Drug delivery to the specific site of action is known as active targeting. This phenomenon is principally based on the recognition of molecular patterns using a ligand that can identify its specific receptors. This type of targeting is indeed important for those drugs that have serious side effects, such as tumor-targeting drugs. Due to the non-target effect, healthy tissues are also at a high risk of damage along with cancer cells during anti-cancer therapies. Hence, targeting the drug to the specific tumor site and increasing internalization is crucial for a successful anti-cancer therapy with fewer side effects.

To overcome the bottleneck of various biological barriers, many efficient pharmaceutical tools have been designed for the targeted delivery of chemotherapeutic drugs [1]. There are different systems to transfer drugs at the site of action like the distribution of the drug as free drugs, by active targeting, or by passive targeting [2]. The therapeutic efficiency of the drug depends upon the availability of the drug at the site of the tumor, whatever way is utilized for its transportation, but active targeting provides ease in the uptake of API by tumor cells directly [3]. Passive targeting also helps the drug to localize at the area of the tumor but it cannot support the uptake of the drug by the tumor itself. Active targeting can be enhanced by nanoparticle encapsulation of anti-cancer drugs. Nanocarriers have drug moieties either conjugated to the surface or encapsulated within them. Nanotechnology has featured striking advantages, including a high concentration of drugs at the targeted sites, enhanced solubility, and drug internalization. The nanoscale size, bigger surface area and ability to activate only targeted molecules make nanocarriers the best agents for active tumor targeting [1].

Active targeting at the specific tumor site can be achieved by focusing the receptors or protein biomarkers on the cancerous cells that are overexpressed in various tumors. Researchers have identified several such cell surface receptors and antigens, many of which are being identified by ligands of drug-loaded nanocarriers for active targeting of the cancer cell. As soon as the nanocarriers are injected into the bloodstream, their opsonization takes place to make large aggregates. Subsequently, these aggregates are recognized and uptaken by the reticuloendothelial system (RES), which determined their pharmacokinetic fate. RES uptake of nanocarriers must be avoided to retain longer in blood circulation [4]. For this purpose, the nanocarriers are being ornamented with such ligands/moieties able to recognize the tumor cell-expressed receptors or the components of the tumor microenvironment (TME), which is the basis of active tumor targeting.

While encapsulation of drugs in nanocarriers, the following concerns should be in focus to make them potential anti-cancer agents:

DOI: 10.1201/9781003363958-6

1. They should remain stable till reaching the point of action, i.e., tumor site.
2. They should protect themselves from the RES and mononuclear phagocyte system.
3. They should be accumulated in TME.
4. They should be able to penetrate the tumor cells and interstitial fluid of TME with high affinity or pressure, respectively.
5. It should reach the site of action and interact with the targeted cells exclusively.

Active tumor targeting can be broadly subdivided into two groups; targeting the tumor cell and targeting TME [5–7]. Components of an active targeting moiety include a ligand on the nanocarrier, the targeted cells/receptors, the nanocarrier, and a chemotherapeutic drug. These components are discussed below.

5.2 LIGANDS FOR ACTIVE TARGETING

A ligand is a molecule that identifies and attaches to the target antigen or receptors on certain cells or tissue components. This binding interaction between the ligand and receptor is exploited to create the ligand-installed nanocarriers. An ideal ligand for targeted delivery should possess specific binding, high avidity, compatibility for chemical modification, and the possibility to be synthesized in sufficient amounts [8].

5.2.1 ANTIBODIES AND THEIR FRAGMENTS AS TARGETING LIGANDS

Antibodies (Abs) represent one of the natural ligands most frequently used to adorn the nanocarriers. They are Y-shaped glycoproteins that are released by the immune system in response to an antigen. Due to the presence of epitope interacting sites, they exhibit exceptionally high affinity and specificity for antigens hence resulting in an improved pharmacokinetic profile [9, 10]. Their huge size and extensive systemic circulation time, however, limit their usage against solid tumors [11]. Since smaller Ab fragments have greater diffusion rates and hence better cellular absorption, they are preferable over full-length Abs. Owing to advances in protein engineering, it has become possible to create customized small fragment Abs possessing intended pharmacological effects and tailored properties. For example, Fabs, bispecific Abs, single-chain variable fragment (ScFv), bifunctional Abs, nanobodies, mini bodies, and diabodies [12, 13]. When introducing the small Ab fragments on the nanocarrier, their affinity for the target antigen must be examined since a low affinity might result in reverse diffusion to the vasculature and, ultimately, removal by renal excretion [14].

5.2.2 PROTEINS AS TARGETING LIGANDS

Proteins can also be exploited as targeting ligands for nanocarriers, e.g., human serum albumin and transferrin. The expression of these receptors is higher (up to 100-fold) in cancer cells as compared to normal cells. Due to the higher expression in tumor cells, the ligands of these receptors act as a promising targeting moiety that can be conjugated with nanocarriers to deliver therapeutics [9].

5.2.3 APTAMERS AS TARGETING LIGANDS

The word "aptamer" is derived from the Latin word "Aptus", which means "to fit" [15]. Aptamers are short-chain, single-stranded nucleotides (DNA or RNA) with a 3D structure that has a high affinity to bind with a specific targeting moiety. These emerging molecules have high specificity and stability even under high temperatures. The flexible conformation of these ligands allows them to identify several biomolecules, including proteins, phospholipids, and oligosaccharides. The aptamer binding with specific receptors leads to receptor-mediated endocytosis, which ultimately causes the release of drugs from nanocarriers. Aptamers are usually selected from a random pool of single-stranded oligonucleotides by using technology systematic evolution of ligands by exponential enrichment (SELEX) after which the aptamer is purified and amplified to produce a high-affinity molecule [16]. Aptamer-functionalized nanocarriers are internalized into the cell by clathrin-mediated endocytosis [17].

They have received a great deal of attention for the development of biosensors, drug delivery, and target imaging agents. To date, various high-affinity aptamers have been identified against a wide range of target molecules, such as peptides, proteins, drugs, metal ions, and even viruses and complete cells [18]. They offer certain advantages, such as their small size, ease of penetration, thermostability, minimal immunogenicity, efficient synthesis, and ability to recognize multiple tumor targets [9]. AS1411 is an example of an aptamer that interacts with the nucleolin, a nonribosomal nucleolar protein overexpressed on the surface of different cancer cells. Hence, AS1411 aptamers can target and limit the growth of a wide range of cancer cells exhibiting overexpression of nucleolin. Currently, Mucagen is the only aptamer-based therapeutic that has been approved by the FDA for the treatment of age-related muscular degeneration, however, many others are being investigated in clinical trials. In addition to cancer, aptamers have also been used to treat obesity, diabetes mellitus, cardiovascular, immunological, bone, and infectious diseases [19, 20].

5.2.4 SMALL MOLECULES AS TARGETING LIGANDS

Various small molecules such as sugars (lactobionic acid and galactose) and vitamins (folic acid, biotin) are also used as a ligand for active targeting. The sugar ligands have a high affinity for asialoglycoprotein receptors (ASGPR) that are overexpressed on the surface of the tumor cell membrane. Hence, lactobionic acid-installed nanocarriers have been associated with an improved targeted delivery due to ASGPR-mediated endocytosis that delivers the drug under an increased level of matrix metalloproteinases or glutathione and leads to cell apoptosis [21].

Among vitamins, folic acid is considered an important targeting ligand. Folic acid is indispensable for the synthesis of purines and pyrimidines and is also required by tumor cells. It shows a high affinity for folic acid receptors, upregulated in numerous carcinomas including lung, breast, colorectal, and ovarian cancers. Other vitamins commonly used for active targeting are biotin, thiamine, and vitamin B_{12} [21–23].

5.3 ACTIVE TARGETING OF CANCER CELLS

Targeted tumor cells mean targeting the cell surface tumor-specific receptors on either cancer cells or tumor endothelial cells and targeting the internal cell organelles [1]. However, the specific receptors must be overexpressed on the surface of target cells, while having a reduced expression on neighboring cells, to create additional binding sites for ligands and achieve specificity.

5.3.1 CANCER CELL SURFACE RECEPTORS-MEDIATED ACTIVE TARGETING

The internalization of the drug occurs via receptor-mediated endocytosis when a specific ligand present on the nanocarriers attaches to the targeted receptor on the cell. Subsequently, this endocytic vesicle fuses with lysosomes or other cell organelles to release the drug molecules into the cell [24, 25]. Target receptors that facilitate the phagocytosis of drug-loaded nanocarriers include folate receptors, transferrin receptors, growth factor receptors, and various other receptors that are frequently overexpressed on the tumor cells.

5.3.1.1 Folate Receptors

Folate receptors (FR) belong to glycoprotein and bind to folic acid (FA), which is necessary for the synthesis of DNA nucleotide bases. These receptors occur in three isoforms: FRα, FRβ, and FRγ where FRα is significantly over-expressed in various cancers like kidney cancers, lung cancers, and breast cancers [26, 27]. During cancer development, the loosening of tight junctions between the cells results in the alteration in cell morphology. Consequently, the FR becomes accessible to the folic acid nanocarriers over the entire cell surface [28, 29]. Nanocarriers with conjugated FA are transported into the cell by endocytosis after being captured by FR. The drug is then released into the tumor cell where it induces cell death.

5.3.1.2 Transferrin Receptors

Transferrin (Tf), also a glycoprotein, binds to transferrin receptors (TfR) and is responsible for iron transportation. The transferrin-transferrin receptor complex after endocytosis forms an endosomal compartment that releases iron after maturation. These receptors are extensively over-expressed in various cancers to accommodate the requirement of iron for rapid cell growth during tumorigenesis [30]. Luckily these receptors are also present in endothelial cells of brain capillaries, which makes them an attractive target for delivering chemotherapeutic agents [31]. One of the reasons for the failure of chemotherapeutic agents' blood–brain barrier, which serves as an obstacle for various drugs to be transferred to the brain [32].

5.3.1.3 Human Epidermal Growth Factor Receptors

The human epidermal growth factor receptor (HER) is involved in the pathogenesis of many tumors. This receptor is found to be over-expressed in pancreatic, renal, colon, breast, liver, head and neck, brain and ovarian cancers [33, 34]. It plays a significant role in the activation of many cellular signaling pathways that lead to cell growth, proliferation, survival, and differentiation. This activation is manifested by tyrosine kinase activity, which makes this receptor a suitable target in drug-resistant cancers. Tyrosine kinase inhibitors (TKI) are mostly implicated in the nanocarriers that are developed to target the HER receptor family.

5.3.1.4 Epidermal Growth Factor Receptor

Epidermal growth factor receptor (EGFR) is overexpressed in various types of cancers. It is activated when it binds to the epidermal growth factor (EGF), transforming growth factor (TGFα), betacellulin, epiregulin, and amphiregulin. After activation, it initiates a cascade of signaling pathways that are responsible for cell growth, proliferation, angiogenesis, and invasion making EGFR a suitable candidate for active targeting [1]. Active targeting of EGFR may include direct blocking of the receptor by monoclonal antibody to inhibit the signaling cascade, application of TKIs, which bind to the intracellular domain of the receptor to obstruct the signaling pathway, and administration of the anti-cancer drug, which is transported to the cell via receptor-mediated endocytosis [1, 35].

5.3.1.5 Cluster of Differentiation Receptors

Various studies have reported the potential role of a cluster of differentiation (CD) receptors such as CD22, CD36, CD44, and CD133 in the metastasis of cancers. CD44 receptors have been widely studied for active targeting via nanocarriers. Activation of CD44 results from its binding with hyaluronic acid (HA) that causes activation of receptors leading to invasion and metastasis [36]. The receptor can also bind with surface-expressed matrix metalloproteases [37].

5.3.1.6 Estrogen Receptors

Estrogen is a steroid hormone and it plays an important role in the progression of breast, endometrial, and ovarian cancers. It functions after binding with one of the two surface-expressed estrogen receptors (ERα or ERβ). More than 80% of breast cancers are classified as ERα positive tumors, which makes it an ideal receptor for actively targeting breast cancers. ER is targeted via estrogen-tagged nanocarriers with encapsulated anti-tumor drugs; this drug, for example, doxycycline can be either alone or conjugated with estrogen where the estrogen-conjugated drug is released in the intracellular compartment to bind with the ER present on the nuclear membrane, which supports the entry of the drug into the nucleus [38].

5.3.1.7 Integrin Receptors

Integrin receptors are expressed on the cell surfaces with intramembrane and cytoplasmic domains. They occur as a heterodimer of two subunits α and β. The cytoplasmic domain of integrins is attached to focal adhesion kinase (FAK) and Src kinase which upon activation initiate the cascade of signaling events responsible for cell migration, survival, and growth. The extracellular domain not only maintains the cell-to-cell connection but also interacts with ECM. Integrins have an affinity to conjugate with ligands containing the RGD (arginine-glycine aspartic acid-D-tyrosine-lysine) domains and disintegrin and metalloproteases (ADAM8, 10 and 17) [39, 40]. Targeting integrins via peptides containing the RGD domain results in greater cellular uptake of the nanocarriers. Due to their overexpression in various cancers, integrins are also considered a suitable targeting moiety for anti-cancer therapy.

5.3.1.8 Other Receptors

There are many other receptors and surface-expressed proteins that are being over-expressed in cancer cells and can be used as specific targets for the active targeting of anti-cancer drugs. Among these, biotin-specific receptors, insulin and insulin-like growth factor (IGF) receptors, chemokines, interleukins, and metalloproteases have been explored for active targeting. Surface-expressed proteins are actively targeted by using antibody-tagged nanocarriers [41].

5.3.2 Cancer Cell Organelle-Mediated Active Targeting

Delivery of anti-cancer drugs to the cytoplasm is not always sufficient to attain the maximum therapeutic efficacy, as long as it reaches its ultimate target site. The bioactive molecules may face several challenges like enzymatic degradation and limitation like toxicity when released in the cytoplasm. Therefore, to overcome this challenge, subcellular targeting is employed [42]. Mitochondria, lysosomes, Golgi apparatus, endoplasmic reticulum, and nuclei are the main targeting organelles in this strategy, which is also beneficial to surmount the drug resistance and recurrence of cancers.

5.3.2.1 Mitochondria Targeting

Mitochondria are the powerhouse of cells and are the main producers of ATP. It is also responsible for activating the signaling pathway associated with cell apoptosis. Tumor development results in the dysfunction of mitochondria. As a result, the cell is shifted to the glycolysis pathway to circumvent its need for energy. This shifting of energy production pathway is the result of a mutation of a tumor suppressor gene, p53. The mitochondrial membranes possess highly negative potential, which can attract positively charged moieties. Drugs with a positive charge like triphenylphosphonium (TPP) can easily penetrate the mitochondrial membranes [43]. The nanocarriers are designed for multi-stage targeting, first to reach and get internalized into the tumor cell by ligand-receptor conjugation and afterward, the drug is released in mitochondria causing the activation of the programmed cell death pathway [44].

5.3.2.2 Lysosome Targeting

Lysosomes, the digestive compartments of the cell, are crucial for their significant role in degradation, repair, and cell death signaling. Moreover, lysosomes are associated with cancer progression by promoting cell survival, drug resistance, and metastasis. Therefore, targeting lysosomes of the tumor cells is a promising approach for cancer therapy. The acidic environment of lysosomes is manipulated for the delivery of pH-dependent anti-cancer drugs. Lysosomes can be directly targeted by enhancing the pH sensitivity of the drug molecules, which are encapsulated in nanocarriers and internalized into the cell via receptor-mediated endocytosis [45].

5.3.2.3 Endoplasmic Reticulum Targeting

The endoplasmic reticulum (ER) plays a significant role in the synthesis, folding, and trafficking of proteins. ER is a sensitive organelle, as a slight dysfunctioning, such as protein misfolding or stress may lead to disrupted cell signaling, which has been reported in cancers along with other serious ailments [46]. The ER can be targeted by anti-cancer drugs, which may cause ER stress that activates the caspase8-mediated cell death process. ER also serves as a site for peptide delivery, ultimately promoting the presentation of these peptides to the antigen-containing cells that cause the anti-cancer activity. Nanocarriers transported the drug into the cells by endocytosis and the drug is localized to ER-derived through peptides such as pardaxin, which is selectively accumulated in ER enhancing the release of calcium followed by ER stress, ROS production, mitochondrial dysfunctioning, and ultimately cell death [1].

5.3.2.4 Golgi Body Targeting

Golgi bodies can be targeted similarly to ER, creating the Golgi stress resulting in misfolding of proteins. The pH-sensitive nanocarriers are designed to exploit the acidic environment of the Golgi bodies. More recently, photodynamic therapy was used to actively target Golgi bodies of cancer cells to induce apoptosis by causing Golgi stress and ROS production [47].

5.3.2.5 Nucleustargeting

Nucleus is considered the brain of the cell, controlling cell processes, such as reproduction, cell cycle, and metabolism. The transportation of small molecules between cytoplasm and nucleus takes place through either nuclear pore complex (NPC) or diffusion. However, for the transportation of large molecules through NPC, a nucleus localization sequence should be attached to the transported molecule. This sequence at first interacts and binds with a cytoplasmic transporter, importinα followed by binding to importinβ, which then passes through NPC and localizes in the nucleus [48]. Nucleus localization is important for the action of certain anti-cancer drugs such as doxorubicin which involves oxidative DNA damage within the nucleus [3].

5.3.3 TUMOR MICROENVIRONMENT-MEDIATED ACTIVE TARGETING

The tumor microenvironment sensitivity plays an important role in the selection of targeted drug delivery systems as there are differences between the tumor microenvironment and normal tissues surrounding the tumor. It mainly helps out the drug delivery system in a way that it makes the environment a little acidic, hypoxic, and other differences that the delivery system would focus to target specifically cancerous extracellular matrix (ECM) and the normal tissues remain safe. TME is based on the role of different cells and their interaction with one another to make TME so influential in the control of tumor progression. These components include stromal cells, cancer-associated fibroblasts (CAF), tumor-associated macrophages (TAM), immune cells, and ECM [1].

ECM plays a pivotal role in the progression of the tumor by changes not only in its composition but also in its density. These changes help the tumor to spread, grow, proliferate, and invade. Similarly, the stiffness of ECM makes drugs difficult to reach cell surface receptors resulting in treatment failure [49]. It is essential to maintain homeostasis in the ECM so that penetration of the drug at the site of action becomes easy and this becomes possible through strict control of the enzymatic processes of ECM components [50]. The hypoxic environment of ECM degrades it and enhances tumor development. CAFs induce hypoxia within the TME and cause stiffness and degradation of ECM. This may provide various strategies for treating cancers by controlling ECM density, composition, and homeostasis [51]. Control of ECM in favor of tumor reduction can be possible by controlling various factors like reduction in TME hypoxia, reprogramming of TAMs and CAFs, and through inhibitors of TGF-β and metalloproteases [52].

5.3.3.1 Cancer-Associated Fibroblasts Targeting

CAFs play a vital role in the proliferation and invasion of cancer by providing various oncogenic signals mainly by synthesizing fibroblast activation protein (FAP) that is protease in nature and cleaving collagen and gelatin as a result of TME remodeling takes place. There is no precise role of FAP in a normal cell while it is overexpressed in different cancerous ailments, i.e., colon, breast, lung, and ovarian cancers. Blockage of enzymatic activity of FAP can be a source of active targeting for controlling CAFs.

5.3.3.2 Angiogenesis Targeting

It is either a new vessel formation in the tumor as it gets progressed or an extension of vessels from existing vessels. Tumor growth can be inhibited by controlling mediators of angiogenesis. As the tumor progresses it spreads various factors among them vascular endothelial growth factor (VEGF) and platelet-derived growth factor (PDGF) play a critical role in the spread and development of tumors. VEGFA causes endothelial cell migration, proliferation, vascular permeability, and tube formation that leads to a progression of cancer while VEGFC and VEGFD play critical roles in cancerous conditions of the lymphatic system, i.e., lymphangiogenesis and lymph node metastases. The role of VGFB is not clearly defined. Survival of endothelial cells is under the control of PDGF, which also controls the signaling of VEGF. Active targeting of any of these receptors via nanocarriers may result in the dissociation of metastasis and hamper tumor progression.

5.3.3.3 TGF-β Targeting

TGF-β plays its role by promoting angiogenesis through activation of fibroblast growth factor that leads to the secretion of VEGF that results in proliferation and growth of the tumor by MAPK pathway. Inhibition of TGF-β binding to its receptor leads to a significant approach to controlling tumor growth.

5.3.3.4 Fibroblast Growth Factor Targeting

Fibroblast growth factor (FGF) has two subtypes FGF1 and FGF2. These growth factors not only regulate endothelial cell proliferation and migration but also stimulates the process of angiogenesis through their binding to tyrosine kinase receptors. The therapeutic target is the inhibition of FGF receptor-mediated signaling those results in not only an antitumor effect but also antiangiogenic action.

5.3.3.5 Notch Signaling Pathway Targeting

The notch signaling pathway regulates genetically the process of differentiation not only in embryonic stages but also in adult life and this control is important for cell-to-cell communication. Similarly, this pathway plays an important role in angiogenesis as the tumor progresses [53]. DLL4 (delta-like ligand 4) is a ligand for notch signaling and targeting this ligand results in a hyperproliferative response in endothelial cells that cause an increase in vascularity that weakens the vessels and shows antiangiogenic effects. Notch inhibitors inhibit stem cell proliferation either single or in combination with other anti-cancer drugs [54].

5.3.3.6 Angiopoiten/TIE Receptor Pathway Targeting

These angiopoietins (ANG-1 to ANG-4) are ligands that bind on tie receptors (TIE1 and TIE2) and control endothelial cell functions, their growth, stabilization, and maintenance and as a result, they control vascular permeability and angiogenesis, and inflammatory responses [55]. Therefore, TIE receptors are one of the appropriate targets for inhibiting anti-cancer therapy to inhibit angiogenesis. Many drugs are in clinical trials that act as inhibitors on these receptors and can be promising anti-cancer agents [56].

5.3.3.7 Targeting Cell Adhesion to the ECM

The extracellular matrix (ECM) is one of the most important components playing a crucial role in the malignant transformation of cells. The stiffness of ECM helps tumors to propagate and spread. It also serves as a signaling molecule for migration, adhesion, and invasion of cancers [57]. There are 300 different components of ECM, including interstitial matrix (fibronectin, elastin, collagen) laminins, integrins, hyaluronic acid, and many others [58]. Activation of these components may result in the invasion, adhesion, and migration of cancer. In inactive vessels, integrins interact with the basal membrane, thereby maintaining vascular quiescence. During angiogenesis, integrins are essential for endothelial cell migration, proliferation, and survival. Similarly, FAK is involved in cell spreading, adhesion, motility, survival, and cell cycle progression, and has been shown to play a role in tumor angiogenesis. Pharmacological inhibition of the FAK pathway reduces tumor growth. These molecules can be targeted in both tumor cells and endothelial cells to achieve the desirable anti-cancer effects [59]. Various receptors with their targeting ligand, anti-tumor drug, and nanocarriers are listed in Table 5.1.

TABLE 5.1
Actively Targeted Nanocarriers

Nanocarriers	Ligand	Receptor/ Antigen	Drug	Cancer Cells
Liposome	Folic acid	Folate receptor	DOX	Nasopharengyeal carcinoma cells [60]
Liposome	Folic acid	Folate receptor	Mitomycin-c prodrug + DOX	Prostate-specific membrane antigen-positive tumor cells [28]
Liposomes	Folic acid	Folate receptor	Celastrol + Irinotecan	MCF-7 and MDA-MB-231 cells [61]
Bifunctional Fe_3O_4 magnetic nanoparticles	Folic acid	Folate receptor	DOX	KB cells [62]
PEG and PEI co-coated iron oxide nanoparticles	Folic acid	Folate receptor	DOX	MCF-7 [63]
magnetic nanoparticles	Folic acid	Folate receptor	DOX	MDA-MB-231 cells [64]
Polydopamine (PDA)- modified mesoporous silica nanoparticles (MSNs)	Folic acid	Folate receptor	DOX	Hela cells [65]
Gold nanoparticles	Folic acid	Folate receptor	Curcumin	Breast cancer cells [66]
Gold nanprods and liposomal nanocoomplex	Folic acid	Folate receptor	DOX	Breast cancer cells [67]
poly(lactic-co-glycolide) (PLGA) nanoparticles	Transferrin	Transferrin receptors	PTX (paclitaxel)	Breast cancer cell lines (MCF-7) [68]

TABLE 5.1 (Continued)
Actively Targeted Nanocarriers

Nanocarriers	Ligand	Receptor/ Antigen	Drug	Cancer Cells
chitosan coated γ-Fe$_2$O$_3$ nanocarriers	Transferrin	Transferrin receptors	DOX + Rhodamine B isothiocyanate	Imaging and targeting human brain tumor U251 MG cells [69]
PEG coated MSNs	Transferrin	Transferrin receptors	DOX	HT29 and MCF-7 [70]
Polymer (chitosan PLGA) coated MSNs	Transferrin	Transferrin receptors	gemcitabine	Pancreatic cancer cells (MIA PaCa-2 cells) [71]
RBC membrane coated PLGA nanoparticles	Transferrin	Transferrin receptors	DOX + Methylene blue	Photodynamic & anti-tumor effect on HeLa and MCF-7 cells [72]
Solid lipid nanoparticles	Anti-EGFR antibody	EGFR	Carmustine	Glioblastoma cells [73]
Fe3O4 loaded polymeric micelle	Anti-EGFR mAb	EGFR	Cetuximab	A431 cells [74]
pH-sensitive liposomes	Anti-EGFR antibody	EGFR	gemcitabine	Breast cancer cells [75]
PLGA nanoparticles	Anti-EGFR antibody	EGFR	gemcitabine	Pancreatic cancer [76]
lipid polymeric nanoparticle (LPNs)	Anti-EGFR antibody	EGFR	Cisplatin + DOX	Lung carcinoma [77]
Iron oxide nanoparticles	Anti-EGFR antibody	EGFR		Cancer detection via MRI [78]
pH-sensitive double-emulsion nanocapsules + magnetic nanoparticles	anti-HER2 antibody	HER2	DOX + PTX	SKBR3 breast cancer cells [79]
PEI and PLGA nanoparticles	Anti-HER2 mAb (Trastuzumab)	HER2	PTX	BT-474 [80]
PLGA-PLA nanoparticles	Single chain anti-HER2 mAb	HER2	Docetaxel	BT-474 [81]
Immunoliposomes	Anti-HER2 antibody	HER2	PTX + Rapa	SK-BR-3 [82]
PEG gold nanoparticles	Anti-HER2 mAb (Trastuzumab)	HER2	DOX	SK-BR-3 [83]
Fe$_3$O$_4$ nanoparticles	Anti-HER2/neu peptide	HER2	PTX	SK-BR-3 [84]
PEG-modified Au-Fe3O4 nanoparticles	Anti-HER2 mAb (Trastuzumab)	HER2	Oxaliplatin	SGC-7901 (human gastric cancer cells) [85]
Liposomes	Anti-HER2 antibody	HER2	DOX	BT-474 & SK-BR-3 cells [86]
amphiphilic core-shell polymeric nanocarrier	Hyaluronic acid (HA)	CD44	DOX + Cyclopamine	MCF-7 cells [87]
Liposome	Anti-CD44 mAb	CD44	DOX	Hepatocellular carcinoma [88]
Fe$_3$O$_4$ magnetic nanoparticles	Anti-CD44 antibody	CD44	Gemcitabine	Panc-1 and MDA-MB-231 [89]
superparamagnetic iron oxide nanoparticles	Hyaluronic acid (HA)	CD44	Photothermal effect	MRI and photothermal effect on MDA-MB-231 [90]
Carbon dots	Hyaluronic acid (HA)	CD44	DOX	4T1 cells [91]

(Continued)

TABLE 5.1 (Continued)
Actively Targeted Nanocarriers

Nanocarriers	Ligand	Receptor/ Antigen	Drug	Cancer Cells
Superparamagnetic iron oxide/mesoporous silica nanoparticles	pH-responsive anti-CD44 conjugate	CD44	Oxaliplatin	HCT-116 cells [92]
pH-sensitive liposomes	Estrone	Estrone receptors	DOX	MCF-7 [93]
Stealth liposome	Estradiol	Estrogen receptor	Anti-cancer gene	Breast cancer cells [94]
Glycol chitosan nanoparticles	Estrone	Estrogen receptor	PTX	MCF-7 cells [95]
Polymerosome	Estradiol	Estrogen receptor	DOX	Breast cancer cell [96]
Chitosan nanoparticles	Estrone	Nuclear and cellular Estrogen receptors	DOX	MCF-7 cells [97]
Micelles	Cyclic RGD peptide	$\alpha_v\beta_3$ integrin	PTX	Glioblastoma cells [98]
Human serum albumin nanoparticles	RGD	$\alpha_v\beta_3$ integrin	Resveratrol	Ovarian cancer cells [99]
PLGA-chitosan nanoparticles	RGD	$\alpha_v\beta_3$ integrin	Cisplatin/PTX	Lung cancer cell lines (A549, H1299, H1975) [100]
Fluorescent nanoparticles	RGD	$\alpha_v\beta_3$ integrin	Epirubicin	Imaging & targeting esophageal cancer [101]
Chitosan nanoparticles	RGD	$\alpha_v\beta_3$ integrin	Raloxifene	Breast cancer cells (4T1, MBA-MD-231) [102]
Mesoporous silica nanoparticles	T22 peptide	CXCR4	DOX	Lymphoma cells [103]
Polymeric nanoparticles	LFC131 peptide	CXCR4	Epirubicin	HepG2 cells [104]
PLGA cellulose nanoparticles	LFC131 peptide	CXCR4	DOX	BT-549-Luc cells [105]
Liposomes	Anti-CXCR4 antibody	CXCR4	DOX	HCC1500 and MDA-MB-175VII cells [106, 107]
Dextran nanoparticles	Anti-LHRH peptide	LHRH receptors	Cisplatin	MCF-7 cells [107]
Human serum albumin nanoparticles	Anti-LHRH peptide	LHRH receptors	Methotraxate	T47D cells [108]
Liposomes	Anti-LHRH peptide	LHRH receptors	Mitoxantrone	MCF-7 cells [109]
human serum albumin nanoparticles	Biotin	Biotin receptor	Methotraxate	4T1 cells [110]
Hexagonal zinc oxide nanodisc	Biotin	Biotin receptor	DOX	Breast cancer cells [111]
Carboxy methyl chitosan nanoparticles	Biotin	Biotin receptor	DOX + Tariquidar	MCF-7 cells [112]
Liposomes	IL-13	IL-13	DOX	Brain cancer cells [113]
Mesoporous silica nanoparticles	Anti-IL-13 peptide	IL-13	DOX	Human glioma cells (U251 cells) [114]
Liposomes	Atherosclerotic plaque-specific peptide-1	IL-4 receptor	DOX	Colorectal cancer cells [115]

TABLE 5.1 (Continued)
Actively Targeted Nanocarriers

Nanocarriers	Ligand	Receptor/ Antigen	Drug	Cancer Cells
PEG coated liposomes	Sgc8 aptamer		FITC-dextran	CCRF-CEM cells [116]
Liposome	TLS1c aptamer		Cabazitaxel	[117]
Liposome	AS1411 aptamer		5-fluorouracil	Basal cell carcinoma [118]
PLA-PEG micelles		PSMA	DOX	Prostate cancer cells [119, 120]
Composite micelles	AS1411 aptamer		DOX	Breast cancer cells [120]
PLGA-PEG nanocarriers	A10 2'-fluoropyrimidine RNA aptamer	PSMA	Docetaxel	Prostate cancer cells [121]
PLGA-PEG nanocarriers	Wy5a aptamer		Docetaxel	castration-resistant prostate cancer [122]
Hollow gold nanosphere	39-mer RNA aptamer	CD30 receptor	DOX	Lymphoma tumour cells [123]
Gold nanoparticles	AS1411 aptamer		DOX	breast cancer and uveal melanoma cells [123]
Gold modified pH sensitive liposomes	AS1411 aptamer			SGC-7901 cells [124]
Iron oxide nanoparticles	Anti-FGFR1 aptamer	FGFR1		Human osteosarcoma cells [125]
Silicon oxide nanoparticles	Sgc8 aptamer		FITC & DOX	Hela cells [126]
PEG-coated magnetic mesoporous silicon oxide nanoparticles	AS1411 aptamer	[126]	DOX	MCF-7 [127]
mesoporous silicon oxide nanoparticles	Triphenylphosphonium (TPP) + hyaluronic acid	Nucleus CD44	DOX	Breast cancer cells [128]
Gold nanostars	TPP + HA	Nucleus CD44	DOX	SCC-7 and MCF-7 cells [129]
30 nm gold nanoparticles	RGD peptide	Nucleus $\alpha_v\beta_6$ integrin	DOX	Human oral squamous carcinoma cells [116]

REFERENCES

1. Dutta, B., K.C. Barick, and P.A. Hassan, *Recent advances in active targeting of nanomaterials for anticancer drug delivery. Advances in Colloid and Interface Science*, 2021. **296**: p. 102509.
2. Clemons, T.D., et al., *Distinction between active and passive targeting of nanoparticles dictate their overall therapeutic efficacy. Langmuir*, 2018. **34**(50): pp. 15343–15349.
3. Attia, M.F., et al., *An overview of active and passive targeting strategies to improve the nanocarriers efficiency to tumour sites. J Pharm Pharmacol*, 2019. **71**(8): pp. 1185–1198.
4. Gref, R., et al., *'Stealth'corona-core nanoparticles surface modified by polyethylene glycol (PEG): influences of the corona (PEG chain length and surface density) and of the core composition on phagocytic uptake and plasma protein adsorption. Colloids and Surfaces B: Biointerfaces*, 2000. **18**(3–4): pp. 301–313.
5. Torchilin, V.P., Nanoparticulates as drug carriers. 2006: Imperial College Press.
6. Ding, L., et al., *Size, shape, and protein corona determine cellular uptake and removal mechanisms of gold nanoparticles. Small*, 2018. **14**(42): pp. 1801451.

7. Manzanares, D. and V. Ceña, *Endocytosis: the nanoparticle and submicron nanocompounds gateway into the cell. Pharmaceutics*, 2020. **12**(4): p. 371.

8. Das, M., C. Mohanty, and S.K. Sahoo, *Ligand-based targeted therapy for cancer tissue. Expert Opinion on Drug Delivery*, 2009. **6**(3): pp. 285–304.

9. Khan, N., R.K. Dhritlahre, and A. Saneja, *Recent advances in dual-ligand targeted nanocarriers for cancer therapy. Drug Discovery Today*, 2022. **27**(8): pp. 2288–2299.

10. Bazak, R., et al., *Cancer active targeting by nanoparticles: a comprehensive review of literature. Journal of Cancer Research and Clinical Oncology*, 2015. **141**(5): pp. 769–784.

11. Ahmad, E., et al., *Ligand decorated biodegradable nanomedicine in the treatment of cancer. Pharmacological Research*, 2021. **167**: p. 105544.

12. Dhritlahre, R.K. and A. Saneja, *Recent advances in HER2-targeted delivery for cancer therapy. Drug Discovery Today*, 2021. **26**(5): pp. 1319–1329.

13. Alibakhshi, A., et al., *Targeted cancer therapy through antibody fragments-decorated nanomedicines. Journal of Controlled Release*, 2017. **268**: pp. 323–334.

14. Chen, W., Y. Yuan, and X. Jiang, *Antibody and antibody fragments for cancer immunotherapy. Journal of Controlled Release*, 2020. **328**: pp. 395–406.

15. Filippi, L., O. Bagni, and O. Schillaci, *Re:"Sgc8-c aptamer as a potential theranostic agent for hemato-oncological malignancies" by Sicco et al. Cancer Biotherapy & Radiopharmaceuticals*, 2020. **35**(8): pp. 626–626.

16. Fu, Z. and J. Xiang, *Aptamer-functionalized nanoparticles in targeted delivery and cancer therapy. International Journal of Molecular Science*, 2020. **21**(23): p. 9123.

17. Yoon, S. and J.J. Rossi, *Aptamers: Uptake mechanisms and intracellular applications. Advanced Drug Delivery Reviews*, 2018. **134**: pp. 22–35.

18. Mokhtarzadeh, A., et al., *Aptamers as smart ligands for nano-carriers targeting. TrAC Trends in Analytical Chemistry*, 2016. **82**: pp. 316–327.

19. Zhu, M. and S. Wang, *Functional nucleic-acid-decorated spherical nanoparticles: preparation strategies and current applications in cancer therapy. Small Science*, 2021. **1**(3): p. 2000056.

20. Guan, B. and X. Zhang, *Aptamers as versatile ligands for biomedical and pharmaceutical applications. International Journal of Nanomedicine*, 2020. **15**: p. 1059.

21. Dai, L., et al., *Tumor therapy: Targeted drug delivery systems. Journal of Materials Chemistry B*, 2016. **4**(42): pp. 6758–6772.

22. Tagde, P., et al., *Recent advances in folic acid engineered nanocarriers for treatment of breast cancer. Journal of Drug Delivery Science and Technology*, 2020. **56**: p. 101613.

23. Yu, B., et al., *Receptor-targeted nanocarriers for therapeutic delivery to cancer. Molecular Membrane Biology*, 2010. **27**(7): pp. 286–298.

24. Kaasgaard, T. and T.L. Andresen, *Liposomal cancer therapy: Exploiting tumor characteristics. Expert Opinion on Drug Delivery*, 2010. **7**(2): pp. 225–243.

25. Hirsjarvi, S., C. Passirani, and J.-P. Benoit, *Passive and active tumour targeting with nanocarriers. Current Drug Discovery Technologies*, 2011. **8**(3): pp. 188–196.

26. Chen, C., et al., *Structural basis for molecular recognition of folic acid by folate receptors. Nature*, 2013. **500**(7463): pp. 486–489.

27. Assaraf, Y.G., C.P. Leamon, and J.A. Reddy, *The folate receptor as a rational therapeutic target for personalized cancer treatment. Drug Resistance Updates*, 2014. **17**(4–6): pp. 89–95.

28. Patil, Y., et al., *Targeting of folate-conjugated liposomes with co-entrapped drugs to prostate cancer cells via prostate-specific membrane antigen (PSMA). Nanomedicine: Nanotechnology, Biology and Medicine*, 2018. **14**(4): pp. 1407–1416.

29. Soe, Z.C., et al., *Folate receptor-mediated celastrol and irinotecan combination delivery using liposomes for effective chemotherapy. Colloids and Surfaces B: Biointerfaces*, 2018. **170**: pp. 718–728.

30. Byrne, J.D., T. Betancourt, and L. Brannon-Peppas, *Active targeting schemes for nanoparticle systems in cancer therapeutics. Advanced Drug Delivery Reviews*, 2008. **60**(15): pp. 1615–1626.

31. Jefferies, W.A., et al., *Transferrin receptor on endothelium of brain capillaries. Nature,* 1984. **312**(5990): pp. 162–163.

32. Groothuis, D.R., *The blood-brain and blood-tumor barriers: a review of strategies for increasing drug delivery. Neuro-oncology*, 2000. **2**(1): pp. 45–59.

33. Minner, S., et al., *Low activated leukocyte cell adhesion molecule expression is associated with advanced tumor stage and early prostate-specific antigen relapse in prostate cancer. Human Pathology,* 2011. **42**(12): pp. 1946–1952.

34. Zimmermann, T.S., et al., *RNAi-mediated gene silencing in non-human primates. Nature,* 2006. **441**(7089): pp. 111–114.

35. Nguyen, P.V., et al., *Nanomedicines functionalized with anti-EGFR ligands for active targeting in cancer therapy: biological strategy, design and quality control. International Journal of Pharmaceutics,* 2021. **605**: p. 120795.

36. Senbanjo, L.T. and M.A. Chellaiah, *CD44: a multifunctional cell surface adhesion receptor is a regulator of progression and metastasis of cancer cells. Frontiers in Cell and Developmental Biology,* 2017. **5**: p. 18.

37. Argenziano, M., et al., *Developing actively targeted nanoparticles to fight cancer: focus on Italian research. Pharmaceutics,* 2021. **13**(10): p. 1538.

38. Kurmi, B.D., et al., *Molecular approaches for targeted drug delivery towards cancer: a concise review with respect to nanotechnology. Journal of Drug Delivery Science and Technology,* 2020. **57**: p. 101682.

39. Awan, T., et al., *Expression of the metalloproteinase ADAM8 is upregulated in liver inflammation models and enhances cytokine release in vitro. Mediators of Inflammation,* 2021. **11**: p. 6665028.

40. Siney, E.J., et al., *Metalloproteinases ADAM10 and ADAM17 mediate migration and differentiation in glioblastoma sphere-forming cells. Molecular Neurobiology,* 2017. **54**(5): pp. 3893–3905.

41. Alawak, M., et al., *ADAM 8 as a novel target for doxorubicin delivery to TNBC cells using magnetic thermosensitive liposomes. European Journal of Pharmaceutics and Biopharmaceutics,* 2021. **158**: pp. 390–400.

42. Rajendran, L., H.J. Knölker, and K. Simons, *Subcellular targeting strategies for drug design and delivery. Nature Reviews Drug Discovery,* 2010. **9**(1): pp. 29–42.

43. Buchke, S., et al., *Mitochondria-targeted, nanoparticle-based drug-delivery systems: therapeutics for mitochondrial disorders. Life,* 2022. **12**(5): p. 657.

44. Tabish, T.A. and M.R. Hamblin, *Mitochondria-targeted nanoparticles (mitoNANO): An emerging therapeutic shortcut for cancer. Biomaterials and Biosystems,* 2021. **3**: p. 100023.

45. Ellegaard, A.M., P. Bach, and M. Jäättelä, *Targeting cancer lysosomes with good old cationic amphiphilic drugs. Reviews of Physiology, Biochemistry and Pharmacology,* 2021. **185**: pp. 107–152.

46. Ozcan, L. and I. Tabas, *Role of endoplasmic reticulum stress in metabolic disease and other disorders. Annual Review of Medicine,* 2012. **63**: pp. 317–328.

47. Liu, M., et al., *Golgi apparatus-targeted aggregation-induced emission luminogens for effective cancer photodynamic therapy. Nature Communications,* 2022. **13**(1): p. 2179.

48. Fagotto, F., U. Glück, and B.M. Gumbiner, *Nuclear localization signal-independent and importin/karyopherin-independent nuclear import of β-catenin. Current Biology,* 1998. **8**(4): pp. 181–190.

49. Najafi, M., B. Farhood, and K. Mortezaee, *Extracellular matrix (ECM) stiffness and degradation as cancer drivers. Journal of Cell Biochemistry,* 2019. **120**(3): pp. 2782–2790.

50. Insua-Rodríguez, J. and T. Oskarsson, *The extracellular matrix in breast cancer. Advanced Drug Delivery Reviews,* 2016. **97**: pp. 41–55.

51. Barbazán, J. and D. Matic Vignjevic, *Cancer associated fibroblasts: Is the force the path to the dark side? Current Opinion in Cell Biology,* 2019. **56**: pp. 71–79.

52. Raskov, H., et al., *Cancer-associated fibroblasts and tumor-associated macrophages in cancer and cancer immunotherapy. Front Oncology,* 2021. **11**: p. 668731.

53. Yin, L., O.C. Velazquez, and Z.-J. Liu, *Notch signaling: Emerging molecular targets for cancer therapy. Biochemical Pharmacology,* 2010. **80**(5): pp. 690–701.

54. Venkatesh, V., et al., *Targeting notch signalling pathway of cancer stem cells. Stem Cell Investigation,* 2018. **12**(5): p. 5.

55. Akwii, R.G. and C.M. Mikelis, *Targeting the angiopoietin/tie pathway: prospects for treatment of retinal and respiratory disorders. Drugs,* 2021. **81**(15): pp. 1731–1749.

56. Saharinen, P., L. Eklund, and K. Alitalo, *Therapeutic targeting of the angiopoietin–TIE pathway. Nature Reviews Drug Discovery,* 2017. **16**(9): pp. 635–661.

57. Huang, J., et al., *Extracellular matrix and its therapeutic potential for cancer treatment. Signal Transduction and Targeted Therapy,* 2021. **6**(1): p. 153.

58. Naba, A., et al., *The extracellular matrix: tools and insights for the "omics" era. Matrix Biology*, 2016. **49**: pp. 10–24.

59. Jurj, A., et al., *The extracellular matrix alteration, implication in modulation of drug resistance mechanism: Friends or foes? Journal of Experimental & Clinical Cancer Research*, 2022. **41**(1): p. 276.

60. Watanabe, K., M. Kaneko, and Y. Maitani, *Functional coating of liposomes using a folate–polymer conjugate to target folate receptors. International Journal of Nanomedicine*, 2012. **7**: p. 3679.

61. Soe, Z.C., et al., *Folate receptor-mediated celastrol and irinotecan combination delivery using liposomes for effective chemotherapy. Colloids and Surfaces B: Biointerfaces*, 2018. **170**: pp. 718–728.

62. Rana, S., et al., *Folic acid conjugated Fe_3O_4 magnetic nanoparticles for targeted delivery of doxorubicin. Dalton Transactions*, 2016. **45**(43): pp. 17401–17408.

63. Huang, Y., et al., *Superparamagnetic iron oxide nanoparticles conjugated with folic acid for dual target-specific drug delivery and MRI in cancer theranostics. Materials Science and Engineering: C*, 2017. **70**: pp. 763–771.

64. Angelopoulou, A., et al., *Folic acid-functionalized, condensed magnetic nanoparticles for targeted delivery of doxorubicin to tumor cancer cells overexpressing the folate receptor. ACS Omega*, 2019. **4**(26): pp. 22214–22227.

65. Cheng, W., et al., *pH-sensitive delivery vehicle based on folic acid-conjugated polydopamine-modified mesoporous silica nanoparticles for targeted cancer therapy. ACS Applied Materials & Interfaces*, 2017. **9**(22): pp. 18462–18473.

66. Mahalunkar, S., et al., *Functional design of pH-responsive folate-targeted polymer-coated gold nanoparticles for drug delivery and in vivo therapy in breast cancer. International Journal of Nanomedicine*, 2019. **14**: p. 8285.

67. Min, H.-K., et al., *Folate receptor-targeted liposomal nanocomplex for effective synergistic photothermal-chemotherapy of breast cancer in vivo. Colloids and Surfaces B: Biointerfaces*, 2019. **173**: pp. 539–548.

68. Sahoo, S.K. and V. Labhasetwar, *Enhanced antiproliferative activity of transferrin-conjugated paclitaxel-loaded nanoparticles is mediated via sustained intracellular drug retention. Molecular Pharmaceutics*, 2005. **2**(5): pp. 373–383.

69. Soe, Z.C., et al., *Transferrin-conjugated polymeric nanoparticle for receptor-mediated delivery of doxorubicin in doxorubicin-resistant breast cancer cells. Pharmaceutics*, 2019. **11**(2): p. 63.

70. Venkatesan, P., et al., *Redox stimuli delivery vehicle based on Transferrin-Capped MSNPs for targeted drug delivery in cancer therapy. ACS Applied Bio Materials*, 2019. **2**(4): pp. 1623–1633.

71. Saini, K. and R. Bandyopadhyaya, *Transferrin-conjugated polymer-coated mesoporous silica nanoparticles loaded with gemcitabine for killing pancreatic cancer cells. ACS Applied Nano Materials*, 2019. **3**(1): pp. 229–240.

72. Bidkar, A.P., P. Sanpui, and S.S. Ghosh, *Transferrin-conjugated red blood cell membrane-coated poly (lactic-co-glycolic acid) nanoparticles for the delivery of doxorubicin and methylene blue. ACS Applied Nano Materials*, 2020. **3**(4): pp. 3807–3819.

73. Kuo, Y.-C. and C.-T. Liang, *Inhibition of human brain malignant glioblastoma cells using carmustine-loaded catanionic solid lipid nanoparticles with surface anti-epithelial growth factor receptor. Biomaterials*, 2011. **32**(12): pp. 3340–3350.

74. Liao, C., et al., *Targeting EGFR-overexpressing tumor cells using Cetuximab-immunomicelles loaded with doxorubicin and superparamagnetic iron oxide. European Journal of Radiology*, 2011. **80**(3): pp. 699–705.

75. Kim, I.-Y., et al., *Antitumor activity of EGFR targeted pH-sensitive immunoliposomes encapsulating gemcitabine in A549 xenograft nude mice. Journal of Controlled Release*, 2009. **140**(1): pp. 55–60.

76. Aggarwal, S., S. Yadav, and S. Gupta, *EGFR targeted PLGA nanoparticles using gemcitabine for treatment of pancreatic cancer. Journal of Biomedical Nanotechnology*, 2011. **7**(1): pp. 137–138.

77. Nan, Y., *Lung carcinoma therapy using epidermal growth factor receptor-targeted lipid polymeric nanoparticles co-loaded with cisplatin and doxorubicin. Oncology Reports*, 2019. **42**(5): pp. 2087–2096.

78. Salehnia, Z., et al., *Synthesis and characterisation of iron oxide nanoparticles conjugated with epidermal growth factor receptor (EGFR) monoclonal antibody as MRI contrast agent for cancer detection. IET Nanobiotechnology*, 2019. **13**(4): pp. 400–406.

79. Chiang, C.-S., et al., *Enhancement of cancer therapy efficacy by trastuzumab-conjugated and pH-sensitive nanocapsules with the simultaneous encapsulation of hydrophilic and hydrophobic compounds.* Nanomedicine: Nanotechnology, Biology and Medicine, 2014. **10**(1): pp. 99–107.

80. Yu, K., et al., *Enhanced delivery of Paclitaxel using electrostatically-conjugated Herceptin-bearing PEI/PLGA nanoparticles against HER-positive breast cancer cells.* International Journal of Pharmaceutics, 2016. **497**(1–2): pp. 78–87.

81. Le, T.T.D., et al., *Evaluation of anti-HER2 scFv-conjugated PLGA–PEG nanoparticles on 3D tumor spheroids of BT474 and HCT116 cancer cells.* Advances in Natural Sciences: Nanoscience and Nanotechnology, 2016. **7**(2): p. 025004.

82. Eloy, J.O., et al., *Anti-HER2 immunoliposomes for co-delivery of paclitaxel and rapamycin for breast cancer therapy.* European Journal of Pharmaceutics and Biopharmaceutics, 2017. **115**: pp. 159–167.

83. You, J.O., P. Guo, and D.T. Auguste, *A drug-delivery vehicle combining the targeting and thermal ablation of HER2+ breast-cancer cells with triggered drug release.* Angewandte Chemie International Edition, 2013. **52**(15): pp. 4141–4146.

84. Mu, Q., et al., *Anti-HER2/neu peptide-conjugated iron oxide nanoparticles for targeted delivery of paclitaxel to breast cancer cells.* Nanoscale, 2015. **7**(43): pp. 18010–18014.

85. Liu, D., et al., *Target-specific delivery of oxaliplatin to HER2-positive gastric cancer cells in vivo using oxaliplatin-au-fe3o4-herceptin nanoparticles.* Oncology Letters, 2018. **15**(5): pp. 8079–8087.

86. Farasat, A., et al., *Effective suppression of tumour cells by oligoclonal HER2-targeted delivery of liposomal doxorubicin.* Journal of Liposome Research, 2019. **29**(1): pp. 53–65.

87. Hu, K., et al., *Hyaluronic acid functional amphipathic and redox-responsive polymer particles for the co-delivery of doxorubicin and cyclopamine to eradicate breast cancer cells and cancer stem cells.* Nanoscale, 2015. **7**(18): pp. 8607–8618.

88. Wang, L., et al., *CD44 antibody-targeted liposomal nanoparticles for molecular imaging and therapy of hepatocellular carcinoma.* Biomaterials, 2012. **33**(20): pp. 5107–5114.

89. Aires, A., et al., *Multifunctionalized iron oxide nanoparticles for selective drug delivery to CD44-positive cancer cells.* Nanotechnology, 2016. **27**(6): p. 065103.

90. Yang, R.-M., et al., *Hyaluronan-modified superparamagnetic iron oxide nanoparticles for bimodal breast cancer imaging and photothermal therapy.* International Journal of Nanomedicine, 2017. **12**: p. 197.

91. Li, J., et al., *Facile strategy by hyaluronic acid functional carbon dot-doxorubicin nanoparticles for CD44 targeted drug delivery and enhanced breast cancer therapy.* International Journal of Pharmaceutics, 2020. **578**: p. 119122.

92. Tabasi, H., et al., *pH-responsive and CD44-targeting by Fe3O4/MSNs-NH2 nanocarriers for Oxaliplatin loading and colon cancer treatment.* Inorganic Chemistry Communications, 2021. **125**: p. 108430.

93. Paliwal, S.R., et al., *Estrogen-anchored pH-sensitive liposomes as nanomodule designed for site-specific delivery of doxorubicin in breast cancer therapy.* Molecular Pharmaceutics, 2012. **9**(1): pp. 176–186.

94. Reddy, B.S. and R. Banerjee, *17β-Estradiol-associated stealth-liposomal delivery of anticancer gene to breast cancer cells.* Angewandte Chemie, 2005. **117**(41): pp. 6881–6885.

95. Yang, H., C. Tang, and C. Yin, *Estrone-modified pH-sensitive glycol chitosan nanoparticles for drug delivery in breast cancer.* Acta Biomaterialia, 2018. **73**: pp. 400–411.

96. Mamnoon, B., et al., *Hypoxia-responsive, polymeric nanocarriers for targeted drug delivery to estrogen receptor-positive breast cancer cell spheroids.* Molecular Pharmaceutics, 2020. **17**(11): pp. 4312–4322.

97. Kurmi, B.D., R. Paliwal, and S.R. Paliwal, *Dual cancer targeting using estrogen functionalized chitosan nanoparticles loaded with doxorubicin-estrone conjugate: a quality by design approach.* International Journal of Biological Macromolecules, 2020. **164**: pp. 2881–2894.

98. Zhan, C., et al., *Cyclic RGD conjugated poly (ethylene glycol)-co-poly (lactic acid) micelle enhances paclitaxel anti-glioblastoma effect.* Journal of Controlled Release, 2010. **143**(1): pp. 136–142.

99. Long, Q., et al., *RGD-conjugated resveratrol HSA nanoparticles as a novel delivery system in ovarian cancer therapy.* Drug Design, Development and Therapy, 2020. **14**: p. 5747.

100. Babu, A., et al., *Chemodrug delivery using integrin-targeted PLGA-Chitosan nanoparticle for lung cancer therapy.* Scientific Reports, 2017. **7**(1): pp. 1–17.

101. Fan, Z., et al., *Near infrared fluorescent peptide nanoparticles for enhancing esophageal cancer therapeutic efficacy. Nature Communications*, 2018. **9**(1): pp. 1–11.
102. Yadav, A.S., et al., *RGD functionalized chitosan nanoparticle mediated targeted delivery of raloxifene selectively suppresses angiogenesis and tumor growth in breast cancer. Nanoscale*, 2020. **12**(19): pp. 10664–10684.
103. De La Torre, C., et al., *Gated mesoporous silica nanoparticles using a double-role circular peptide for the controlled and target-preferential release of doxorubicin in CXCR4-expresing lymphoma cells. Advanced Functional Materials*, 2015. **25**(5): pp. 687–695.
104. Di-Wen, S., et al., *Improved antitumor activity of epirubicin-loaded CXCR4-targeted polymeric nanoparticles in liver cancers. International Journal of Pharmaceutics*, 2016. **500**(1–2): pp. 54–61.
105. Chittasupho, C., P. Kewsuwan, and T. Murakami, *CXCR4-targeted nanoparticles reduce cell viability, induce apoptosis and inhibit SDF-1α induced BT-549-Luc cell migration in vitro. Current Drug Delivery*, 2017. **14**(8): pp. 1060–1070.
106. Guo, P., et al., *Using breast cancer cell CXCR4 surface expression to predict liposome binding and cytotoxicity. Biomaterials*, 2012. **33**(32): pp. 8104–8110.
107. Li, M., et al., *LHRH-peptide conjugated dextran nanoparticles for targeted delivery of cisplatin to breast cancer. Journal of Materials Chemistry B*, 2014. **2**(22): pp. 3490–3499.
108. Taheri, A., et al., *Enhanced anti-tumoral activity of methotrexate-human serum albumin conjugated nanoparticles by targeting with luteinizing hormone-releasing hormone (LHRH) peptide. International Journal of Molecular Sciences*, 2011. **12**(7): pp. 4591–4608.
109. Zhang, L., et al., *Pharmacokinetics, distribution and anti-tumor efficacy of liposomal mitoxantrone modified with a luteinizing hormone-releasing hormone receptor-specific peptide. International Journal of Nanomedicine*, 2018. **13**: pp. 1097–1105.
110. Taheri, A., et al., *Use of biotin targeted methotrexate–human serum albumin conjugated nanoparticles to enhance methotrexate antitumor efficacy. International Journal of Nanomedicine*, 2011. **6**: p. 1863.
111. Patra, P., et al., *Simple synthesis of biocompatible biotinylated porous hexagonal ZnO nanodisc for targeted doxorubicin delivery against breast cancer cell: In vitro and in vivo cytotoxic potential. Colloids and Surfaces B: Biointerfaces*, 2015. **133**: pp. 88–98.
112. Wu, J.-L., et al., *Biotinylated carboxymethyl chitosan/CaCO$_3$ hybrid nanoparticles for targeted drug delivery to overcome tumor drug resistance. RSC Advances*, 2016. **6**(73): pp. 69083–69093.
113. Madhankumar, A.B., et al., *Interleukin-13 receptor-targeted nanovesicles are a potential therapy for glioblastoma multiforme. Molecular Cancer Therapeutics*, 2006. **5**(12): pp. 3162–3169.
114. Wang, Y., et al., *Tumor cell targeted delivery by specific peptide-modified mesoporous silica nanoparticles. Journal of Materials Chemistry*, 2012. **22**(29): pp. 14608–14616.
115. Yang, C.-Y., et al., *Interleukin-4 receptor-targeted liposomal doxorubicin as a model for enhancing cellular uptake and antitumor efficacy in murine colorectal cancer. Cancer Biology & Therapy*, 2015. **16**(11): pp. 1641–1650.
116. Kang, H., et al., *A liposome-based nanostructure for aptamer directed delivery. Chemical Communications,* 2010. **46**(2): pp. 249–251.
117. Cheng, Y., et al., *Cabazitaxel liposomes with aptamer modification enhance tumor-targeting efficacy in nude mice. Molecular Medicine Reports*, 2019. **19**(1): pp. 490–498.
118. Cadinoiu, A.N., et al., *Aptamer-functionalized liposomes as a potential treatment for basal cell carcinoma. Polymers*, 2019. **11**(9): p. 1515.
119. Xu, W., et al., *Aptamer-conjugated and doxorubicin-loaded unimolecular micelles for targeted therapy of prostate cancer. Biomaterials*, 2013. **34**(21): pp. 5244–5253.
120. Li, X., et al., *Targeted delivery of anticancer drugs by aptamer AS1411 mediated Pluronic F127/cyclodextrin-linked polymer composite micelles. Nanomedicine: Nanotechnology, Biology and Medicine*, 2015. **11**(1): pp. 175–184.
121. Farokhzad, O.C., et al., *Targeted nanoparticle-aptamer bioconjugates for cancer chemotherapy in vivo. Proceedings of National Academy of Sciences USA*, 2006. **103**(16): pp. 6315–6320.
122. Fang, Y., et al., *Aptamer-conjugated multifunctional polymeric nanoparticles as cancer-targeted, MRI-ultrasensitive drug delivery systems for treatment of castration-resistant prostate cancer. Biomed Research International*, 2020. **25**: p. 9186583.

123. Zhao, N., et al., *An ultra pH-sensitive and aptamer-equipped nanoscale drug-delivery system for selective killing of tumor cells. Small*, 2013. **9**(20): pp. 3477–3484.

124. Ding, X., et al., *Designing aptamer-gold nanoparticle-loaded pH-sensitive liposomes encapsulate morin for treating cancer. Nanoscale Research Letters*, 2020. **15**(1): p. 68.

125. Jurek, P.M., et al., *Anti-FGFR1 aptamer-tagged superparamagnetic conjugates for anticancer hyperthermia therapy. International Journal of Nanomedicine*, 2017. **12**: pp. 2941–2950.

126. Zhu, C.-L., et al., *An efficient cell-targeting and intracellular controlled-release drug delivery system based on MSN-PEM-aptamer conjugates. Journal of Materials Chemistry*, 2009. **19**(41): pp. 7765–7770.

127. Sakhtianchi, R., et al., *Pegylated magnetic mesoporous silica nanoparticles decorated with AS1411 Aptamer as a targeting delivery system for cytotoxic agents. Pharmaceutical Development and Technology*, 2019. **24**(9): pp. 1063–1075.

128. Naz, S., et al., *Enzyme-responsive mesoporous silica nanoparticles for tumor cells and mitochondria multistage-targeted drug delivery. International Journal of Nanomedicine*, 2019. **14**: p. 2533.

129. Cao, W., et al., *Folic acid-conjugated gold nanorod@ polypyrrole@ Fe$_3$O$_4$ nanocomposites for targeted MR/CT/PA multimodal imaging and chemo-photothermal therapy. RSC Advances*, 2019. **9**(33): pp. 18874–18887.

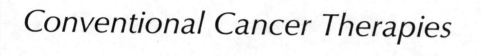

Conventional Cancer Therapies

6 Oral Anticancer Therapies

*Ayesha Saeed, Liaqat Hussain, Hua Naranmandura,
Qian Qian Wang, Muhammad Yasir Ali,
Ummaima Shahzad, and Ijaz Ali*

6.1 INTRODUCTION

Cancer has been very common around the world and holds great diversity. The proper formation of deoxyribonucleotide triphosphates and their exact positioning on the DNA is highly important for normal cell formation. Alteration in its sequences can cause several genetic diseases like cancer, type 1 diabetes, Alzheimer's disease, Down's syndrome [1], and familial hypercholesterolemia [2]. There are particular genes that regulate normal cell formation. In cancer cells, the genes that suppress tumor growth have a higher level of methylation and are silenced. As a result, uncontrolled replication occurs [3]. Cancer cells have more nutrient uptake, e.g., glucose and glutamine. Glucose metabolism occurs by the Warburg effect where it is converted to pyruvate without using oxygen, and further this pyruvate is converted to lactate and is secreted from the cell [4]. In cancerous cells, either too many copies of a healthy gene are formed or mutations in the amino acid sequence occur or gene expression is altered. Different chemotherapeutic agents work at different phases of replication and cause "cell cycle arrest". Two things can happen then, either the cell is repaired by DNA repair enzymes or apoptosis occurs and the cell dies. The main targets of most cancer chemotherapeutic agents are the enzymes involved in cellular replication called "the replitase complex" or other receptors like receptors from the tyrosine kinase family. The enzymes in the complex are thymidylate synthetase, dihydrofolate reductase, ribonucleotide reductase, nucleoside-5′ phosphate kinase, thymidine kinase, and tyrosine kinases [5, 6]. Oral anticancer drugs can be described as chemotherapeutic agents and targeted therapy. General chemotherapeutic agents work by acting on uncontrollably dividing cells while target therapy agents work by specifically acting on cells with defined mutations. Alopecia or hair loss is a very common side effect of these anticancer drugs as their main targets are actively proliferating cells and hair follicles have a very high turnover rate, but it is reversible. Myelosuppression is another major toxic effect of many chemotherapeutic agents.

6.2 ANTIMETABOLITES

6.2.1 FOLATE ANTAGONISTS

These three drugs act as folate inhibitors namely methotrexate (oral + parenteral), pemetrexed (parenteral), and pralatrexate (parenteral). These drugs enter the cell via a reduced folate carrier (RFC). It gets converted into a more effective form via the enzyme folypolyglutamate synthase (FPGS). The drug methotrexate possesses a great affinity for dihydrofolate reductase (DHFR) approximately 50,000 times more than other substances [7]. These drugs are folic acid analogs, specifically targeting DHFR and thymidylate synthetase (TS) used in DNA synthesis, replication, RNA, and

DOI: 10.1201/9781003363958-8

protein synthesis. The DHFR is used in the synthesis of thymidine monophosphate, guanosine, and adenosine [8]. Once inhibited, the enzyme requires a very large amount of natural folic acid to free itself from methotrexate.

Methotrexate is S-phase selective. Leucovorin (folinic acid, calcium folinate, citrovorum factor) is used to reverse the effects of methotrexate and initiates protein synthesis up to a certain level but it will not initiate DNA synthesis [7, 8]. The major target of pemetrexed is TS [8]. It also inhibits DHFR (Figure 6.1), GART (glycinamide ribonucleotide formyl transferase), and AICART (aminoimidazole carboxamide ribonucleotide formyl transferase). Pemetrexed polyglutamate, formed by the action of FPGS, is 60 times more potent than pemetrexed itself [9]. Methotrexate is used to treat choriocarcinoma [7], brain tumor, bladder cancer, acute lymphocytic leukemia, Burkitt's lymphoma in children, breast cancer, neck cancer [8], and non-Hodgkin's lymphoma. Resistance to these drugs develops due to lower expression of FGPS, RFC, overexpression of γ-glutamyl hydrolase, DHFR, and TS [9].

Methotrexate has inconsistent absorption and is distributed among the body tissues including intestinal epithelium, liver, kidney, skin, and "pleural effusion and ascites". It has 50% plasma-protein binding, an 8–10 hour half-life, and is mostly excreted in the urine. A little amount is also hydroxylated (7-hydroxymethotrexate) [8, 9].

The common side effects of methotrexate and pemetrexed are nausea, vomiting, diarrhea, mouth inflammation, hair loss, hypersensitivity, bone marrow depression, and megaloblastic anemia. These may also cause GIT bleeding [7, 8]. Folate antagonists should be carefully used in patients with mild-to-moderate liver or kidney dysfunction [8, 10]. Concomitant administration of methotrexate with the NSAIDs, cephalosporin, omeprazole, penicillin, sulfonamides, and warfarin may induce its toxicity. The salicylates or dicumarol reduces protein binding of methotrexate. Methotrexate increases the cytotoxic effects of 5-FU [7, 8].

6.2.2 PURINE ANTAGONISTS

Oral purine antagonists include 6-mercaptopurine (6-MP), 6-thioguanine (6-TG), and azathioprine (Figure 6.2). These prodrugs are phosphorylated and metabolized by the enzyme

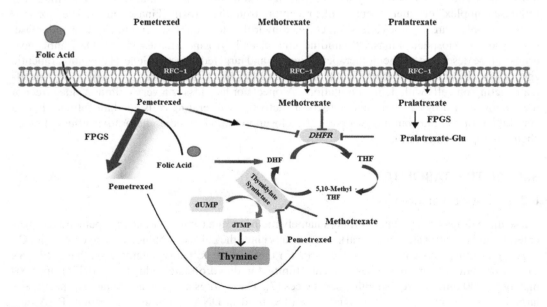

FIGURE 6.1 Mechanism of action of folate antagonists.

hypoxanthine-guanine phosphoribosyl transferase (HGPRT) and exert antitumor effects. It inhibits 5-phosphoribosyl-1-pyrophosphate amido-transferase (PRPP), blocks the *de novo* purine synthesis, incorporates these metabolites into DNA as false purine bases, and inhibits DNA synthesis [9]. 6-MP is also metabolized by thiopurine methyl transferase [7].

The 6-MP and 6-TG are particularly used in combination to treat childhood acute leukemia and choriocarcinoma. Azathioprine mainly acts as an immunosuppressant [7, 8]. Lower expression of HGPRT, reduced transport of drug across the membrane, or cross-resistance in both 6-MP and 6-TG can create resistance against the drugs [9]. 6-MP has inconsistent absorption when given orally. It is broadly distributed among the body tissue but does not penetrate CSF, 20–30% drug is plasma protein bound. Inactive metabolites of 6-MP are formed via methylation through hepatic enzymes, and almost 50% of it gets excreted via the kidneys. 6-TG also shows inconsistent absorption but the absorption is increased if it is taken on an empty stomach. 6-TG shows a wide distribution in bone marrow cells, and peripheral blood cells and can penetrate the placenta but not the blood–brain barrier. Inactive metabolites of this drug are formed via deamination mainly but also by methylation, and the elimination occurs via urine and feces [9].

The common adverse effects include a slow progression of myelosuppression (mild to moderate in the case of 6-MP but it is dose-limiting with 6-TG). 6-MP has greater potential than 6-TG to cause nausea, vomiting (mild), and jaundice. Both 6-MP and 6-TG cause hyperuricemia and immunosuppression, which makes the patient more prone to infection [7, 9]. High doses of 6-MP cause diarrhea, light sensitivity, and hypersensitivity [9]. These drugs must be used carefully in patients suffering from liver or kidney dysfunction [10]. Co-administration of 6-MP with warfarin reduces the effects of warfarin while allopurinol potentiates its toxic effects. When 6-MP is given with sulfonamides, bone marrow suppression is intensified [9].

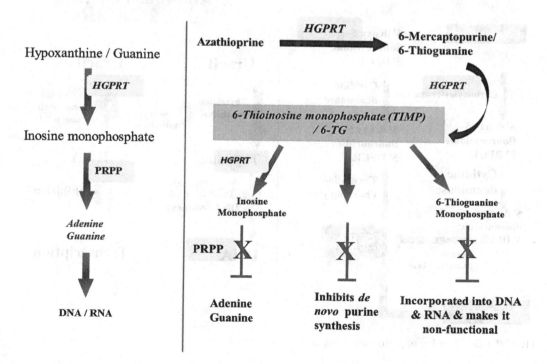

FIGURE 6.2 General mechanism of DNA synthesis vs competitive inhibition by purine antagonists.

6.2.3 PYRIMIDINE ANTAGONISTS

Oral pyrimidine antagonists include capecitabine [8] and doxyfluridine [7]. Capecitabine is used in metastatic breast cancer as well as in colorectal cancer [8]. It is used as an adjunct in stage 3 colon cancer [9]. Doxyfluridine is also used in the treatment of breast cancer and metastatic gastrointestinal, pancreatic, and liver cancers [7].

Doxyfluridine is primarily metabolized in the liver into 5'-deoxy-5-flourocytidine then into 5'-deoxy-5-flourouridine (5'-DFUR). The 5'-DFUR is taken up by tumor cells and is converted into 5-FU (Figure 6.3) by thymidine phosphorylase (tumor cells specifically contain a high concentration of thymidine phosphorylase) [8, 9]. The 5-FU blocks TS and inhibits methylation of uracil (thymine). Doxyfluridine prodrug bypasses the degrading enzyme (dihydropyrimidine dehydrogenase) [7]. TS is more active in S-phase [9]. Metabolism of capecitabine occurs via carboxylesterase, cytidine deaminase, thymidine phosphorylase, and dihydropyrimidine dehydrogenase [9].

Lower expression of TS, reduced incorporation of 5-flourouracil into DNA and RNA, and reduction in the binding affinity of TS due to mutation can create resistance [9] and overexpression of 5-FU degrading enzyme (dihydropyrimidine dehydrogenase) can create resistance against drugs of this class [7].

Capecitabine has fast oral absorption. Its peak plasma levels are obtained in approximately 90 minutes, it is 60% plasma protein bound and is mainly excreted via the kidneys. It should be taken on an empty stomach. Major adverse effects induced by capecitabine are diarrhea and hand–foot syndrome while doxyfluridine causes myelosuppression, hearing loss, diarrhea, inflammation in the

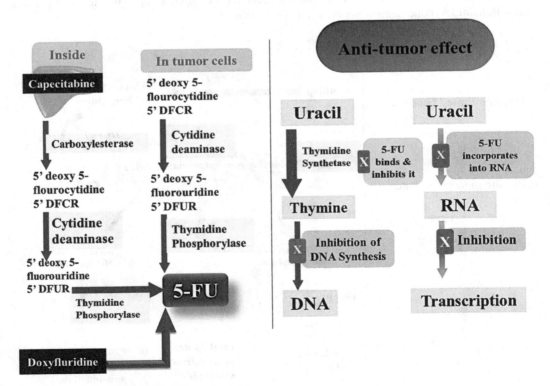

FIGURE 6.3 Working of pyrimidine antagonists.

mouth, and neuritis [7]. Other side effects include bone marrow depression, chest pain, soreness and inflammation in the mouth [8], nausea, and vomiting [9].

Concomitant administration of these drugs with warfarin exacerbates anticoagulant effects [8, 9]. Capecitabine's bioavailability increases when it is used with antacids (aluminum/magnesium hydroxide) [9].

6.3 ALKYLATING AGENTS

These are mostly cell cycle non-specific (active in all phases) and bind with the DNA at different sites, e.g., sulfhydryl, carboxyl, hydroxyl, amino, or phosphate groups, but the seventh position of thioguanine residues is more prone to alkylating agents [7, 9].

6.3.1 CYCLOPHOSPHAMIDE

This prodrug inhibits DNA synthesis by cross-linking the DNA. At low doses, it acts as an immunomodulator and boosts the effector T-cells as well as targets suppressive regulatory immune cells. Its active metabolites aldophosphamide, phosphoramide mustard, and acrolein are formed via the cytochrome P450 (CYP450) enzymes [7, 9]. It is well absorbed and well distributed among body tissues including CSF as well in saliva and milk. It has almost 90% bioavailability. It has a minimal plasma protein binding as compared to its active metabolite phosphoramide mustard. It has a half-life of 4–6 hours and is mainly excreted in the urine [9].

Resistance against cyclophosphamide develops due to reduced cellular uptake, reduced expression of CYP450 enzymes, higher activity of DNA repairing enzymes, and overexpression of sulfhydryl proteins [9]. Phenobarbital, phenytoin, or other drugs inducing the CYP450 system enhances the metabolism of chlorambucil that can reach toxicity level. It increases the effect of anticoagulants. When given with digoxin, it enhances digoxin's metabolism [9].

Bladder toxicity including hemorrhagic cystitis, dysuria, increased urination, and bladder fibrosis can be caused by cyclophosphamide, hence it must be carefully given to patients with kidney dysfunction [9]. Fluid intake is maintained to prevent bladder toxicity or the detoxifying drug "mesna (mercaptoethane sulfonate)" is given along with it [8, 11]. Other side effects are hyperpigmentation on nails and skin, nausea and vomiting occurring within 2–4 hours, alopecia, infection risk, and high dose causes thrombocytopenia and reduced bone marrow activity [9, 10]. It can also lead to ADH secretion syndrome, cardiac, and lung impairment [11].

6.3.2 CHLORAMBUCIL

It is a nitrogen mustard analog that works as a bi-functional agent by making cross-links with both DNA strands and thus inhibits its synthesis. In chronic lymphatic leukemia, it is used as the drug of choice for long-term maintenance therapy. It is slow acting and particularly used in lymphatic leukemia [7, 9].

Resistance for chlorambucil develops due to reduced cellular uptake of the drug, reduced expression of CYP 450 enzymes, higher activity of DNA repairing enzymes, and overexpression of sulfhydryl proteins [9]. The drug possesses 75% bioavailability when taken with food and maximum plasma levels are obtained within 1–2 hours. It is highly protein bound, its metabolism occurs via the CYP 450 enzymes and is excreted in the urine [9]. Its adverse effects include anemia, GI upset, leucopenia, neutropenia, thrombocytopenia, epilepsy, bone, marrow disorder [9], and alopecia [10]. It can rarely cause skin reactions, cystitis, respiratory, liver, and movement disorders [10].

6.3.3 MELPHALAN

It is another nitrogen mustard analog that works as a bi-functional agent by making cross-links with the DNA and thus inhibits its synthesis [9]. Reduced cellular uptake, reduced expression of cytochrome P450 enzymes, or higher activity of DNA-repairing enzymes can cause resistance against it. Overexpression of sulfhydryl proteins will lead to the inactivation of the drug [9].

It has inconsistent absorption and it should be taken on an empty stomach. It is well distributed among the body tissues and almost 80–90% is plasma protein bound. The half-life of melphalan is approximately 60–90 minutes and 25–30% of it is excreted within 1 day and up to 50% of the drug gets excreted through feces in 6 days [9]. Its adverse effects include anemia, GI upset, alopecia, thrombocytopenia, nausea, vomiting, diarrhea, and leucopenia [10].

6.3.4 LOMUSTINE

This prodrug can cross the blood–brain barrier as it is highly lipid soluble and is a nitrosourea compound [7]. Lomustine is converted to its active metabolites, which alkylates DNA and hence prevents replication and synthesis of RNA and proteins. It also causes protein carbamoylation. This alkylating agent is particularly used in the treatment of brain tumors [8]. Resistance against this drug develops due to reduced cellular uptake, reduced expression of CYP 450 enzymes, higher activity of DNA repairing enzymes, and overexpression of sulfhydryl proteins, which leads to its inactivation [9].

It should be given on an empty stomach. It has fast and complete absorption and is widely distributed among the body tissues and CSF as well [9, 8]. It is metabolized by CYP 450 enzymes and has a half-life of approximately 72 hours [9]. Common adverse effects of lomustine include leucopenia, nausea, diarrhea, and vomiting. Other side effects are anemia, GI upset, thrombocytopenia, lethargy, loss of vision (irreversible) [10], bone marrow depression [7], and hair loss (not common) [9]. It must be avoided during breastfeeding, pregnancy, and in patients with kidney dysfunction [10]. It is contraindicated in celiac disease [10] and is used as a second-choice drug to imatinib in chronic bone marrow tumors (myelogenous leukemias) [7].

6.3.5 BUSULFAN

This bi-functional drug interacts and forms cross-links via thiol groups and nucleic acids between DNA–DNA strands and DNA–proteins. Hence, retarding further replication processes, RNA, and protein synthesis [9]. Resistance to busulfan occurs due to reduced cellular uptake, reduced expression of CYP 450 enzymes, higher activity of DNA repairing enzymes, and high thiol content inside the cell [9].

It has good oral bioavailability and is almost 30% plasma protein bound. It is well distributed among the body tissues including the CSF and also crosses placental barriers. It is metabolized by CYP 450 enzymes and is mainly excreted via the kidneys. Almost 50–60% of the drug is excreted within 48 hours of administration. Its metabolism is enhanced by circadian rhythm, i.e., in younger patients increased clearance is seen in the evening time [9]. Its common side effects include respiratory fibrosis, skin pigmentation, bone marrow suppression, diarrhea, vomiting, and amenorrhea [7–10].

6.3.6 ALTRETAMINE (HEXAMETHYL MELAMINE HMA)

This prodrug is a triazine derivative. Its actual mechanism of action is not known yet but it acts like other alkylating agents and prohibits further replication [9]. It is used to treat recurring ovarian cancer, as a palliative therapy [7]. In advanced-stage or consistent ovarian cancer, altretamine is used as a first-line therapy in combination with cisplatin or other alkylating agents [9].

It has immense first-pass metabolism and is well distributed among body tissues, particularly those with high-fat content. It is metabolized via CYP 450 enzymes into pentamethyelamine and tetramethylmelamine and excreted primarily via the kidneys [9]. The common side effects include myelosuppression, ataxia, confusion, hallucinations [7], nausea, vomiting, hypersensitivity, and flu-like syndrome [9].

6.3.7 Temozolomide

It is also a triazine derivative. It is converted into its active metabolites via chemical transformation at normal pH. The active metabolite, methyltriazeno-imidazole carboxamide (MTIC) causes methylation of the nucleic acid at the O-6 and N-7 positions of guanine. It retards further DNA replication, RNA, and protein synthesis [8]. It inhibits DNA-repairing enzymes like O6-alkylguanine-DNA alkyltransferase (AGAT). It is used in metastatic melanoma, glioblastoma multiforme, and astrocytoma because it reaches the CSF [8].

Mutations in base excision repair (BER), mismatch repair genes (MMR), or overexpression of mitogen-activated protein kinase 1 can cause resistance against temozolomide [9]. It has a fast and excellent absorption but it should be taken on an empty stomach. Its bioavailability is nearly 100%, and almost 30–40% reaches CSF and is weakly plasma protein bound. It is primarily metabolized by hydrolysis but a very little amount via CYP 450 enzymes and is mainly excreted in urine with 2 hours half-life [9]. Its common side effects include myelosuppression, nausea, vomiting (mild-to-moderate), hair loss, cough, joint pain, anorexia, dyspnea, muscle weakness, and edema. It should be carefully given to patients with severe liver and kidney impairment and is contraindicated during pregnancy and breastfeeding. Sun exposure must be avoided for several days after its consumption [7, 9, 10].

6.4 ANTI-MICROTUBULE AGENTS

6.4.1 Estramustine

The estramustine phosphate is a combination of normustine linked with estradiol, which is devoid of alkylating effects but possesses weak estrogen-like effects [7]. It is used to treat metastatic prostate cancer, only when the treatment with hormonal therapy stops working [7, 9]. It inhibits the arrangement of the mitotic spindle (Figure 6.4). Mitotic spindle formation is interrupted as estramustine binds with the β-tubulin and inhibits their binding and arrangement, hence hindering the formation of microtubules [7].

It has fast and excellent absorption (about 70–75%) when given orally. The estramustine phosphate is hydrophilic and gets de-phosphorylated in the GI tract. It undergoes hepatic metabolism, which results in the formation of active and inactive metabolites [7, 9]. It is mainly excreted from the body via feces. Its common adverse effects include nausea, vomiting, gynecomastia, and diarrhea. Some rare and uncommon side effects are bone marrow suppression, hypersensitivity, and heart disease complications [7, 9]. It is particularly contraindicated in patients with severe heart, kidney, or liver disease [9].

6.5 TOPOISOMERASE INHIBITORS

The DNA is relaxed and un-winded at a particular point for cellular replication or transcription. This induces supercoiling, which adds-up stress to the DNA strands. To reduce this pressure, topoisomerases induces cut in DNA to reduce the number of twists [8]. Topoisomerase I removes one twist by cutting at a certain point in one strand and the next twists are transiently cut via topoisomerase II at both strands of DNA. Topoisomerase II relaxes supercoils, both DNA strand breaks, reduce the tension, and re-joins them. By inhibiting these enzymes, topoisomerase inhibitors cause

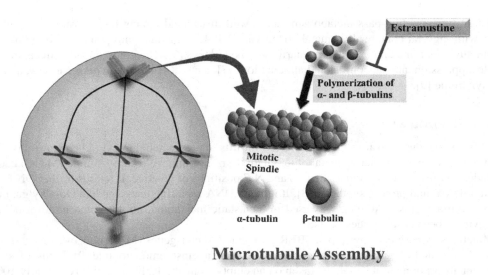

FIGURE 6.4   Estramustine's mechanism of action.

DNA breaks, either because the DNA cannot reduce the tension due to supercoiling or because the broken strands cannot re-join again [8].

6.5.1 TOPOTECAN

Topotecan is a topoisomerase I inhibitor. It is derived semi-synthetically from alkaloids (camptothecin) obtained from a tree named Camptotheca acuminata [8, 9]. It acts at the S-phase and causes cell cycle arrest at G_2-phase by inhibiting the re-joining of the DNA strand [8, 9]. It enhances the expression of the Bax gene (a pro-apoptotic gene) [12], which belongs to the Bcl-2 gene family and induces its pro-apoptotic effects [13]. The BAK gene also gets activated, making the mitochondrial membrane more permeable and releasing cytotoxic contents into the cytoplasm, which ultimately leads to cell death [14]. In metastatic ovarian cancer, if the primary treatment fails, topotecan is used. It is also used in the treatment of "small cell lung cancer" [8].

Resistance against topotecan increases if the target enzyme (topoisomerase I) has reduced expression, mutations, and possesses less affinity for the drug, or with increased drug efflux from the tumor cells [9]. It has fast oral absorption, and peak plasma levels are achieved within an hour with almost 40% bioavailability. The active form, topotecan lactone, (stable in acidic pH), is hydrolyzed to inactive carboxylate form. A small amount of topotecan is metabolized via the CYP 450 enzymes. It is mainly excreted in urine and has a 3-hour half-life [9]. Its common adverse effects are myelosuppression, diarrhea, anorexia, abdominal pain, alopecia, and transient elevation of bilirubin [7–9].

6.5.2 ETOPOSIDE

Etoposide is a topoisomerase II inhibitor. It is derived semi-synthetically from alkaloids (podophyllotoxins) obtained from a tree named Podophyllum peltatum and has a metal-like taste [8, 9]. Topoisomerase II induces a double-strand break during DNA replication, transcription, chromatin remodeling, and DNA repair by performing catenation/decatenation or by knotting/unknotting. Etoposide poisons the topoisomerase-cleaved DNA complex and inhibits DNA religation. This drug and all of its metabolites introduce DNA double-stranded breaks (DSBs) and the accretion of

DSBs will trigger cell apoptosis. Even if a cell manages to survive, then gene translocation occurs with faulty events, which result in the development of abnormal cells and carcinogenesis occurs [15, 16].

It is used to treat lung cancer, Hodgkin's lymphoma, testicular tumors, and non-Hodgkin's lymphoma. Resistance against etoposide occurs if the target enzyme has less affinity for the drug, or due to increased drug efflux, and hyperactivity of DNA repairing enzymes [9]. Studies have found that when four particular genes, the CSMD3 gene, PCLO gene, RYR1 gene, and EPB41L3 gene, get mutated, it results in resistance development against etoposide [17].

It has inconsistency absorption. Almost 50% of the drug is orally absorbed, so the dose needs to be doubled. Almost 50% of the drug is excreted via the kidneys and it has a 3–10 hour half-life [9]. One of its common side effects is myelosuppression, which results in leukopenia more prominently than thrombocytopenia [8]. Mild to moderate GI symptoms including nausea and vomiting, hair loss, and anorexia are also seen commonly.

6.6 ANTI-METABOLITE AGENTS

6.6.1 HYDROXYUREA

The nucleotide bases (purines and pyrimidines) are very essential as these are used to make DNA and RNA. The bases are attached to the ribose sugar and are converted to their deoxyribose form for the synthesis of DNA by using enzymes. The enzyme ribonucleotide reductase (RNR) along with the coenzyme thioredoxin converts the ribonucleosides into deoxyribonucleosides. The hydroxyurea (hydroxycarbamide) binds to the β-subunit of the RNR enzyme and inhibits (dNTP's) formation [18]. If a cell fails to maintain the required number of dNTPs, which is very essential in the S-phase, the DNA polymerase functions are disturbed and cell cycle arrest occurs [19]. The cell cannot survive as the DNA strand breaks and eventually dies [18]. Hydroxyurea does not initiate a cytotoxic effect on neutrophils in sickle cell disease patients [20].

It is used as a monotherapy and is more effective in treating advanced-stage chronic myeloid leukemia (CML) and produces lesser side effects [21]. It is considered a first choice agent for CML [21]. It is very effective in increasing Hb levels in the fetus with sickle cell disease [22]. It is also used with radiation therapy [6] and to treat thrombocytosis, polycythemia vera, and refractory ovarian cancer [9].

Hydroxyurea shows resistance if there is overexpression of the target enzyme ribonucleotide reductase [9]. It has a fast oral absorption with approximately 80–90% oral bioavailability. Peak plasma levels are achieved in 60–90 minutes. It is broadly distributed among the body tissues including CSF and pleural effusion. Its common side effects are myelosuppression, hair loss, GI upset including nausea, vomiting, mucositis, and hyperpigmentation of the skin [10].

A few examples of antimetabolites, alkylating agents, anti-microtubule agents, topoisomerase inhibitors, and anti-metabolite agents are listed in Table 6.1.

6.7 RETINOIDS

6.7.1 TRETINOIN

The nuclear receptors are found inside the cells and perform very important functions by binding to the DNA and controlling the expression of particular genes. Hence, these receptors act as transcription factors. Two of the nuclear receptors are the retinoic acid receptor or RAR [23] and the retinoid X receptor or RXR [24]. RXR combines and forms heterodimers and homodimers with other nuclear receptors leading to the control of transcription suppression or activation [24]. Retinoids bind to the RAR receptors and are involved in cellular differentiation, apoptosis, and cell growth. Retinol (vitamin A) is metabolized and converted into its active form retinoic acid and its derivatives;

TABLE 6.1
A Few Examples of Drugs with their Cellular Interactions

Class	Sub-class	Drug	Myelosuppression	Cell Cycle Specificity	Emesis	Pregnancy and Breastfeeding
Antimetabolites	Folate antagonists	Methotrexate	Dose-limiting	S-phase	Mild	Avoid during pregnancy and discontinue during breastfeeding
	Purine antagonist	6-mercaptopurine	Mild to moderate	S-phase	Moderate	
		6-thioguanine	Dose-limiting	S-phase	Mild	
		Azathioprine	Dose-limiting	S-phase	Moderate	
	Pyrimidine antagonist	Capecitabine	Mild to moderate	S-phase	Mild	
		Doxyfluridine				
Alkylating agents	Nitrogen mustard analogs	Mechlorethamine	Dose-limiting	Active in all phases	High	
		Cyclophosphamide	Dose-limiting	Active in all phases	High	
		Chlorambucil	Dose-limiting	Active in all phases	Mild	
		Melphalan	Dose-limiting	Active in all phases	Moderate	
Alkylating agents	Nitrosoureas	Lomustine	Dose-limiting	Active in all phases	High	
	Ethylenimine	Altretamine	Dose-limiting	Active in all phases	Moderate	
	Triazine derivative	Temozolomide	Dose-limiting	Active in all phases	Mild to moderate	
	Methyl hydrazine	Procarbazine	Dose-limiting	Active in all phases	Moderate	
Antimicrotubule agents	Estrogen ester	Estramustine	Rare	M-phase	Mild	
Topoisomerase inhibitors	Topoisomerase I inhibitor	Topotecan	Dose-limiting	S-to-G_2 phase	Mild to moderate	
	Topoisomerase II inhibitor	Etoposide	Dose-limiting	S-to-G_2 phase	Mild to moderate	
Antimetabolites	Ribonucleotide reductase inhibitor	Hydroxyurea	Dose-limiting	S-phase	Mild	Avoid during pregnancy and discontinue during breastfeeding

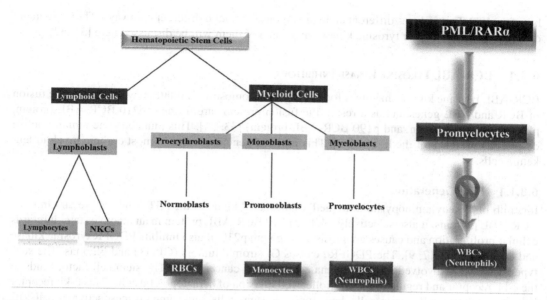

FIGURE 6.5 Tretinoin's mechanism of action.

all-trans-retinoic acid (ATRA), 9 cis retinoic acid (9-Cis RA), and 13 cis-retinoic acids (13-Cis RA) [24]. When a ligand binds, the co-repressor attached to the RARα is displaced and transcription is initiated (Figure 6.5). While in the absence of a ligand, the transcription is inhibited via co-repressor [25]. PML gene encodes for PML protein, which acts as a tumor suppressor protein [26] and RARα regulates normal and controlled cell division and differentiation [27]. It inhibits uncontrolled cellular proliferation [26]. One formulation is the retin-A micro gel pump.

In acute promyelocytic leukemia, the genetic translocation occurs at chromosome 15 and 17 (PML-RARα Complex), which makes it dysfunctional [27] and cellular maturation and differentiation are inhibited [25]. ATRA is highly effective in promyelocytic leukemia [28]. It binds to the disrupted RA receptor and initiates various functions by binding to the cellular retinoic acid binding protein (CRABP) inside the cytoplasm [25, 29]. It causes cellular maturation and later on the matured cell dies [25]. It also induces degradation of the fusion gene PML/RARα and hence causes temporary but prolonged remission of undifferentiated cells [27, 30]. Tumor cells develop resistance against ATRA but the fusion gene being thermo-sensitive destabilizes at mild hyperthermia [28].

Peak plasma levels of tretinoin are achieved within first 60–120 minutes. It is highly plasma protein bound (albumin mostly) and is metabolized via the CYP 450 enzyme. It is primarily excreted in the urine and a small amount is also excreted in the feces [24]. The common adverse effects are xerostomia, dry nose, itching, elevation of transaminases, retinoic acid syndrome with pericardial and pleural effusion, pyrexia, headache, and confusion [7, 9]. Tretinoin shows interaction with the drugs, which are CYP 450 inducers. Co-administration with vitamin A supplements induces tretinoin toxicity [9].

6.8 TYROSINE KINASE INHIBITORS

Tyrosine kinases are a large family of enzymes including epidermal growth factor receptor (EGFR) or human epidermal receptor (HER), vascular endothelial growth factor receptor (VEGFR), platelet-derived growth factor receptors (PDGFR), insulin receptor (IR), Trk receptor, fibroblast growth factor receptor (FBGF), and mesenchymal-epithelial transition factor receptor (c-MET), which activates various proteins via signal transduction cascades. It activates different proteins via phosphorylation, by using ATP. This induces different cellular responses through different pathways. There are many different types of receptor tyrosine kinases and some of them will be discussed here [31, 32].

6.8.1 BCR-ABL Tyrosine Kinase Inhibitors

BCR-ABL tyrosine kinase enzyme is formed due to chromosomal mutation, which causes the fusion of BCR and ABL genes and as a result, the fusion proteins are formed (p210 BCR-ABL protein, p230 BCR-ABL protein, and p190 BCR-ABL protein) [33, 34]. This mutated gene remains active despite the presence of the ligand [33]. This mutated gene is present in most chronic myeloid leukemia cells.

6.8.1.1 First Generation

Imatinib or "phenylaminopyrimidine methansulfonate" binds to the ATP binding site and inhibits BCR-ABL proteins, it also selectively inhibits p210 BCR-ABL protein in an inactive state. It retards cellular proliferation and causes apoptosis. Along with p210, it also inhibits PDGFR tyrosine kinase and c-kit receptors [7, 9]. The PDGFRα causes GI stromal tumors (GISTs) and gliomas. The subtype PDGFRβ is involved in myofibroma and myeloid cancers [35]. The stem cell factor binds to the c-kit receptor and regulates the controlled cell division of hematopoietic cells. This c-kit receptor is present in mast cells, germ cells, hematopoietic stem cells, and some GI mesenchymal cells. Its overexpression, underexpression, or mutations can cause, for example, leukemia, GI stromal cell tumors, bone marrow cancer, lung, and prostate cancer [36].

6.8.1.2 Second Generation

Dasatinib and nilotinib are the second generation inhibitors of BCR-ABL tyrosine kinase receptor (TKR). These agents are used when imatinib resistance develops. Dasatinib is a selective and potent inhibitor of BCR-ABL and binds to the receptor in both active and inactive states [37]. These drugs are also used in acute and chronic leukemia [38]. Both dasatinib and nilotinib also inhibit PDGFR-β and c-kit tyrosine kinase receptors [9]. Nilotinib is way more effective as compared to imatinib (20–50 times more effective).

Imatinib's resistance occurs when there is overexpression or mutation of the BCR-ABL gene. Overexpression of protein p170 hinders nilotinib and imatinib from retaining in the tumor cells [34]. Overexpression or mutations in the c-kit also results in the development of resistance. All three drugs possess excellent oral bioavailability and are highly plasma protein bound. Imatinib and nilotinib are mainly metabolized by CYP 3A4 enzymes and most of the drug is excreted in feces [9, 37]. The elimination half-life of nilotinib is 15–17 hours [9].

The common adverse effects of these drugs are GI symptoms like nausea, diarrhea, vomiting, and myelosuppression (thrombocytopenia, anemia, neutropenia) [7, 9, 10]. Imatinib also causes transient swelling of the eye socket and ankle, pleural effusion, and weight gain [9].

Imatinib and nilotinib interact with the drugs, which are either CYP3A4 inducers or inhibitors of CYP3A4 enzymes. The inhibitors of CYP3A4 like ketoconazole and itraconazole reduce the metabolism of imatinib and nilotinib, and hence, their concentration in the body increases. Similarly, the metabolism of these drugs is enhanced if given concomitantly with the inducers of CYP3A4 like rifampin, phenobarbital, phenytoin, St. John's Wort, and carbamazepine [37].

6.8.2 EGFR Tyrosine Kinase Inhibitors

The EGF receptors or HER (human epidermal growth factor receptors) have four subtypes. These membrane receptors are involved in the control and regulation of many different functions including gene expression, cellular growth, maturation, migration, differentiation, as well as cell survival [39]. All these processes occur via a stream of signaling pathways, which activate several important proteins and molecules [40]. Mutations in EGFR results in drastic changes [39]. Its hyper-activation could be ligand dependent or independent, depending upon the mutation. It occurs either due to augmentation of the EGFR gene, reduced expression, or down-regulation of DNA-repairing genes like BRCA1 [40]. There are four types of EGFR receptors including ErbB1 or EGFR1/HER1, ErbB2 or EGFR2/HER2, ErbB3 or EGFR3/HER3 and ErbB4 or EGFR4/HER4 [41]. For example, mutations in HER2 results in the development of breast cancer, and in HER1, this leads to development of lung cancer. The receptor HER2 activates when it forms a dimer with the other HER receptor, mostly with HER3 [41]. Both tyrosine kinase inhibitors (TKIs) and monoclonal antibodies inhibit EGFR receptors but the TKIs are more effective than monoclonal antibodies [42].

6.8.2.1 First Generation

Gefitinib, erlotinib, and icotinib are the first generation EGFR inhibitors [43, 44]. These drugs potentially inhibit EGFR with a mutation in exon 21(L858R) or EGFR having exon 19 omitted [42]. Gefitinib binds selectively to the ATP binding site of the EGFR receptor (ErbB receptor), more precisely ErbB1. It reversibly binds to this site and retards its activation and further signaling cascade [45, 42]. It inhibits tumor cell replication in different tumor types like breast cancer, lung cancer (non-small cell) [9, 42], ovarian, colorectal, and prostate cancer [42]. Erlotinib is used in the treatment of breast cancer, lung cancer (non-small cell), skin cancer, ovary cancer, and head and neck cancer [42]. Even a novel compound called SP101 is derived from gefitinib, which has the potential to inhibit the surviving protein and potentiate apoptosis [46]. The surviving protein protects a cell from programmed death (apoptosis) [46, 47].

Gefitinib possesses slow oral absorption and is almost 60% orally bioavailable. Peak plasma levels are achieved within 3–7 hours [9, 45]. This drug is highly plasma protein-bound and its metabolism occurs via Cytochrome P450 System mainly by CYP3A4 and some amount of the drug is metabolized by CYP2D6 and CYP3A5. It is mainly excreted via feces and a very little amount gets excreted in urine [9, 45]. Erlotinib also possesses approximately 60% bioavailability. Its bioavailability is enhanced when given with food [48]. It is highly bound to plasma proteins, primarily metabolized by CYP3A4 and a little amount is metabolized via CYP1A1 and CYP1A2. The major route of elimination is via feces and a small amount is excreted in urine [48].

6.8.2.2 Second Generation

Afatinib and dacomitinib are the second generation EGFR TK inhibitors and work by irreversibly binding to the receptors [49–51]. They block various EGFR receptors including HER2, HER4, and EGFR1. Their use is significant in treating non-small cell lung cancer (NSCLC) (even with T790M) as compared to other chemotherapeutic options and when the first generation EGFR inhibitors are not effective anymore. These are also used to treat breast, head, and neck cancer [49]. Dacomitinib is used to treat NSCLC, more precisely, the metastatic one [50].

Resistance to the first generation EGFR inhibitors occurs when the enzyme is mutated. An example of the mutation is the T790M mutation, which makes the receptor have more affinity for ATP as compared to the EGFR inhibitors [45]. Resistance against first and second generation EGFR inhibitors also develops when tumor cells initiate signaling via other pathways, mutations in both KRAS and BRAF [45]. Enhanced activity of the mTOR signaling pathway also causes resistance to afatinib. Resistance to dacomitinib develops due to cMET amplification or overexpression [9].

Afatinib has good oral bioavailability and is highly plasma protein bound. It is mainly metabolized via CYP 3A4 enzyme and is excreted via feces with a very little amount excreted through urine. It has a terminal half-life of approximately 37 hours [9]. Dacomitinib has very good oral bioavailability, is widely distributed among the body tissues and is highly plasma protein bound. Steady-state concentration is achieved in a span of 14 days and plasma half-life is approximately 70 hours. It is hepatically metabolized via CYP 2D6 enzyme, following conjugation and oxidation, into

O-desmethyl dacomitinib. The major route of elimination is via feces and a little amount is excreted in urine [50].

The common and transient adverse effects of all these drugs include hypersensitivity, GI symptoms are nausea and vomiting, which is mild [48]. Other adverse effects are transient increase in serum transaminases, conjunctivitis caused by first generation EGFR inhibitors and afatinib [9]. Both first and second generation drugs cause anorexia and fatigue [50]. Dacomitinib also frequently causes diarrhea [50]. All these drugs have teratogenic effects.

First generation EGFR inhibitors' and afatinib's metabolism is enhanced when CYP3A4 inducers are given concomitantly like phenytoin, phenobarbital, carbamazepine, dilantin, rifampicin, and St. John's Wort [45]. CYP 3A4 inhibitors like ketoconazole, itraconazole, clarithromycin, and erythromycin reduce gefitinib and afatinib's metabolism. Warfarin's metabolism is reduced when it is given with first generation EGFR inhibitors and afatinib [48]. Afatinib also interacts with inducers or inhibitors of p-glycoprotein [8]. PPIs decrease dacomitinib's bioavailability but it is not altered by antacids or H2-receptor blockers. CYP 2D6 substrates and dacomitinib should not be used simultaneously as this can potentiate the toxic effects of dacomitinib [50].

6.8.2.3 Third Generation

Osimertinib is the third generation EGFR inhibitor and works by irreversibly binding to the EGFR receptor by making covalent bonds [41, 51]. It is used as a first line agent for malignant lung cancer (non-small cell) having EGFR mutations like L858R or exon 19 deletions and second line agent for T790M mutation [41]. Lapatinib, another drug of this generation, inhibits two EGFR receptors EGFR1 and EGFR2 by reversibly binding to the ATP binding site. It binds to the receptor in an inactive form and slowly dissociates from it. It is used to treat breast cancer and brain malignancy associated with it. It is used as a first line agent in postmenopausal women with breast cancer [52].

Resistance to osimertinib develops when C797S mutations occur as it prevents the drug from making covalent bonds with the receptor [41]. Amplification of cMET or EGFR receptor's overexpression or amplification also induces resistance to osimertinib and lapatinib [9, 53]. Osimertinib possesses good bioavailability, it is widely distributed among body tissues and is highly plasma protein bound [9, 54]. It is primarily metabolized by CYP 3A4 enzyme and is converted into two active metabolites AZ5104 and AZ7550 with a half-life of almost 50 hours. Both drugs are primarily eliminated via feces [52, 54]. Lapatinib's absorption fluctuates in patients and fat-containing food enhances its bioavailability. It is widely distributed among the body tissues and reaches CSF [52]. It is highly plasma protein bound and peak plasma levels are obtained within 3–6 hours. It is metabolized primarily via CYP 3A4 [52] and a little amount by CYP3A5, and CYP2C19 enzymes [55].

The common side effects of osimertinib and lapatinib are mild to moderate nausea, vomiting, diarrhea, and skin rash. Other side effects of osimertinib are tiredness, loss of appetite, and cough. Lapatinib also causes restlessness, bone-marrow suppression with anemia, mild to moderate increase in serum transaminases level, hypersensitivity, and hand–foot syndrome [9, 54]. Osimertinib and lapatinib are readily metabolized when given with CYP 3A4 inducers like phenytoin, carbamazepine, rifampin, St. John's Wort, and phenobarbital [52, 54]. The CYP3A4 inhibitors like erythromycin, ketoconazole, itraconazole, and clarithromycin enhances toxic effects of these drugs [9, 52].

6.8.3 MULTIPLE KINASE INHIBITORS

Sorafenib was first used to treat renal cancer but later on it was approved to treat differentiated thyroid cancer, hepatocellular, and refractory prostate cancer [56, 57]. It targets VEGFR, PDGFR more precisely PDGFR-β and RAFs (BRAF, CRAF, and mutated BRAF) [57]. Sunitinib is also a first generation multiple TK inhibitor which targets VEGFR1-2-3, PDGFR more precisely PDGFR-α and β, neurotropic factor receptors and stem cell receptors. It is used in kidney cancers in both advanced and metastatic forms [58, 59]. Pazopanib is a multiple tyrosine kinase inhibitor that inhibits VEGFR1,2,3, FGFR1 and 3, PDGFR-α and β, IL- 2 receptors, stem cell receptor c-kit, and is used in renal cancer and soft tissue sarcoma. By binding to ATP binding site, it prevents tumor vessel formation [60].

Resistance to sorafenib develops because of the overexpression of targeted receptors, the growth and proliferation of tumor cells via other signaling pathways [9]. Resistance to sunitinib and pazopanib develops due to overexpression, hyper-activation or mutations in target enzymes, signal transduction via other signaling mechanisms, e.g., mTOR pathway, increased gene transcription, etc. [9, 59].

Sorafenib is readily absorbed [9]. It should be taken on an empty stomach as fat-containing food alters its bioavailability. It is highly plasma protein bound, metabolism occurs via oxidation through CYP 3A4 enzyme, and glucuronidation occurs via UGT1A9. Sorafenib and pazopanib are primarily excreted in feces. Sorafenib's half-life is 25–48 hours [57, 61]. Sunitinib is slowly absorbed and primarily metabolized by CYP 3A4 enzyme [59]. Pazopanib is orally well-absorbed [9], food increases its absorption and bioavailability [62]. It is highly plasma protein bound (mostly albumin), mainly metabolized via CYP 3A4 enzyme [62].

Common side effects of sorafenib are hypersensitivity specifically on hand and foot, and reduced weight [57]. Sorafenib, sunitinib, and pazopanib cause BP elevation, bleeding, fatigue, nausea, and diarrhea [9, 57, 59, 61]. Sunitinib and pazopanib also cause hand–foot syndrome, mucositis, and cough [59]. VEGF usually maintains nitric oxide level, which causes blood vessel relaxation and BP reduction. Sorafenib and sunitinib inhibits VEGFR, which causes BP elevation due to reduced nitric oxide [58]. Pazopanib causes hypertension, hair color change, increased ALT, and hypersensitivity [61].

Antihypertensive agents reduce sorafenib's metabolism and potentiates its toxic effects. Carbamazepine, phenobarbital, and other inducers of CYP 3A4 can reduce the bioavailability of sorafenib and sunitinib [58]. The co-administration of CYP 3A4 inhibitors with sunitinib or pazopanib exaggerates their toxic effects [9, 62]. The CYP3A4 inducers enhance pazopanib's metabolism and decrease its bioavailability. Avoid using these drugs in patients with Gilbert's syndrome as they exaggerate hyper-bilirubinemia in these patients [62].

REFERENCES

1. Asim, A., et al., *"Down syndrome: An insight of the disease"*. Journal of Biomedical Science, 2015. **22**(1): p. 41.

2. Henderson, R., et al., *The genetics and screening of familial hypercholesterolaemia*. Journal of Biomedical Science, 2016. **23**(1): pp. 1–12.

3. Singh, N., et al., *Clinical significance of promoter methylation status of tumor suppressor genes in circulating DNA of pancreatic cancer patients*. Journal of Cancer Research and Clinical Oncology, 2020. **146**(4): pp. 897–907.

4. Sun, L., et al., *Metabolic reprogramming for cancer cells and their microenvironment: Beyond the Warburg effect*. Biochimica et Biophysica Acta (BBA)-Reviews on Cancer, 2018. **1870**(1): pp. 51–66.

5. Lui, D.T., A.C. Lee, and K.C. Tan, *Management of familial hypercholesterolemia: current status and future perspectives*. Journal of the Endocrine Society, 2021. **5**(1): p. bvaa122.

6. Kapor, S., V. Čokić, and J.F. Santibanez, *Mechanisms of hydroxyurea-induced cellular senescence: an oxidative stress connection?* Oxidative Medicine and Cellular Longevity, 2021. **2021**: p. 7753857.

7. Tripathi, K., *Essentials of Medical Pharmacology*. 8 ed. 2019. Jaypee Brothers Medical Publishers: New Delhi.

8. Whalen, K., C. Feild and R. Radhakrishnan, *Lippincott Illustrated Reviews: Pharmacology*. 7 ed. 2019. Lippincott Illustrated Reviews: Philadelphia.

9. Chu, E. and V.T. DeVita, *Physicians' Cancer Chemotherapy Drug Manual*. 21 ed. 2019. Jones and Bartlett Learning: Burlington.

10. *BNF 82 September 2021–March 2022*. 2021: BMJ Group, Pharmaceutical Press.

11. Katzung, B. G., et al., *Katzung & Trevor's Pharmacology: Examination & Board Review,* 13 ed. 2021. McGraw Hill: New York.

12. Liu, Z., et al., *Topotecan inhibits metastasis of non-small cell lung cancer by regulating epithelial-mesenchymal transition. European Journal of Medicinal Chemistry Reports,* 2022. **5**: p. 100051.

13. Maes, M.E., C.L. Schlamp, and R.W. Nickells, *BAX to basics: How the BCL2 gene family controls the death of retinal ganglion cells. Progress in Retinal and Eye Research,* 2017. **57**: pp. 1–25.

14. Zhang, Y., et al., *Plasma membrane changes during programmed cell deaths. Cell Research,* 2018. **28**(1): pp. 9–21.

15. Zhang, W., et al., *Etoposide, an anticancer drug involved in therapy-related secondary leukemia: Enzymes at play. Translational Oncology,* 2021. **14**(10): p. 101169.

16. Montecucco, A., F. Zanetta, and G. Biamonti, *Molecular mechanisms of etoposide. EXCLI Journal,* 2015. **14**: pp. 95–108.

17. Qiu, Z., et al., *A novel mutation panel for predicting etoposide resistance in small-cell lung cancer. Drug Design, Development and Therapy,* 2019. **13**: pp. 2021–2041.

18. Aye, Y., et al., *Ribonucleotide reductase and cancer: biological mechanisms and targeted therapies. Oncogene,* 2015. **34**(16): pp. 2011–2021.

19. Xu, Y.-j., A. Singh, and G.M. Alter, *Hydroxyurea induces cytokinesis arrest in cells expressing a mutated sterol-14α-demethylase in the ergosterol biosynthesis pathway. Genetics,* 2016. **204**(3): pp. 959–973.

20. Pedrosa, A.M., L. Leal, and R.P.G. Lemes, *Effects of hydroxyurea on cytotoxicity, inflammation and oxidative stress markers in neutrophils of patients with sickle cell anemia: dose-effect relationship. Hematology Transfusion and Cell Therapy,* 2021. **43**(4): pp. 468–475.

21. Al-Amleh, E.K., et al., *Investigation of the effect of imatinib and hydroxyurea combination therapy on hematological parameters and gene expression in chronic myeloid leukemia (CML) patients. Journal of Clinical Medicine,* 2022. **11**(17): pp. 4954.

22. Dong, M. and P. McGann, *Changing the clinical paradigm of hydroxyurea treatment for sickle cell anemia through precision medicine. Clinical Pharmacology & Therapeutics,* 2020. **109**: pp. 73–81.

23. Zhao, L., S. Zhou, and J.-Å. Gustafsson, *Nuclear receptors: recent drug discovery for cancer therapies. Endocrine Reviews,* 2019. **40**(5): pp. 1207–1249.

24. Hunsu, V.O., et al., *Retinoids as chemo-preventive and molecular-targeted anti-cancer therapies. International Journal of Molecular Sciences,* 2021. **22**(14): p. 7731.

25. Schenk, T., S. Stengel, and A. Zelent, *Unlocking the potential of retinoic acid in anticancer therapy. British Journal of Cancer,* 2014. **111**(11): pp. 2039–2045.

26. Liquori, A., et al., *Acute promyelocytic leukemia: a constellation of molecular events around a single PML-RARA fusion gene. Cancers,* 2020. **12**(3): p. 624.

27. Borges, G.S.M., et al., *All-trans retinoic acid in anticancer therapy: how nanotechnology can enhance its efficacy and resolve its drawbacks. Expert Opinion on Drug Delivery,* 2021. **18**(10): pp. 1335–1354.

28. Wang, Q.-q., et al., *Hyperthermia promotes degradation of the acute promyelocytic leukemia driver oncoprotein ZBTB16/RARα. Acta Pharmacologica Sinica,* 2022. **44**(4): pp. 822–831.

29. Giuli, M.V., et al., *Current trends in ATRA delivery for cancer therapy. Pharmaceutics,* 2020. **12**(8): p. 707.

30. Maimaitiyiming, Y., et al., *Hyperthermia selectively destabilizes oncogenic fusion proteins destabilizing the PML/RARα oncofusion by hyperthermia. Blood Cancer Discovery,* 2021. **2**(4): pp. 388–401.

31. Yamaoka, T., et al., *Receptor tyrosine kinase-targeted cancer therapy. International Journal of Molecular Sciences,* 2018. **19**(11): p. 3491.

32. Zhang, Y., et al., *Function of the c-met receptor tyrosine kinase in carcinogenesis and associated therapeutic opportunities. Molecular Cancer,* 2018. **17**(1): p. 45.

33. Koyama, D., et al., *AMP-activated protein kinase activation primes cytoplasmic translocation and autophagic degradation of the BCR-ABL protein in CML cells. Cancer Science,* 2021. **112**(1): pp. 194–204.

34. Zhu, H.-Q. and F.-H. Gao, *Regulatory molecules and corresponding processes of BCR-ABL protein degradation. Journal of Cancer,* 2019. **10**(11): p. 2488.

35. Guérit, E., et al., *PDGF receptor mutations in human diseases. Cellular and Molecular Life Sciences,* 2021. **78**(8): pp. 3867–3881.

36. Liang, J., et al., *The C-kit receptor-mediated signal transduction and tumor-related diseases. International Journal of Biological Sciences,* 2013. **9**(5): pp. 435–443.

37. Levêque, D., et al., *Clinical pharmacokinetics and pharmacodynamics of dasatinib. Clinical Pharmacokinetics,* 2020. **59**(7): pp. 849–856.

38. Nekoukar, Z., M. Moghimi, and E. Salehifar, *A narrative review on adverse effects of dasatinib with a focus on pharmacotherapy of dasatinib-induced pulmonary toxicities. Blood Research,* 2021. **56**(4): pp. 229–242.

39. Sigismund, S., D. Avanzato, and L. Lanzetti, *Emerging functions of the EGFR in cancer. Molecular Oncology,* 2018. **12**(1): pp. 3–20.

40. Hsu, J.L. and M.C. Hung, *The role of HER2, EGFR, and other receptor tyrosine kinases in breast cancer. Cancer and Metastasis Reviews,* 2016. **35**(4): pp. 575–588.

41. Roskoski, R., *Small molecule inhibitors targeting the EGFR/ErbB family of protein-tyrosine kinases in human cancers. Pharmacological Research,* 2019. **139**: pp. 395–411.

42. Sabbah, D.A., R. Hajjo, and K. Sweidan, *Review on epidermal growth factor receptor (EGFR) structure, signaling pathways, interactions, and recent updates of EGFR inhibitors. Current Topics in Medicinal Chemistry,* 2020. **20**(10): pp. 815–834.

43. Pilotto, S., et al., *Outcomes of first-generation EGFR-TKIs against non-small-cell lung cancer harboring uncommon EGFR mutations: a post hoc analysis of the BE-POSITIVE study. Clinical Lung Cancer,* 2018. **19**(1): pp. 93–104.

44. He, Q., et al., *Comparison of first-generation EGFR-TKIs (gefitinib, erlotinib, and icotinib) as adjuvant therapy in resected NSCLC patients with sensitive EGFR mutations. Translational Lung Cancer Research,* 2021. **10**(11): pp. 4120–4129.

45. Rawluk, J. and C.F. Waller, *Gefitinib,* in *Small Molecules in Oncology,* U.M. Martens, Editor. 2018, Springer: Cham. pp. 235–246.

46. Wang, S.-P., et al., *A novel EGFR inhibitor suppresses survivin expression and tumor growth in human gefitinib-resistant EGFR-wild type and -T790M non-small cell lung cancer. Biochemical Pharmacology,* 2021. **193**: p. 114792.

47. Li, D., C. Hu, and H. Li, *Survivin as a novel target protein for reducing the proliferation of cancer cells. Biomedical Reports,* 2018. **8**(5): pp. 399–406.

48. Abdelgalil, A.A., H.M. Al-Kahtani, and F.I. Al-Jenoobi, *Chapter Four – Erlotinib,* in *Profiles of Drug Substances, Excipients and Related Methodology,* H.G. Brittain, Editor. 2020, Academic Press: Cambridge. pp. 93–117.

49. Wecker, H. and C.F. Waller, *Afatinib,* in *Small Molecules in Oncology,* U.M. Martens, Editor. 2018, Springer: Cham. pp. 199–215.

50. Shirley, M., *Dacomitinib: First global approval. Drugs,* 2018. **78**(18): pp. 1947–1953.

51. Westover, D., et al., *Mechanisms of acquired resistance to first- and second-generation EGFR tyrosine kinase inhibitors. Annals of Oncology,* 2018. **29**: pp. i10–i19.

52. Voigtlaender, M., T. Schneider-Merck, and M. Trepel, *Lapatinib,* in *Small Molecules in Oncology,* U.M. Martens, Editor. *2018,* Springer: Cham. pp. 19–44.

53. Ramalingam, S.S., et al., *Osimertinib as first-line treatment of EGFR mutation-positive advanced non-small-cell lung cancer. Journal of Clinical Oncology,* 2018. **36**(9): pp. 841–849.

54. Malapelle, U., et al., *Osimertinib,* in *Small Molecules in Oncology,* U.M. Martens, Editor. 2018, Springer: Cham. pp. 257–276.

55. Rodseeda, C., et al., *Inhibitory effects of Thai herbal extracts on the cytochrome P450 3A-mediated the metabolism of gefitinib, lapatinib and sorafenib. Toxicology Reports,* 2022. **9**: pp. 1846–1852.

56. Escudier, B., F. Worden, and M. Kudo, *Sorafenib: Key lessons from over 10 years of experience. Expert Review of Anticancer Therapy,* 2019. **19**(2): pp. 177–189.

57. Abdelgalil, A.A., H.M. Alkahtani, and F.I. Al-Jenoobi, *Chapter Four – Sorafenib,* in *Profiles of Drug Substances, Excipients and Related Methodology.* 2019, Academic Press: Cambridge. pp. 239–266.

58. Randrup Hansen, C., et al., *Effects and side effects of using sorafenib and sunitinib in the treatment of metastatic renal cell carcinoma. International Journal of Molecular Sciences,* 2017. **18**(2): p. 461.

59. Nassif, E., et al., *Sunitinib in kidney cancer: 10 years of experience and development. Expert Review of Anticancer Therapy*, 2017. **17**(2): pp. 129–142.
60. Miyamoto, S., et al., *Drug review: pazopanib. Japanese Journal of Clinical Oncology*, 2018. **48**(6): pp. 503–513.
61. Verheijen, R.B., et al., *Clinical pharmacokinetics and pharmacodynamics of pazopanib: towards optimized dosing. Clinical Pharmacokinetics*, 2017. **56**(9): pp. 987–997.
62. Thorn, C.F., et al., *PharmGKB summary: pazopanib pathway, pharmacokinetics. Pharmacogenetics and Genomics*, 2017. **27**(8): p. 307.

7 Parenteral Anticancer Therapies

Mishal Fatima, Liaqat Hussain, Yasen Maimaitiyiming, Hua Naranmandura, Ayesha Saeed, Yang Chang, Muhammad Yasir Ali, and Ummaima Shahzad

7.1 INTRODUCTION

None of the cancer chemotherapeutic drugs available in the market is devoid of toxicity. The natural compounds obtained from medicinal plants have become more important in this context for the treatment of cancer. According to the WHO, plant-derived medications are used to treat 80% of the world's population, particularly those in impoverished nations [1].

Historically, the foundation of cancer treatment has been based on the idea that tumor cells frequently go through the cell cycle and are more sensitive than normal cells to interference with DNA production and mitosis. Some of the earliest medications to be evaluated as chemotherapeutic agents were antimetabolites, which include analogs of endogenous folates, purine, and pyrimidine and act as inhibitors of the enzymes responsible for nucleotide synthesis [2].

Following these and other discoveries, various types of anti-cancer medications have been synthesized that target DNA synthesis and cell division, DNA damage, and chromosomal instability to encourage cytotoxicity and programmed cell death (apoptosis). Unfortunately, these medications have a limited therapeutic window since they can also affect healthy cells that regularly divide [2]. The ultimate goal of cancer chemotherapy is to synthesize medications that specifically target particular cancer cells using advancements in cell biology [3].

7.2 THE GENESIS OF CANCER

A typical cell transforms into a diseased cell as a result of one or more transformations in its DNA. These can be acquired or gained, generally through openness to infections or cancer-causing agents (for example, tobacco items, asbestos). A genuine model is bosom malignant growth; ladies who acquire a solitary flawed duplicate of both of the growth silencer genes; BRCA1 and BRCA2 have an essentially expanded hazard of creating bosom malignant growth. Notwithstanding, carcinogenesis is a compile multistage process, generally including multiple hereditary changes as well as other, epigenetic factors (hormonal, co-cancer-causing agent and growth advertiser impacts, and so on) that do not themselves produce disease, however, they enhance the probability that the hereditary mutation(s) will ultimately bring about disease. There are two primary classifications of relevant hereditary change:

1. The conversion of proto-oncogenes to oncogenes. Proto-oncogenes have typically a role in controlling cell division.

DOI: 10.1201/9781003363958-9

2. The inactivation of growth silencer genes. Ordinary cells contain elements that are named growth silencer elements and transformations of these elements are engaged with a wide range of malignant growths. The genetic abnormality of these growth silencer elements is responsible for oncogenesis. Around 30 growth silencer elements and 100 prevailing oncogenes have been distinguished [4].

7.3 THE CELL CYCLE STAGES

Numerous cytotoxic agents act by disrupting DNA. Their harmfulness is most prominent during the S stage. Different agents, such as the vinca alkaloids and Texans, block the development of a mitotic spindle formation in the M stage. These agents are best on cells entering mitosis. Human tumors generally vulnerable to chemotherapy are those having a high level of multiplying cells. Below are the various cell cycle stages that are the target of cancer chemotherapy:

- Growth phase, where the cell is getting ready for DNA synthesis (G1).
- DNA synthesis stage (S).
- Growth stage where the cell is preparing itself for mitosis (G2).
- The mitotic stage (M) cell division stage.

7.4 GENERAL TOXICITY OF CYTOTOXIC DRUGS

1. Bone marrow depression brings about agranulocytosis, granulocytopenia, thrombocytopenia, and plastic frailty.
2. Oral depression: the oral mucosa is especially vulnerable to cytotoxic medications because of high epithelial cell turnover. The gums and oral mucosa are routinely exposed to a minor injury, and breaks are normal during biting. Thrombocytopenia may cause draining gums. Xerostomia due to the medication might cause dental carries.
3. Gonads inhibition of gonadal cells causes oligozoospermia in males; hindrance of ovulation and amenorrhea in females.
4. Cancer-causing nature; secondary malignant growths, particularly leukemias, lymphomas, and histolytic growths show up with more noteworthy recurrence numerous years later after treatment with cytotoxic medications. This might be expected to the wretchedness of cell interceded and humoral obstructing factors against neoplastic.
5. Various anti-cancer drugs are responsible for complex toxic reactions, such as neuropathy by vincristine, cardiomyopathy by doxorubicin, cystitis, and alopecia by cyclophosphamide [5].

7.5 PARENTERAL CHEMOTHERAPEUTICS AGENTS

7.5.1 Anti-Metabolites

7.5.1.1 Methotrexate

The antimetabolites are antagonists of folic acid (methotrexate), purine (mercaptopurine, thioguanine), or pyrimidine and share structural similarities with natural substances (fluorouracil, cytarabine, gemcitabine). Cell cycle non-specific (CCNS) antineoplastic agents called antimetabolites primarily affect the S-phase of the cell cycle. Antimetabolites not only have cytotoxic effects on the neoplastic cells but also immunosuppressive effects [6].

Dihydrofolate reductase (DHFR) is inhibited by methotrexate. It suppresses DHFR, which inhibits the production of thymidylate, purines, nucleotides, serine, and methionine [1]. Methotrexate is usually used orally, but can also be administered intravenously, intramuscularly, or intrathecally. The medication is poorly soluble in lipids and does not pass the blood–brain barrier. Methotrexate provides good tissue absorption, except for the CNS. Its plasma concentrations decrease after intravenous administration in a triphasic fashion, with extended terminal clearance because of enterohepatic circulation. Its clearance is done by renal function and is mainly excreted in urine [7].

Methotrexate is an effective treatment for several types of leukemia, choriocarcinoma, lymphoma, sarcoma, testicular growths, and lung cancer. High-dose methotrexate therapy requires serum blood concentration monitoring and the use of folinic acid "rescue".

It has several significant medication interactions. Drugs that are highly plasma protein-bound, such as salicylates, sulfonamides, and phenytoin, may displace methotrexate from its protein-binding sites, resulting in increased toxicity [8]. The principal toxicity of methotrexate is on bone marrow and intestinal epithelium. Patients who are febrile may be at risk of spontaneous bleeding or life-threatening illness and may require prophylactic platelet transfusions and broad-spectrum antibiotics [9]. Long-term methotrexate use has resulted in hepatotoxicity as well as lung infiltrates and fibrosis [3].

7.5.1.2 Fludarabine

This newer purine antimetabolite is intracellularly phosphorylated to its active triphosphate form. The active form inhibits DNA polymerase and ribonucleotide reductase interferes with DNA repair and integrates it to produce dysfunctional DNA [3].

Fludarabine is delivered intravenously rather than orally because intestinal bacteria split off the sugar to produce a very poisonous metabolite. It is partially eliminated by urinary excretion [10]. It is used to treat relapsed chronic lymphatic leukemia. Fludarabine injection is also used to treat non-Hodgkin's lymphoma (NHL; cancer that begins in a type of white blood cell that normally fights infection) and mycosis fungoides (a type of lymphoma that affects the skin) [5]. When abciximab is taken with fludarabine, the risk or severity of bleeding can be enhanced [11]. Chills, fever, myalgia, arthralgia, vomiting after injection, as well as myelosuppression are common side effects. Some other serious side effects include hearing loss, chest pain, and peeling or blistering skin. Fludarabine injection can cause damage to the central nervous system [3,12].

7.5.1.3 Cladribine

It has a similar mechanism of action to fludarabine, but to become cytotoxic it must be phosphorylated to a nucleotide. It prevents elongation because it is incorporated into the 3'-terminus of DNA. It has an impact on DNA repair and is a potent ribonucleotide reductase inhibitor [13, 14]. This drug is administered as a single, continuous infusion. Cladribine circulates throughout the body, including the cerebrospinal fluid (CSF) [10]. This drug is mainly used in hairy cell leukemia, chronic lymphocytic leukemia, non-Hodgkin lymphoma, and also in multiple sclerosis (MS), which is a central nervous system immune-mediated inflammatory demyelinating disease [15].

Cladribine showed serious side effects in clinical trials including lymphopenia and infections. Some of the additional side effects include headaches, herpetic infections or complications, nasopharyngitis, rashes, and alopecia [3].

7.5.1.4 5-Fluorouracil (5-FU)

5-FU inhibits thymidylate synthase, and its metabolites are integrated into DNA and RNA. As a result, DNA synthesis, function, and RNA processing, are all inhibited [16]. It is administered intravenously as a bolus injection or as a continuous injection for days to weeks. Dose reduction is required for patients with hepatic dysfunction or in patients with a genetic deficiency of dihydropyridine dehydrogenase. The drug penetrates the tissues and is metabolized mainly by the liver, kidneys, and lungs. It is then converted into fluoro-β-alanine and excreted by urine [7]. In normal tissues, concomitant administration of allopurinol and fluorouracil inhibits the intracellular formation of fluorouridine monophosphate from fluorouracil [17].

Cancers of the bladder, breast, colon, esophagus, head and neck, liver, and ovary are treated with fluorouracil. For superficial basal cell carcinoma and keratosis, this medication can be used topically [3]. The main unwanted effects of 5-FU include gastrointestinal epithelial damage and myelotoxicity. Other side effects can be cardiotoxicity, alopecia, cerebellar syndrome, visual changes myelosuppression, nematotoxicity, and neurotoxicity.

7.5.1.5 Cytarabine

In the body, this cytidine analog is phosphorylated to the corresponding nucleotide, which inhibits DNA synthesis. Cytarabine triphosphate inhibits DNA polymerase and prevents the production of cytidilic acid. Its incorporation into DNA, however, is now thought to be more important for the expression of its cytotoxicity [18].

When administered intravenously, the drug is rapidly removed from the bloodstream by deamination in the liver, with a plasma half-life ranging from 5 to 20 minutes. With these characteristics, continuous infusion is frequently the preferred mode of administration. Cytarabine is a polar nucleoside drug used for the treatment of myeloid leukemia and non-Hodgkin's lymphoma [19]. It is also useful in the treatment of acute myeloid leukemia (AML), meningeal leukemia, and acute lymphoblastic leukemia [20]. When adalimumab is combined with cytarabine, the risk or severity of adverse effects can be increased [21]. Major side effects are on the bone marrow and gastrointestinal tract. It also induces myelosuppression, hepatotoxicity, kidney disease, neurologic toxicity, and vomiting [22].

7.5.1.6 Azacitidine

Azacitidine is activated into the nucleotide metabolite azacitidine triphosphate and incorporated into RNA to inhibit RNA processing and function [10]. 5-Azacytidine is rapidly deaminated by cytidine deaminase after subcutaneous administration. The effects of aza-nucleosides last for many hours due to the formation of intracellular nucleotides that become incorporated into the DNA [9].

Azacitidine is used in the treatment of patients suffering from myelodysplastic syndromes (MDS)/acute myeloid leukemia (AML) [23]. It induces myelosuppression, neutropenia, renal failure, thrombocytopenia, constipation, and renal toxicity [24].

7.5.1.7 Gemcitabine

Gemcitabine (deoxycytidine analog) is converted into the active metabolite forms, i.e., diphosphate and triphosphate nucleotide. Gemcitabine diphosphate reduces the amount of deoxyribonucleoside triphosphate needed for DNA synthesis by appearing to block ribonucleotide reductase [9]. It is infused intravenously and is then deaminated to difluoro deoxyuridine, which is non-cytotoxic and excreted in the urine [10].

This drug was initially approved for pancreatic cancer and is now widely used in the treatment of malignancies, pancreatic cancer, non-small cell lung cancer, and a variety of solid tumors [25]. Myelosuppression and primarily thrombocytopenia is the dose-limiting side effect of gemcitabine. Transient febrile reactions and a flu-like syndrome, as well as rare cases of pulmonary toxicity, have also been reported. Other common side effects include alopecia, capillary leak syndrome, hyperglycemia edema, rash, and flu-like syndrome [26].

7.5.1.8 Mercaptopurine

This is an extremely potent anti-cancer drug. It inhibits the conversion of inosine monophosphate to adenine and guanine nucleotides, which after being synthesized in the body to the corresponding mono ribonucleotides, are the building blocks for RNA and DNA. This drug is also incorporated into dysfunctional RNA and DNA [27].

Mercaptopurine is easily absorbed when taken orally but extensively undergoes the first pass of metabolism by the liver. Its plasma half-life after intravenous injection is approximately 90 minutes. The drug is metabolized in the liver via methylation and the hepatic enzyme xanthine oxidase. 6-MP is particularly useful in childhood acute leukemia, and choriocarcinoma, and has been used in some solid tumors as well [5].

Its main toxic effect is bone marrow depression, which takes time to develop. It also causes a high rate of reversible jaundice and hyperuricemia, which can be treated with allopurinol. But allopurinol inhibits the enzyme xanthine oxidase. To avoid toxicity in patients who are also taking allopurinol, the usual dose of 6-MP should be reduced by 75%. This is significant because allopurinol pretreatment is used to reduce the risk of acute uric acid nephropathy caused by rapid tumor lysis syndrome in leukemia patients [28]. Other common side effects include nausea, vomiting, pancreatitis, myelosuppression, increased risk of infection, rash, and gastrointestinal upset [29].

7.5.1.9 Clofarabine

Clofarabine is converted intracellularly by deoxycytidine kinase to the 5-monophosphate metabolite, which is then converted to the active 5-triphosphate form via monophosphokinases and diphosphokinases. Clofarabrine 5-triphosphate prevents DNA synthesis by inhibiting ribonucleotide reductase and DNA polymerases [30]. This drug is administered intravenously and it is bound to plasma proteins, especially to albumin. According to 24-hour urine collections in pediatric studies, 49–60% of the dose is excreted unchanged in the urine. The half-life of this drug is 5.2 hours.

Clofarabrine is approved for the treatment of pediatric patients who have relapsed or are refractory to at least two prior treatment regimens for acute lymphocytic leukemia. It is also being researched for other cancers, such as the treatment of acute myeloid leukemia in adults. The main side effects are nausea, vomiting, hematologic toxicity, febrile neutropenia, hepatobiliary toxicity, infections, and renal toxicity. Myelosuppression, a clinical syndrome of hypotension, tachyphemia, pulmonary edema, organ dysfunction, and fever are the primary toxicities [32].

7.5.1.10 Nelarabine

Nelarabine is a prodrug of 9-beta-d-arabinofuranosylguanine, a deoxyguanosine analog (ara-G). It is demethylated to ara-G and activated to ara-GTP, an active 5-triphosphate. The active ara-G is incorporated into the DNA, inhibiting DNA synthesis and causing cell death. It has been approved for use in patients with relapsed/refractory acute T-cell leukemia (20% complete responses) and closely related T-cell lymphoblastic lymphoma [9].

The combination of nelarabine and adenosine deaminase inhibitors, such as pentostatin, should be avoided with it, because it may result in a decrease in nelarabine conversion to its active substrate, lowering efficacy and potentially changing the adverse effect profile of both drugs. A major side effect of nelarabine that has resulted in a "black box" warning involves neurologic events such as severe somnolence, convulsions, peripheral neuropathies, and paralysis. Fatigue, bone marrow suppression, gastrointestinal side effects, and some pulmonary complaints of cough and dyspnea are also possible. Patients receiving nelarabine have occasionally reported blurred vision [32].

7.5.1.11 Pentostatin

It can inhibit RNA synthesis, and its triphosphate derivative is also incorporated into DNA, causing strand breaks. Although the precise mechanism of cytotoxicity is unknown, the antineoplastic effect in hairy cell leukemia and T-cell lymphomas is likely due to an imbalance in purine nucleotide pools [9].

Pentostatin is rapidly distributed to all the body tissues after administration and plasma half-life ranges from 2.6 to 9.4 hours, with the majority of the drug recovered in the urine unchanged. It has been utilized to treat a variety of lymph proliferative conditions. It is specifically used to treat shaggy cell leukemia, and completely eradicates the disease in 33 to 92% of patients [33]. It also produces complete remissions (58%) and partial responses (28%) in patients with hairy cell leukemia [9].

Pentostatin can cause severe even fatal pulmonary toxicity when combined with fludarabine phosphate [9]. Its toxicity varies with dose, with acute renal failure and CNS side effects being the most severe.

7.5.2 ANTI-TUMOR ANTIBIOTICS

7.5.2.1 Doxorubicin, Daunorubicin, Idarubicin, and Epirubicin

The most commonly used drugs in this class are doxorubicin and daunorubicin, but newer analogs (e.g., epirubicin, idarubicin) have lower hepatic and cardiac toxicity. The anthracycline (doxorubicin, idarubicin, and epirubicin) intercalates inside DNA bases, breaking DNA strands and preventing transcription and translation. They inhibit topoisomerase II, which damages DNA and induces apoptosis. Anthracyclines are the CCNS drugs [34].

These drugs are administered intravenously, because they are inactivated in the GI tract, and bind to plasma proteins as well as other tissues, but they do not cross the blood–brain barrier. The primary route of elimination is biliary excretion [10]. Doxorubicin is quickly removed from the plasma and accumulates in the tissues. Its urinary excretion is low, rarely accounting for more than 10% of the administered dose, biliary excretion on the other hand is high. Epirubicin is metabolized in the liver but also outside the liver. The biliary system eliminates the majority of epirubicin metabolites, but up to 20% to 30% are also eliminated in the urine.

Streptomyces peucetius produces the red antibiotic doxorubicin. It is the most widely used anthracycline, with proven activity in acute leukemia, lymphomas, sarcomas, and a variety of carcinomas. Liposomal formulations of doxorubicin are available [7]. Epirubicin is a semi-synthetic doxorubicin derivative that is approved for use in breast cancer patients and also shows activity in gastric and esophageal cancers, as well as soft tissue sarcomas. Epirubicin has also been studied for its potential intravenous use in superficial bladder cancer. Idarubicin is used to treat acute myelogenous leukemia and certain types of lymphoma [35, 36]. Daunorubicin is an anthracycline (anti-microbial) used to treat different sorts of tumors [37].

Concurrent dexrazoxane administration with doxorubicin may reduce troponin T-elevations and prevent later cardiotoxicity [9]. Cardiotoxicity is a unique adverse effect of both doxorubicin and daunorubicin. This can manifest acutely within 2–3 days, causing ECG changes, arrhythmias, and hypotension, all of which are reversible, or it can manifest gradually, resulting in congestive heart failure (CHF) [10]. Epirubicin has primarily been used as part of a regimen for adjuvant therapy for breast carcinoma. Other indications include gastroesophageal carcinoma, pancreatic carcinoma, hepatic carcinoma, and bladder carcinoma. Alopecia, skin and oral mucosal hyperpigmentation, painful oral ulcers, and fever are some of the common adverse effects [38].

7.5.2.2 Bleomycin

Bleomycin was initially isolated from the cultures of *Streptomyces verticillus* and is frequently used as an anti-tumor specialist for the treatment of numerous sorts of dangerous tumors [39]. It is a glycopeptide mixture that produces free radicals, binds to DNA, causes strand breaks, and inhibits DNA synthesis. Bleomycin is a cell cycle-specific (CSS) drug that acts during the G2 phase of the tumor cell cycle [40].

It must be administered parenterally. Although tissues' amino peptidases inactivate it, some renal clearance of intact drugs occurs [10]. This drug is used by dermatologists as a treatment for various skin cancers, squamous cell carcinoma, testicular cancer, and warts [39]. Patients who smoke are more likely to develop pneumonic complications as a result of bleomycin [41].

The side effects include bleomycin pulmonary toxicity (BPT), pulmonary fibrosis, fever, hyper-keratosis, hyper-pigmentation, and cerebral edema [41]. Some severe side effects are mucocutaneous toxicity, pulmonary fibrosis, and myelosuppression. Bleomycin injection can cause allergic and hypertensive reactions [5].

7.5.2.3 Mitomycin

Streptomyces caespitosus is the source of this drug. Mitomycin is a CCNS drug that is metabolized by liver enzymes to form an alkylating agent that cross-links the DNA [3]. Mitomycin is effective against gastrointestinal, head and neck, breast, cervix, and lung carcinomas when combined with fluorouracil or nitrosoureas. It is also commonly used in the treatment of bladder, gastrointestinal (GI), gastric, anal, and breast cancer [42].

This drug is administered intravenously and quickly eliminated through hepatic metabolism [10]. Mitomycin should not be given to patients with immunosuppression due to bone marrow suppression and is contraindicated in pregnant ladies [43]. Dose-related effects of mitomycin include pulmonary toxicity and hemolytic uremic syndrome. Other toxic effects include myelosuppression, mucositis, anorexia, weariness, and hemolytic-uremic disorder [3].

7.5.3 ALKYLATING AGENTS

Specifically, the N-7 position of guanine is alkylated by these reactive chemical species. It causes base cross-linking, mismatched base pairing, and DNA strand breakage [3].

7.5.3.1 Cyclophosphamide and Ifosfamide

The cytochrome P450 (CYP450) system first bio-transforms these medications into hydroxylated intermediates, which are mostly found in the liver. The hydroxylated intermediates are then broken down into the active substances, phosphoramide mustard and acrolein [10]. The gastrointestinal tract has excellent absorption of cyclophosphamide (almost 100% bioavailability). It is metabolized in the liver to active and inactive metabolites and excreted mainly in the urine. Ifosfamide is primarily metabolized by the CYP450 3A4 and 2B6 iso-enzymes. It is mostly excreted through the kidneys [10].

The applications of cyclophosphamide include ovarian cancer, leukemia, non-Hodgkin's lymphoma, and breast cancer. It is also used in anaphylactic reactions and urinary flow obstructive conditions. The cyclophosphamide analog, ifosfamide has a longer and dose-dependent effect. It has been used to treat bronchogenic, breast, testicular, bladder, head and neck, osteogenic sarcoma, and some lymphomas [44].

Cyclophosphamide metabolism is slowed by chloramphenicol [5]. This drug is also contraindicated in patients with a history of cell carcinoma, ovarian cancer, breast cancer, multiple myeloma, and autoimmune diseases [45]. When combined with cisplatin, ifosfamide is associated with peripheral neuropathy [2]. Hemorrhagic cystitis is a unique toxicity of cyclophosphamide that can result in bladder fibrosis. Adequate hydration, as well as the injection of mesna with a high dose (sodium 2-mercaptoethane sulfonate) neutralizes the toxic metabolites and can help in alleviating this problem. Other toxic effects include cardiotoxicity, rash, alopecia, nausea, vomiting, pulmonary toxicity, and amenorrhea [45]. Ifosfamide is less emetogenic and causes less alopecia than cyclophosphamide. Common side effects of ifosfamide include myelosuppression, ototoxicity, and neurological effects [46].

7.5.4 CARMUSTINE (BCNU)

It decomposes in the body to produce reactive intermediates, that act as classic alkylating agents causing strand breaks and cross-links in the DNA. They also generate isocyanates, which prevent DNA repair and RNA synthesis [47]. This drug is administered intravenously. It is rapidly metabolized and excreted in the urine slowly. This drug is distinguished by lipophilicity and its ability to pass through the blood–brain barrier.

Carmustine (BCNU) is given intravenously over 1–2 hours and is given every 6 weeks. It has been used in the treatment of malignant glioma due to its ability to cross the blood–brain barrier. A carmustine wafer implantable for use as an adjunct to surgery for recurrent glioblastoma multiforme is now available. This drug is also useful in the treatment of brain cancer, lymphoma, and multiple myeloma [48]. It usually causes delayed bone marrow suppression that appears in 3 to 6 weeks and lasts for another 2 to 3 weeks. Other common side effects include nausea and vomiting, which occur in the majority of patients within 2 to 6 hours of administration. Long-term treatment with carmustine resulted in renal failure [3].

7.5.4.1 Dacarbazine

Dacarbazine is an alkylating agent that must be biotransformed into methyltriazeno-imidazole carboxamide (MTIC), an active metabolite. This metabolite is responsible for the drug's activity as an alkylating agent by forming methyl-carbonium ions that can attack the nucleophilic groups in the DNA molecule [49].

Dacarbazine is given intravenously and is cleared from the plasma with a terminal half-life ($t_{1/2}$) of about 5 hours after an initial rapid phase ($t_{1/2}$ of about 20 minutes). In the presence of hepatic or renal disease, the $t_{1/2}$ is prolonged. Tubular secretion excretes nearly half of the compound intact in the urine [10]. Dacarbazine has been used to treat melanoma and Hodgkin's lymphoma. It is modestly effective against malignant melanoma and adult sarcomas. Dacarbazine for malignant melanoma is given for 10 days, and repeated every 28 days; alternatively, it can be given daily for 5 days and repeated every 3 weeks [50]. Its most common side effects are nausea, vomiting, flu-like symptoms, neuropathy, and myelosuppression. Less common side effects include hepatotoxicity, alopecia, facial flushing, neurotoxicity, and dermatological reactions [3].

7.5.4.2 Melphalan

Melphalan is a bi-functional alkylating agent that can be administered intravenously. Through synthetic alkylation, melphalan modifies the DNA nucleotide guanine and creates connections between DNA strands [10]. This is an orally administered bi-functional alkylating agent. Although melphalan can be administered orally, its plasma concentrations may vary from patient to patient due to differences in intestinal absorption and metabolism. Its dose is carefully adjusted by monitoring platelet and white blood cell count. It is excreted mainly by urine [10].

Melphalan (L-phenylalanine mustard) has been used to treat a wide range of solid tumors, including breast and ovarian cancers, as well as multiple myeloma. Melphalan given intravenously has been used to treat rhabdomyosarcoma, lymphomas, multiple myeloma, and neuroblastoma [9]. Cardiotoxicity with melphalan or fludarabine alone has been rare, but severe left ventricular failure developed in 3 of 21 patients treated with a combination of these two drugs [17]. Melphalan has the potential to cause acute interstitial pneumonia with hypoxemia this is most likely due to a hypersensitivity mechanism and should be distinguished from fibrosing pneumonitis, which can also be caused by melphalan. It has been linked to fatal pulmonary fibrosis and atypical epithelial proliferation in patients with multiple myeloma. Its side effects also include myelosuppression, headache, and hypersensitivity [3].

7.5.5 MICROTUBULE INHIBITORS

7.5.5.1 Vincristine, Vinblastine, and Vinorelbine

These are mitotic inhibitors that bind to the micro-tubular protein "tubulin," preventing it from polymerizing and assembling microtubules, causing mitotic spindle disruption, and interfering with cytoskeletal function. The chromosomes fail to separate during mitosis, resulting in metaphase arrest. They act only during the mitotic phase of the cell cycle [51]. These medications must be administered parenterally. Except for the CSF, they can penetrate most tissues. Half-lives of vinblastine and vinorelbine are 24 hours, while vincristine has a longer half-life of about 3 days. They are mostly eliminated through biliary excretion [3].

Asparaginase and vincristine should not be used on the same day because concurrent administration can result in increased vincristine toxicity. The use of itraconazole in conjunction with vincristine increased the risk of neurotoxicity in children and adults with acute lymphoblastic leukemia [17]. Vincristine is a fast-acting drug that can induce remission in children with acute lymphoblastic leukemia but is not suitable for maintenance therapy. Acute myeloid leukemia, Hodgkin's disease, Wilms' tumor, Ewing's sarcoma, neuroblastoma, and lung carcinoma are among the other indications of vincristine. Vinblastine is used for the treatment of Kaposi's sarcoma, testicular carcinoma, and neuroblastoma. Vinorelbine is used in breast cancer, and non-small lung cancer [52].

Vinblastine and vinorelbine can cause diarrhea, alopecia, and bone marrow suppression. Although vincristine does not cause severe myelosuppression, it is neurotoxic and may cause areflexia, peripheral neuritis, and paralytic ileus. Other common side effects of these drugs include depression, agitation, alopecia, vision loss, insomnia, and hallucinations [53].

7.5.5.2 Paclitaxel and Docetaxel

Both of these drugs are active during the G2/M phase of the cell cycle, but unlike vinca alkaloids they promote polymerization and polymer stabilization rather than disassembly, resulting in microtubule accumulation. The overly stable microtubules formed are non-functional, and there is no chromosome desegregation. This causes the cell to die [54].

These agents are metabolized in the liver by the CYP450 system and excreted through the biliary system. Dose reduction is not necessary for patients with renal impairment, but it is recommended in patients with hepatic dysfunction [10]. Trastuzumab clearance was reduced in primates when it was combined with paclitaxel. Paclitaxel is metabolized by the cytochrome P450 iso-enzymes CYP2C and CYP3A4, and drugs that inhibit or induce these isozymes are likely to alter paclitaxel metabolism [17]. Paclitaxel is useful in the treatment of ovarian cancer, and metastatic breast cancer. Docetaxel is commonly used in prostate, breast, GI, and non-small lung cancer [54]. Paclitaxel and docetaxel have dose-limiting toxicity in the form of neutropenia and leukopenia. Alopecia occurs, but vomiting and diarrhea are uncommon [55].

7.5.6 Steroid Hormones and Their Antagonist

7.5.6.1 Leuprolide, Goserelin, and Triptorelin

Gonadotropin-releasing hormone (GnRH) analogs include goserelin and triptorelin. As GnRH analogs, they occupy the GnRH receptor in the pituitary, causing desensitization and, as a result, inhibition of FSH and LH release. Hence, both androgen and estrogen synthesis is decreased [56]. These drugs are administered intravenously. Goserelin is not completely protein bound and by injection, bioavailability is nearly complete. These drugs are metabolized by liver.

GnRH agonists are used in the palliative treatment of advanced prostate cancer and are useful in the treatment of breast cancer. The initial surge of hormone release caused by these agents can cause pain or hypercalcemia at the site of the tumor, a condition known as "tumor flare" [57]. Along with triptorelin and goserelin, leuprolide has been used to delay puberty in transgender youth until they are old enough to begin hormone replacement therapy. In pre- and postmenopausal women, goserelin, a gonadotropin-delivering chemical compound, works by lowering plasma/serum estrogen levels [58]. Triptorelin is useful for the treatment of endometriosis [59].

Adverse effects of these drugs include impotence, hot flashes, tumor flare, hot flashes, erectile dysfunction, and gynecomastia. Long-term use can develop osteoporosis and metabolic changes (hypercholesterolemia and hyperglycemia) [57].

7.5.7   Monoclonal Antibodies

7.5.7.1   Trastuzumab

In breast cancer, gastric cancer, and gastroesophageal disorders, trastuzumab binds to HER2 sites and inhibits the proliferation of cells that over-express the HER2 protein [60]. This drug is administered intravenously.

Patients who had not previously received anthracycline-containing adjuvant chemotherapy were more likely to develop cardiotoxicity when given trastuzumab in combination with doxorubicin or cyclophosphamide [17]. This drug is useful in the treatment of HER-2/neu-receptor-positive breast cancer [61]. Acute toxicity of this antibody includes nausea, vomiting, chills, fever, and headache. The most serious toxicity caused by trastuzumab is congestive heart failure. If anthracycline is used with them, the toxicity is exacerbated [62].

7.5.7.2   Rituximab

The first monoclonal antibody to be approved for the treatment of cancer was rituximab. It is a chimeric monoclonal antibody produced through genetic engineering that targets the CD20 antigen located on the surface of both healthy and cancerous B-cells [63]. Rituximab's FC domain recruits immunological effector functions, such as complement and antibody-dependent, and cell-mediated cytotoxicity of B-cells. The fab domain of rituximab binds to the CD20 antigen on B-lymphocytes [10].

Rituximab is used to treat B-cell malignancies, including low-grade non-Hodgkin's lymphoma and diffuse large B-cell lymphoma. It is also used in B-cell non-Hodgkin's lymphoma, cystic leukemia, and rheumatoid arthritis [64]. A transient flu-like syndrome (50–90%) is a very common side effect, especially after the first rituximab infusion, and is frequently associated with various hypersensitivity-like symptoms (5–20%). Patients with the most severe cytokine release syndrome had dyspnea, bronchospasm, hypoxia, hypotension, urticaria, and angioedema. Other common side effects include fever, chills, hypotension, bronchospasm, and angioedema [3].

7.5.7.3   Bevacizumab

Bevacizumab, a monoclonal antibody, is an intravenous anti-angiogenesis drug. It binds to vascular endothelial growth factor (VEGF) and prevents it from promoting the creation of new blood vessels [65]. Bevacizumab is used as a first-line drug for metastatic colorectal cancer and a variety of solid tumors [66]. Its common side effects include hypertension, GI perforation, wound healing problems, and bleeding [67].

7.5.7.4   Cetuximab

This drug targets the epidermal growth factor receptor (EGFR) on the surface of cancer cells and hinders their proliferation to have an anti-proliferative impact [68]. It is used in combination with irinotecan for metastatic breast cancer, colorectal cancer, and also used in combination with radiation for head and neck cancers [3]. Its primary toxicity is hypersensitivity infusion reaction and skin rash. Other common side effects include electrolyte wasting, and infusion reactions [69].

7.5.8   Platinum Coordination Complexes

7.5.8.1   Cisplatin

It binds to guanine in DNA and creates cross-connections within the strands. The resultant cytotoxic lesions block RNA synthesis and DNA replication [7]. Cisplatin is the most highly protein-bound drug (> 90%), followed by oxaliplatin (85%) and carboplatin (24–50%). It binds to plasma proteins, penetrates tissues, and is excreted unchanged in urine over a 72-hour period. Only a small amount of this drug enters the brain [5].

Concurrent amifostine and cisplatin administration may reduce the cumulative renal toxicity associated with repeated administration in patients with advanced ovarian carcinoma. Cisplatin has found widespread use in the treatment of solid tumors, including metastatic testicular carcinoma in combination with vinblastine and bleomycin, ovarian carcinoma in combination with cyclophosphamide, and bladder carcinoma alone [70].

7.5.8.2 Carboplatin

Carboplatin is a second-generation platinum complex that is intended to maintain anti-tumor efficacy while reducing nephrotoxicity, ototoxicity, and neurotoxicity. Its mechanism of action is the same as that of cisplatin. It binds to the plasma proteins and crosses the blood–brain barrier. Carboplatin is primarily eliminated (about 75%) by glomerular filtration [7].

After administration of the drug, vomiting occurs for 1 hour and continues for as long as 5 days. Other toxicities include ototoxicity with high-frequency hearing loss and tinnitus [10]. Concurrent use of potentially nephrotoxic agents (for example, conventional amphotericin, tacrolimus) with carboplatin should be avoided [17].

This drug is used when patients cannot be energetically hydrated, which most would consider normal for cisplatin treatment [10]. Carboplatin is effective against small cell and non-small cell lung cancer, ovarian cancer, head and neck cancer, and a variety of other cancers. Myelosuppression is its most common dose-limiting side effect, with thrombocytopenia being more severe than leukopenia [9].

7.5.8.3 Oxaliplatin

Oxaliplatin is a platinum derivative of the third generation with the additional mechanism of inhibiting DNA replication and transcription. Approximately 33% to 40% of the oxaliplatin dose is bound to erythrocytes and plasma proteins after intravenous administration. The platinum-containing metabolites of oxaliplatin are primarily excreted in the urine (about 50% of the dose within 3 days), while feces excretion is minor (about 5% of the dose after 11 days) [17]. This drug is used in the treatment of colorectal cancer, gastroesophageal cancer, and pancreatic cancer [10].

Concurrent administration of irinotecan as a 1-hour infusion immediately after a 2-hour infusion of oxaliplatin resulted in more severe hyper-salivation and abdominal pain [17]. Cold-induced peripheral neuropathy is a distinct side effect of oxaliplatin that usually resolves within 72 hours of administration. Neurotoxicity, hepatotoxicity, and myelosuppression are its most common side effects [5].

7.5.9 Topoisomerase Inhibitors

7.5.9.1 Irinotecan

Irinotecan is a semi-synthetic camptothecin derivative. A complex tree found in China called *Camptothecaacuminata* is used to extract camptothecin. This medication specifically inhibits topoisomerase I in the S-phase, which is necessary for DNA replication in human cells [5].

It is a prodrug that is decarboxylated to the active metabolite SN-38 in the liver [5]. Irinotecan is primarily used to treat metastatic/advanced colorectal carcinoma, but it is also used to treat cancers of the lung, cervix, ovary, and stomach. It was mixed with 5-FU and leucovorin. It is also used in the treatment of colorectal malignant growth, little cell cellular breakdown in the lungs, and GI cancers [9].

Potent CYP3A4 inhibitors like ketoconazole and itraconazole reduce the formation of inactive aminopentane-carboxylic acid from irinotecan, resulting in higher concentrations of the active metabolite SN-38 [17]. Diarrhea is its dose-limiting toxicity. Other side effects include neutropenia, thrombocytopenia, hemorrhage, body ache, and weakness. Common side effects include bone marrow suppression, diarrhea, nausea, vomiting, and myelosuppression [3].

7.5.9.2 Topotecan

Topotecan is S-phase specific and inhibits topoisomerase I, which is required for DNA replication in human cells [5]. It is primarily excreted unchanged in the urine. Approximately 49% of the intravenous dose is recovered as the parent drug in the urine and 18% in the feces. Because of its high water solubility, topotecan does not cause urinary toxicity even at high urinary concentrations. Topotecan has a low plasma protein binding (7–35%). Topotecan, unlike many other anti-cancer drugs, can enter the central nervous system. More than 30% of the plasma concentration can be recovered in cerebrospinal fluid if the blood–brain barrier is intact [17].

Topotecan has been approved for the treatment of advanced pretreated ovarian and small-cell lung cancer in several countries. It is also useful in the treatment of metastatic ovarian carcinoma, and headstrong cervical disease. Administration of cisplatin before topotecan has a sequence-dependent effect on topotecan disposition [71]. The toxic effects of topotecan include hemorrhagic cystitis, leukopenia, and thrombocytopenia. Furthermore, during phase I studies, patients experienced sterile hemorrhagic cystitis, myelosuppression, and gastrointestinal side effects. Other toxic effects include myelosuppression, and acute, and delayed diarrhea [9].

7.5.9.3 Etoposide and Teniposide

Etoposide and teniposide are semi-synthetic derivatives of podophyllin, which was isolated from the root of the Indian podophyllum plant originally [17]. Within the tumor cell, etoposide and teniposide interact with topoisomerase II. This nuclear enzyme, which is most active during the late S and G2, phases of the cell cycle, catalyzes the passage of DNA across adjacent strands during cell division. If the tumor cell is exposed to etoposide during this stage, the enzyme-DNA complex is stabilized, resulting in double- and single-strand breaks in DNA as well as cell-cycle arrest.

Etoposide is administered intravenously and reaches the peak plasma concentration. The half-life of etoposide is 7.1 hours. Approximately 96% of the etoposide dose is bound to plasma proteins, with the remaining 4% being unbound. Teniposide undergoes more extensive metabolic degradation than etoposide, yielding the catechol derivative 4'-demethyldeoxypodophyllotoxin [17]. Etoposide is effective in testicular tumors, Hodgkin's disease, other lymphomas, ovarian carcinoma, gastric carcinoma, breast cancer, small-cell, and non-small-cell lung cancers, and cancers of unknown origin, bladder cancer, acute lymphoblastic leukemia, and glioblastoma.

Etoposide serum concentrations increased when etoposide and high-dose cyclosporine were administered together. Etoposide and teniposide are CYP3A4 substrates, and inducers such as carbamazepine, phenobarbital, phenytoin, rifampicin, and St. John's wort increase their clearance rate [17]. A 38-year-old man with advanced testicular cancer experienced hypotension, bronchospasm, and facial flushing after receiving an intravenous infusion of etoposide. Its side effects include myelosuppression, nausea, and vomiting. Exposure to etoposide and teniposide has been linked to an increased risk of developing secondary acute myelogenous leukemia [9].

7.6 CONCLUSION

Despite the fact that "cancer growth" as a disease has not completely been eradicated. It still poses a significant challenge for physicians and future researchers. Patient satisfaction and treatment benefit discussions have taken center stage and continue to be a major source of concern in this therapeutic domain. Given the specific hereditary irregularity present in the cancer cells, much effort is needed towards genotyping of cancer tissue, which can guide optimal pharmaceutical combination for the best benefit of the patient.

REFERENCES

1. Sithranga Boopathy, N. and K. Kathiresan, *Anticancer drugs from marine flora: An overview. Journal of Oncology*, 2010. **2010**.
2. Gaitonde, B.B. *The Pathophysiologic Basis of Drug Therapy*, ed. P. David E. Golan MD. 2014, London: Wolters Kluwer.
3. G.katzungg, B., *Basic and Clinical Pharmacology*. Vol. 12. 2012, New York: The McGraw-Hill Companies.
4. Dales, R.A., *Rang and Dales pharmacology*. Vol. 8. 2016, London: Elsevier Ltd.
5. Tripathi, J. K., *Essentials of Medical Pharmacology*, ed. M. Tripathi. Vol. 6. 2008, New Delhi: Jaypee Brothers Medical Publishers.
6. Kluwer, W., *Handbook of Cancer Chemotherapy*, ed. R.T. Skeel. Vol. 8. 2011, New York: Williams and Wilkins.
7. Rhitter, J. M., L.D. Lewis, and A. Ferro, *A Textbook of Clinical Pharmacology and Therapeutics*. Vol. 5. 2008, London: Hodder Arnold.
8. Hannoodee, M. and M. Mittal, *Methotrexate*, 2021. In StatPearls [Internet]. Treasure Island: StatPearls Publishing.
9. Gillman, G.A., *The Pharmacological Basic of Therapeutics*, ed. P. Laurence L. Brunton. Vol. 13. 2018, New York: McGraw-Hill Education.
10. Whalen, K., *Lippincott Illustrated Reviews: Pharmacology*, ed. P.D. Richard Finkel. 2015, London: Wolters Kluwer.
11. Bethesda, M., *The American Society of Health-System Pharmacists*. 2022.
12. Cunha, J. P., *Antimetabolites*. 2022. In StatPearls [Internet]. Treasure Island: StatPearls Publishing.
13. Clemens, W., H. Wiendl, H.P. Hartung, O. Stuve, and B.C. Kieseier. *Identification of targets and new developments in the treatment of multiple sclerosis--focus on cladribine, Drug Design, Development and Therapy*, 2010. **21**(4): pp. 117–126.
14. Hermann, R., et al., *The clinical pharmacology of cladribine tablets for the treatment of relapsing multiple sclerosis. Clinical Pharmacokinetics*, 2019. **58**(3): pp. 283–297.
15. Dost-Kovalsky, K., et al., *Cladribine and pregnancy in women with multiple sclerosis: the first cohort study. Multiple Sclerosis Journal*, 2022: p. 13524585221131486.
16. Pinedo H.M., and G.F. Peters., *Fluorouracil: biochemistry and pharmacology. Journal of Clinical Oncology*. 1988. **6**(10): pp. 1653–1664.
17. Aronson, J.K. *Meyler's side effect of drugs used in cancer and immunology. Journal of Clinical Oncology*. 2010. Oxford: Elsevier.
18. Faruqi, A. and P. Tadi, *Cytarabine*. 2020. In StatPearls [Internet]. Treasure Island: StatPearls Publishing.
19. Chhikara, B.S. and K. Parang, *Development of cytarabine prodrugs and delivery systems for leukemia treatment. Expert Opinion on Drug Delivery*, 2010. **7**(12): pp. 1399–1414.
20. Reese, N.D. and G.J. Schiller, *High-dose cytarabine (HD araC) in the treatment of leukemias: A review. Current Hematologic Malignancy Reports*, 2013. **8**(2): pp. 141–148.
21. Chu, E., and A.C. Sartorelli, *Cancer Chemotherapy*. 2018, *Lange's Basic and Clinical Pharmacology*, James H. New York: McGraw Hill. pp.948–976.
22. Stentoft, J., *The toxicity of cytarabine. Drug Safety*, 1990. **5**(1): pp. 7–27.
23. Keating, G.M., *Azacitidine. Drugs*, 2012. **72**(8): pp. 1111–1136.
24. Derissen, E.J., J.H. Beijnen, and J.H. Schellens, *Concise drug review: azacitidine and decitabine. The Oncologist*, 2013. **18**(5): pp. 619–624.
25. Wong, A., et al., *Clinical pharmacology and pharmacogenetics of gemcitabine. Drug Metabolism Reviews*, 2009. **41**(2): pp. 77–88.
26. Gupta, N., et al., *Gemcitabine-induced pulmonary toxicity: case report and review of the literature. American Journal of Clinical Oncology*, 2002. **25**(1): pp. 96–100.
27. Seidman, E.G., *Clinical use and practical application of TPMT enzyme and 6-mercaptopurine metabolite monitoring in IBD. Reviews in Gastroenterological Disorders,* 2003. **3**: pp. S30–8.
28. Nielsen, O., B. Vainer, and J. Rask-Madsen, *The treatment of inflammatory bowel disease with 6-mercaptopurine or azathioprine. Alimentary Pharmacology & Therapeutics*, 2001. **15**(11): pp. 1699–1708.

29. Present, D.H., et al., *6-Mercaptopurine in the management of inflammatory bowel disease: short-and long-term toxicity. Annals of Internal Medicine*, 1989. **111**(8): pp. 641–649.
30. Zhenchuk, A., et al., *Mechanisms of anti-cancer action and pharmacology of clofarabine. Biochemical Pharmacology*, 2009. **78**(11): pp. 1351–1359.
31. Kantarjian, H.M., et al., *Clofarabine: past, present, and future. Leukemia & Lymphoma*, 2007. **48**(10): pp. 1922–1930.
32. Sanford, M. and K.A. Lyseng-Williamson, *Nelarabine. Drugs*, 2008. **68**(4): pp. 439–448.
33. Brogden, R.N. and E.M. Sorkin, *Pentostatin. Drugs*, 1993. **46**(4): pp. 652–677.
34. Johnson-Arbor, K. and R. Dubey, *Doxorubicin*. 2017. In StatPearls [Internet]. Treasure Island: StatPearls Publishing.
35. Thorn, C.F., et al., *Doxorubicin pathways: pharmacodynamics and adverse effects. Pharmacogenetics and Genomics*, 2011. **21**(7): p. 440.
36. Zhang, H., et al., *Daunorubicin-TiO2 nanocomposites as a "smart" pH-responsive drug delivery system. International Journal of Nanomedicine*, 2012. **7**: p. 235.
37. Saleem, T. and A. Kasi, *Daunorubicin*. 2020. In StatPearls [Internet]. Treasure Island: StatPearls Publishing.
38. Tacar, O., P. Sriamornsak, and C.R. Dass, *Doxorubicin: an update on anticancer molecular action, toxicity and novel drug delivery systems. Journal of Pharmacy and Pharmacology*, 2013. **65**(2): pp. 157–170.
39. Yamamoto, T., *Bleomycin and the skin. British Journal of Dermatology*, 2006. **155**(5): pp. 869–875.
40. Dorr, R.T. *Bleomycin pharmacology: mechanism of action and resistance, and clinical pharmacokinetics. Seminars in Oncology*. 1992. **19**(2 Suppl 5): pp. 3–8.
41. Brandt, J.P. and V. Gerriets, *Bleomycin*. 2020. In StatPearls [Internet]. Treasure Island: StatPearls Publishing.
42. Khaja, M., et al., *Mitomycin-induced thrombotic thrombocytopenic purpura treated successfully with plasmapheresis and steroid: a case report. Cureus*, 2022. **14**(3): pp. e23525.
43. Sinawe, H. and D. Casadesus, *Mitomycin*. 2020. In StatPearls [Internet]. Treasure Island: StatPearls Publishing.
44. Ogino, M.H. and P. Tadi, *Cyclophosphamide*. 2020. In StatPearls [Internet]. Treasure Island: StatPearls Publishing.
45. Volkmer, B.G., et al., *Cyclophosphamide is contraindicated in patients with a history of transitional cell carcinoma. Clinical Rheumatology*, 2005. **24**(4): pp. 319–323.
46. Skinner, R., et al., *Nephrotoxicity after ifosfamide. Archives of Disease in Childhood*, 1990. **65**(7): pp. 732–738.
47. Steven, H., and Lin, L.R., *Carmustine wafers: Localized delivery of chemotherapeutic agents in CNS malignancies. National Library of Medicine*, 2008. **8**(3): pp. 343–359.
48. Chen, X., et al., *Progress in clinical application of carmustine. Hans Journal of Medicinal Chemistry*, 2018. **6**(4): pp. 97–105.
49. Pourahmad, J., et al., *Biological reactive intermediates that mediate dacarbazine cytotoxicity. Cancer Chemotherapy and Pharmacology*, 2009. **65**(1): pp. 89–96.
50. Liu, Q., et al., *Dacarbazine-loaded hollow mesoporous silica nanoparticles grafted with folic acid for enhancing antimetastatic melanoma response. ACS Applied Materials & Interfaces*, 2017. **9**(26): pp. 21673–21687.
51. Below, J., *Vincristine*. 2019. In StatPearls [Internet]. Treasure Island: StatPearls Publishing.
52. Zhang, Y.-W., et al., *Vinblastine and vincristine. In Natural Small Molecule Drugs from Plants*. 2018, New York: Springer. pp. 551–557.
53. Rosenthal, S. and S. Kaufman, *Vincristine neurotoxicity. Annals of Internal Medicine*, 1974. **80**(6): pp. 733–737.
54. Zhang, Z., L. Mei, and S.-S. Feng, *Paclitaxel drug delivery systems. Expert Opinion on Drug Delivery*, 2013. **10**(3): pp. 325–340.
55. Bergmann, T.K., et al., *Retrospective study of the impact of pharmacogenetic variants on paclitaxel toxicity and survival in patients with ovarian cancer. European Journal of Clinical Pharmacology*, 2011. **67**(7): pp. 693–700.
56. Wilson, A.C., et al., *Leuprolide acetate: a drug of diverse clinical applications. Expert Opinion on Investigational Drugs*, 2007. **16**(11): pp. 1851–1863.

57. Swayzer, D.V. and V. Gerriets, *Leuprolide*, 2021. In StatPearls [Internet]. Treasure Island: StatPearls Publishing.

58. Cheer, S.M., et al., *Goserelin. Drugs*, 2005. **65**(18): pp. 2639–2655.

59. Ploussard, G. and P. Mongiat-Artus, *Triptorelin in the management of prostate cancer. Future Oncology*, 2013. **9**(1): pp. 93–102.

60. Boekhout, A.H., J.H. Beijnen, and J.H. Schellens, *Trastuzumab. The Oncologist*, 2011. **16**(6): pp. 800–810.

61. Garnock-Jones, K.P., G.M. Keating, and L.J. Scott, *Trastuzumab. Drugs*, 2010. **70**(2): pp. 215–239.

62. Keefe, D.L., *Trastuzumab-associated cardiotoxicity. Cancer*, 2002. **95**(7): pp. 1592–1600.

63. Plosker, G.L. and D.P. Figgitt, *Rituximab. Drugs*, 2003. **63**(8): pp. 803–843.

64. Randall, K.L., *Rituximab in autoimmune diseases. Australian Prescriber*, 2016. **39**(4): p. 131.

65. Mukherji, S., *Bevacizumab (avastin). American Journal of Neuroradiology*, 2010. **31**(2): pp. 235–236.

66. Grisanti, S. and F. Ziemssen, *Bevacizumab: Off-label use in ophthalmology. Indian Journal of Ophthalmology*, 2007. **55**(6): p. 417.

67. Gressett, S.M. and S.R. Shah, *Intricacies of bevacizumab-induced toxicities and their management. Annals of Pharmacotherapy*, 2009. **43**(3): pp. 490–501.

68. Lenz, H.-J., *Anti-EGFR mechanism of action: antitumor effect and underlying cause of adverse events. Oncology (Williston Park, NY)*, 2006. **20**(5 Suppl 2): pp. 5–13.

69. Chidharla, A., M. Parsi, and A. Kasi, *Cetuximab*. 2017. In StatPearls [Internet]. Treasure Island: StatPearls Publishing.

70. Gold, J. and A. Raja, *Cisplatin (Cisplatinum)*. 2019. In StatPearls [Internet]. Treasure Island: StatPearls Publishing.

71. Enomoto, Y., et al., *Safety of topotecan monotherapy for relapsed small cell lung cancer patients with pre-existing interstitial lung disease. Cancer Chemotherapy and Pharmacology*, 2015. **76**(3): pp. 499–505.

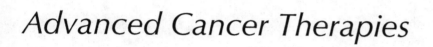

Advanced Cancer Therapies

8 The Advent of Micro- and Nanospheres for Cancer Treatment

Asia Naz Awan, Rabia Iqtadar, Sabahat Abdullah, Muhammad Yasir Ali, and Imran Tariq

8.1 INTRODUCTION

Since the discovery of cancer as a disease, a millennium ago, scientists have extensively investigated treatment regimens that may contribute to the complete recovery of patients from this disease. Cancer treatment is a combination of surgery, radiation, immunotherapy, gene therapy, bone marrow and peripheral blood stem cell transplantation, laser therapy, hyperthermia, photodynamic therapy, classical antitumor drugs, or targeted nanomedicine.

The evolution of nanotechnology has offered new avenues for cancer treatment as it has been evidenced to enhance the cure rates and mitigate severe side effects arising due to the lack of selectivity of conventional anticancer agents for cancer cells (Figure 8.1). Thus, it benefits healthcare practitioners to develop and provide efficient anticancer drugs with a negligible or minimum range of side effects along with the maximum therapeutic value.

8.2 MICROSPHERES AND NANOSPHERES

Spherical drug delivery particles, such as microspheres and nanospheres are increasingly being used for diagnostic and therapeutic purposes. Solid spherical particles having an approximate diameter of 1–1000 microns are characterized as microspheres [1] while the particles from 1–500 nm are nanocarriers [2] with nanospheres in generally the 10–200 nm range [3]. These dimensions must include the suspended drug particles as well. As microspheres and nanospheres differ from each other in dimensions and in turn their application in cancer treatment, both can be used as targeted drug carriers. These materials can be used for encapsulating the drugs/bioactive molecules to be released in a controlled manner. The resulting microspheres are rigid and can be packed to create a porous 3D-structured scaffold together, alone, or in combination with other biomaterials. A variety of drugs may be incorporated within the microspheres owing to their biocompatibility, due to their preparation from biodegradable particles. Microspheres in drug delivery are used for targeted as well as prolonged drug release in the diseased area. It also protects the unstable or pH-sensitive drugs before and after the administration.

8.3 CATEGORIES OF MICRO/NANOSPHERES BASED ON VARIOUS CRITERIA

The prime difference in micro/nanospheres is their dimension (Figure 8.2), hence both can be collectively categorized based on various criteria. This section identifies and explores the classifying categories of micronanospheres.

DOI: 10.1201/9781003363958-11

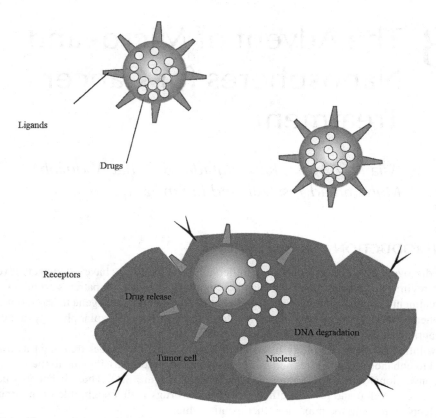

FIGURE 8.1   Nanomedicine drug release at the receptor level.

8.4   TYPES OF MICRO/NANOSPHERES BASED ON THEIR CONFIGURATION

8.4.1   MICRO/NANOSPHERE-INCORPORATING SCAFFOLDS

In this type, the micronanospheres merely serve as one component of the scaffold. The one-component scaffold is mostly inorganic in nature such as a few nanometers of gold nano-spheres are often used to construct gold-nano aggregates for photothermal therapy (PTT) in cancers. These particles are able to adsorb light energy directly or serve as carriers to deliver photoactive agents and are widely explored in photoimmunotherapy (PIT) [4, 5]. Another example is silver nano-spheres are potent bactericides and chemotherapeutic agents. A particle size of approximately 100 nm is more strongly prone to induce these effects than the smaller particles ranging up to 10 nm. These particles have found their applications in improving the resolution of existing imaging techniques or replacing fluorescent molecules as image contrast agents or biosensors [6–8].

8.4.2   MICRO/NANOSPHERE-BASED SCAFFOLDS (BUILDING BLOCKS OF THE SCAFFOLD FRAMEWORK)

In this type of micro- and nanosphere-based scaffolds, the atoms within nanoparticles are carefully ordered with micro- to nanosize dimensions that are rigid and may be packed together, alone or in conjunction with other biomaterials like with lipid, protein, silica, carbon, and metals to produce a structural scaffold. This results in superior materials with greater capabilities. They are able to address long-term issues including drug solubility, systemic distribution, tumor acquired resistance,

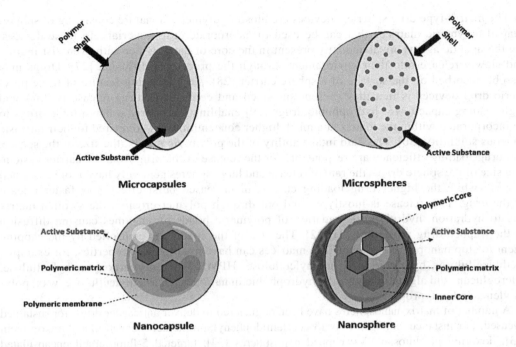

FIGURE 8.2 Morphology of micro/nanosphere and capsule.

TABLE 8.1
Micro/Nanosphere-Based Scaffold Building Blocks for Anticancer Drugs

Type of Nanosphere	Anti-Cancer Drug Loaded on Nanospheres
Lipid-based	Niclosamide [9], floxuridine [10], indirubin [11]
Protein-based	Gemcitabine [12], doxorubicin [13], docetaxel [14],
Carbon-based	5-FU [15], co-delivery of doxorubicin/cisplatin [16], and curcumin/paclitaxel [17]
Metal-based	Gold nanospheres encapsulate doxorubicin [18], methotrexate [19] loaded silver nanospheres, iron oxide nanospheres co-delivers doxorubicin/cisplatin [20]
Silica-based	Doxorubicin [21], gemcitabine [22], and co-delivery of doxorubicin/paclitaxel [23]

and enhance the performance of diagnostic methods in different cancer treatment modalities. Some of these scaffolds for anticancer drugs are summarized in Table 8.1.

8.5 TYPES OF MICRO/NANOSPHERES BASED ON THEIR DRUG LOADING

Some spheres can be classified as matrix systems (monolithic-type) in which the drug is homogeneously dispersed, either dissolved or homogenously suspended [24], while the capsules (reservoir-type) are heterogenous particles where a membrane shell is surrounding the core forming a reservoir [25, 26]. A matrix system is one where the drug is dispersed in very small particles into a solid and homogeneous block of polymer or release-retardant substance. A reservoir system is a macrocapsule, where a big particle of a drug (or many agglomerated particles of the drug) is covered by a polymer or other release-retardant material forming a wall through which the drug must diffuse to be released.

The matrix-type drug spherical devices are mostly polymeric in nature consisting of sphere-shaped polymeric matrices that can be used to incorporate drug materials. In these devices, the therapeutic agents are abundantly present in the core of the polymer with even distribution and slowly release into their environment through the process of diffusion [27]. Drugs may also be adsorbed on the surface of a sphere carrier [28]. An interesting feature of these polymeric drug devices is that they present sustained and controllable drug-release profiles and high-loading capacity for hydrophobic drugs [29] enabling the poorly water-soluble drugs to be incorporated within the matrix at a much higher concentration as compared to their intrinsic aqueous solubility [30]. The fluid intake ability of the polymeric matrix, the size of the sphere, and drug-loading efficiency are responsible for the release of the drug from the carrier system. The size of the sphere drives the rate of release and large spheres generally have more sustained release, while the higher drug loading causes an increased burst effect thus faster release of the drug. This release is mostly carried out through polymer erosion, the swollen matrix due to hydration, hydrolytic degradation of polymeric bonds by enzymes causing diffusion of the trapped drug molecules [31, 32]. The size of the spheres is controlled by the capping agent to stop nanoparticle growth. The matrices can have hydrophilic properties, for example, methylcellulose, hydroxypropyl methylcellulose HPMS, sodium carboxymethylcellulose, scleroglucan, and alginates or may be hydrophobic in nature, such as ethylcellulose, wax, polyethylene, and polypropylene.

A number of matrix-nanospheres have been engineered to deliver anticancer drugs for sustained released. For instance, collagen-poly (3-acrylamidophenylboronic acid) encapsulated doxorubicin [33], doxorubicin chitosan PVP capped nanospheres [34], targeted 5-fluorouracil encapsulated chitosan-carbon spheres [35, 36], cisplatin loaded lipid-chitosan hybrid nanospheres [37], curcumin PEGylated nanospheres coated with iron oxide [38] and cytarabine encapsulated poly (ε-caprolactone) (PCL) matrix based spherical nanoparticles. These reported micro/nanospheres showed a sustained release pattern, preventing the diffusion of drug and water penetration into the core providing long circulating characteristics with fewer side effects.

8.6 TYPES OF MICRO/NANOSPHERES BASED ON ROUTE OF ADMINISTRATION

8.6.1 ORAL ROUTE OF ADMINISTRATION

Polymers are generally used as a building block for the preparation of drug-delivering systems. These polymers confer biodegradability, biocompatibility, long-lasting circulation, and reduced toxicity profile to the micro/nanospheres and to the drugs entrapped. They are also useful delivery systems for an optimized release of the encapsulated drug at site of action.

The advantages of oral drug delivery including ease of use, reliability, and substantial therapeutic efficiency make it a preferred route of administration. However, the oral delivery of chemotherapeutic drugs proposes many challenges, for instance, poor aqueous solubility, membrane permeability, retarded bioavailability due to degradation by chemicals and enzymes. The factors that affect the solubility of a drug are its nature, the polymorphic form, crystalline structure and particle size, and the amount of drug in the pharmaceutical dosage form [39]. The rate-limiting parameter of most anticancer drugs is their release from the pharmaceutical dosage form and in turn their solubility at acidic pH in the gastric environment [40]. These therapeutic agents are dissolved, entrapped, encapsulated, or attached to the matrix of inert polymer, lipid, carbon, lipids, or ceramics including silica, alumina, and calcium phosphate. Biodegradable micro/nanospheres include albumin nanospheres, polypropylene dextran nanospheres, gelatin nano-spheres, modified starch nanospheres, polylactic acid nanospheres, poly-lactic acid (PLA), poly -D- L-glycolide (PLG), poly-D- l-lactide-co-glycolide (PLGA), and poly-cyanoacrylate (PCA).

Doxorubicin a potent anticancer drug shows poor oral bioavailability this challenge is met by encapsulating the drug into amphiphilic PEGylated PLGA nanosphere [41, 42] or cationic nanospherical micelles of PLGA-b-bPEI-b-PLGA that shows increased absorption, prolonged circulation time, and drug penetration into tumor tissues [43]. Similarly, Paclitaxel encapsulated into PLGA-vitE-TPGS [44], 20-80 sized PEG phosphatidylethanolamine nanospheres that increased the water solubility of the drug to 5000 times, showed spontaneous penetration through the interstitium of various tissues, improved permeation efficiency and retention time [45].

8.6.2 LOCAL ROUTE OF ADMINISTRATION

Docetaxel is a commonly used drug for the treatment of breast cancer. Pluronic F108 nanospheres utilize polymeric poly-ε-caprolactone to entrap noninvasive infrared (NIR) dye and the hydrophobic docetaxel molecules for studying the drug localization and cell uptake of spherical nanoparticles in the treatment of breast cancer. The delayed and sustained release of the drug from nanospheres and the localization in the solid tumor cells of the breast and lymphatic system [46]. Spherical micro/nanoparticles acting locally can contribute to the increasing concentration of the drug in the tumor area, decreasing systemic adverse effects, overcome gastrointestinal effects such as incompatibilities and first-pass metabolism.

Catechol-modified chitosan/hyaluronic acid (HA) nanospheres were developed to deliver doxorubicin. These spherical nanoparticles allowed high cellular uptake and excellent adhesion of the carrier to the oral mucosa and sustained local delivery of a drug into the oral cavity. The designed nano-spheres showed potent in vitro anticancer effects against oral carcinoma by inducing apoptosis in cells more extensively compared with free doxorubicin [47]. Cisplatin-loaded poly butyl cyanoacrylate (PBCA) nanospheres were designed through the inflection of temperature and polyethylene glycol (PEG) concentration to improve the cytotoxicity, potency, and drug loading efficiency of cisplatin. These nanospheres are used for the treatment of non-small cell lung cancer [48].

8.6.3 SYSTEMIC ROUTE OF ADMINISTRATION

Systemic administration of the therapeutic agents allows protection from hepatic clearance (first-pass effect) and enzymatic degradation in the gastrointestinal tract, which allows a better pharmacokinetic profile at the cancer site. The drugs may be delivered systemically via a variety of routes such as intravenous, intramuscular, and subcutaneous being the most commonly employed. Other routes are intra-arterial, intrathecal, intraperitoneal, and intravitreal, which are used less frequently.

Synthetic polymers are used predominantly for designing drug carriers. Polymers, such as poly(lactic-co-glycolic acid) (PLGA), poly(lactic acid) (PLA), poly(ethylene glycol) (PEG), poly(methyl methacrylate) (PMMA), poly(ethyleneimine) (PEI), poly(methylene malonate) (PMM), and polyesters have been used to form systemically administered nanoparticles [49]. The surface properties of the polymeric nanoparticles can be altered with numerous moieties, for instance, ligands and drugs, to deliver multimodal treatment. Although synthetic polymers are preferably used, some natural polymers, such as proteins, lipids, polysaccharides, lipids, and polypeptides, have also been utilized [50]. The prime advantage of biopolymers as compared to synthetic polymers is biodegradability due to enzymatic degradation in natural environments, complemented by the release of nonhazardous byproducts that can also be removed biologically [51].

The nanoformulation must be inert and stable for systemic administration. The nanomaterials used must not only protect the drug from the systemic effects of the human body but also impart a controlled release at the tumor site [52]. Moreover, the nanodrug delivery for effective cancer therapies will enter a new era after continuing discoveries in the field of biomarkers and target moieties.

Systemic administration of nanodrugs offers some challenges in terms of possible allergic reactions due to the formulation components. These problems may be addressed by optimizing the formulation characteristics in terms of optimum polymer concentration, surfactant concentration, and the amount of organic solvent as in the case of an intravenous formulation of paclitaxel entrapped in PLGA nanospheres, which is kept free of its non-ionic solubilizer and emulsifier, cremophor EL due to its allergen properties [53].

Another example of a systemic nanodrug is intravitreal topotecan encapsulated in thiolated chitosan nanospheres, which is used for the treatment of retinoblastoma. The nanocarrier improves the effectiveness of the therapy at the tumor site and promotes cell penetration. It also attempts to overcome intravitreal administration challenges, such as poor cellular uptake due to anatomical barriers and the stability of the drug. The surface of the chitosan was modified with the thiol group may enhance the in vivo drug delivery to the target site and improve the management of retinoblastoma [54].

Another nanoformulation, doxorubicin-loaded PEGylated silver nanospheres was designed against breast cancer. This specifically created nanoformulation serves as an effective vehicle for doxorubicin with high drug loading, sustained drug delivery, enhanced synergistic cytotoxicity, and fewer side effects on other healthy cells [55].

8.7 TYPES OF MICRO/NANOSPHERES BASED ON DRUG RELEASE

8.7.1 BIOADHESIVE SPHERES

Micro/nanospheres exhibiting mucoadhesive property, which causes the drug coating on the polymer surface to adsorb to the cancerous organ, resulting in extended delivery of anticancer therapeutic moieties to the tumor site. The surface layer of several organs such as lung airways, gastrointestinal tract, and other tissues with mucosal lining is protected by the viscoelastic mucus. Such organs are not effectively targeted with the microspheres as they may be trapped and removed by the mucus gel. Nanospheres approximating to 200 nm in diameter offer much higher distribution in the mucus, hence the increased tissue penetration as compared to the drug-loaded microspheres as observed in the nanoformulation loaded with budesonide used for the treatment of inflammatory bowel disease in the rodent model. Particle morphology plays an important role in targeting skin tissue for nanodelivery. Cylindrical particles are found to have more distribution in the mucus as compared to the spherical systems. Bioadhesive drug-delivery systems are suitable for drug agents that cannot be administered orally due to hepato-gastric effects. These drug-delivery systems can be controlled by the physicochemical parameters of the polymers in the formulation and also by the nature of the targeted mucosal layer [56].

Polymers that may impart mucoadhesive properties to the drug-delivery system are chitosan, poly(acrylic acid) or carbopol, poly(vinyl pyrrolidone), poly(vinyl alcohol), poly(ethylene glycol), poly(hydroxyethyl methacrylate), etc. The degree of adhesion could be influenced by the hydrophilicity, crosslinking, and swelling ability, molecular weight, spatial orientation, and the concentration of the bioadhesive polymer. It may also be altered by temperature changes, pH, and any supplementary influencing agent in the polymeric dispersion. These polymers have been extensively investigated to facilitate prolonged bioavailability at the tumor site with predictable drug release patterns to improve the efficacy of anticancer agents [56].

Examples of bioadhesive drug-delivery systems containing doxorubicin include maleimide-bearing chitosan, catechol-bearing alginate, PEGylated mucoadhesive nanoparticles, and catechol-modified chitosan/hyaluronic acid (HA) nanospheres. These systems produced an effective cellular uptake of the drug and potent anticancer action in the treatment of bladder cancer [57], non-small-cell lung cancer [58], and oral cancers [47]. The pegylated nanospheres are unique in the fact that they are administered through inhalers and are pH-triggered.

8.7.2 Magnetic Spheres

The spheres containing magnetic particles and having the potential to be utilized for targeted drug delivery are termed as magnetic micro/nanospheres and can be applied for diagnostic procedures as well. These systems are commonly used for magnetic hyperthermia in tumor tissues, though an external magnetic source is required to direct these magnetic drug carriers to the targeted diseased area [59].

Superparamagnetic iron oxide nanoparticles (SPIONs) have been used as a contrast agent for the identification of cell surface markers expressed on tumors and show considerable in vivo activity. Due to the tendency of SPIONs to be absorbed by liver macrophages, polymeric covering was developed to avoid this interaction.

The dual-modal imaging and photothermal effect of hyaluronan (HA)-modified superparamagnetic iron oxide nanoparticles (HA-SPIONs) were investigated for CD44 HA receptor-overexpressing breast cancer. Both in vitro and in vivo results demonstrated that HA-SPIONs exhibited significant negative contrast enhancement on the receptor surface and indicated to have great potential for effective diagnosis and treatment of cancer [60].

The synthesized SPIONs were coated with a fine layer of silica then further modification was done by a polymeric layering of di-carboxylate polyethylene glycol and carboxylate-methoxy polyethylene glycol these nanostructures were co-loaded with doxorubicin and cisplatin these efforts were made to increase the stability, biocompatibility and drug loading capacity of nanospheres pH and NIR irradiation successfully induced the release of both drugs. At the practical dosage, PEGylated silica-coated iron oxide nanospheres (PS-IONs) showed excellent cellular absorption without harming the cell show cytocompatibility and hemocompatibility. PS-IONs are a multifunctional targeted co-delivery system and an acceptable MRI agent with the advantage of utilizing the right combination therapy for the treatment of breast cancer [61].

The magnetic properties of the cobalt reveal that they exhibit a mixture of superparamagnetic and soft ferromagnetic behavior by utilizing this feature superparamagnetic cobalt nanoparticles were designed for the imaging of breast and colon cancer by Raman spectroscopy. A rapid cellular uptake of the cobalt nanospheres was observed as they easily penetrate the cell membrane of cancer cells followed by increased apoptosis. These nanoparticles have minimum cytotoxicity as cobalt is well tolerated by human tissues and can easily be eliminated from the body without accumulating. Raman spectroscopy is a convenient method for investigating the interaction between nanomaterials and cells enabling accurate localization of the cobalt metal nanoparticles in a cellular environment. Laser irradiation of metal nanoparticles locally induces combustion of the cobalt metal nanospheres inside the cells, which opens new routes for cancer phototherapy [62].

8.7.3 Hollow Spheres

The solid metal nanoparticles impart their catalytic characteristics due to the high surface/volume ratio and also due to an increased number of kinetically active moieties on the surface of the metal-nano complex. The confinement cage effect may contribute to enhance catalytic activity by alteration to a hollow or porous morphology of the sphere. These structures may involve single-shell metallic and double-shell bimetallic nanocatalysts or supported inside a porous substrate such as a metalorganic framework, hollow polymer nanofibers, or silica shell coatings of a yolk structure.

Hollow gold nanospheres have been designed among many of the gold nanoparticles with a hollow interior space and robust but thin walls surrounding it. Recent research indicated that these provided high photothermal conversion efficiency in treating cancer cells. Hollow gold nanospheres may be functionalized by biological media, such as polyethylene glycerol, proteins, antibodies, DNA, and drugs and then applied to photothermal therapy, photodynamic therapy, and surface plasmon resonance [63].

8.7.4 MESOPOROUS SPHERES

Mesoporous drug carriers should be able to prevent incorporated drugs to be released into the biological environment before reaching to the targeted area. This function usually requires the capping of the open ends on the surface and the inclusion of targeting ligands on the exterior of nanocarriers. In one of the studies, a mesoporous drug carrier system was synthesized with biocompatible gold nanoparticles as the "hard caps", and folic acid conjugated to the surface for targeting folate receptors, which are overexpressed in the cancer cells (Figure 8.3). Disulfide bonds linking the gold and mesoporous nanoparticles were introduced to the surface as redox-sensitive and chemically removable components. The drug release effects were studied in detail by incorporating the drug in

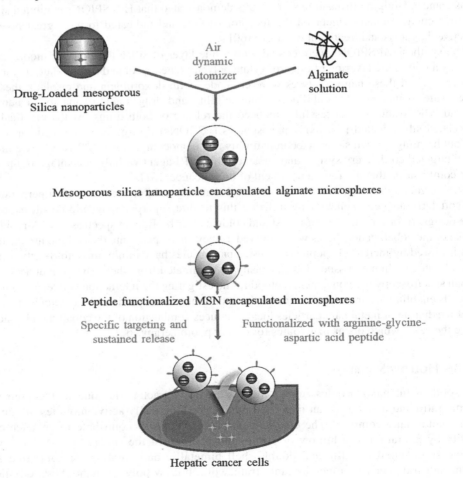

FIGURE 8.3 Mesoporous nanoparticles.

mesoporous silica nanoparticles with hollow structures, large pores mesoporous silica nanoparticles, and typical nanosized pores on the surface [64].

8.7.5 FLOATING SPHERES

Floating micro/nanospheres are meant to release the drugs loaded in them in gastric content. The bulk density of these drug-loaded spheres should be kept lower than the gastric juice so that they can float on the surface, thereby having a prolonged drug release.

The floating drug-delivery system (FDDS) is also called a hydrodynamically balanced system (HBS). FDDS are invented to retain the drug in the stomach thereby also known as a gastroretentive drug delivery system. This system has a lower density than gastric fluids and thus the drug carriers float in the stomach fluid without affecting the gastric emptying and efficiently increase drug bio-availability by prolonging the release period. While the system is floating in the gastric fluid, the drug is released slowly from the system at the desired rate. This system protects those drugs, which are acid labile and have a short half-life. It also improves bioavailability, reduces drug waste, and enhances the residence time of drugs.

The formulation components of floating spheres include chitosan, polyvinyl acetate, eudragit, agar, acrylic resins, and polyacrylates. These polymers in the presence of gastric juices swell to form a colloidal gel barrier from which the drug is released in a controlled manner, the air gets trapped in the swollen polymer, which reduces the density of the system and imparts buoyancy to the microspheres.

In the therapy of pancreatic cancer, floating drug-loaded spheres of paclitaxel were designed by adhering it to gold nanoparticles pre-modified by polydopamine. For structuring this type of drug-delivery system, initially gold nanoparticles and paclitaxel-loaded spheres were developed in which polydopamine was used as a linker to adhere gold nanoparticles to the surface of PLGA microspheres. The designed microspheres exhibited excellent stability in physiological fluids and are suitable for in vivo drug delivery. The combination of drug-loaded polymeric gold microspheres with NIR irradiation can provide a synergistic chemo-photothermal therapy for the treatment of pancreatic cancer [65].

Another example is 5-fluorouracil, a widely used antimetabolite applied as an anticancer agent, possessing poor bioavailability after oral administration. Hollow spheres were designed for use as floating spheres by modification with eudragit to target stomach cancers and increase their localized bioavailability.

8.7.6 RADIOACTIVE MICROSPHERES

Radioactive particles (10–30µm) are used for therapeutic purpose by directly injecting into the veins that are linked to the targeted organ or tissue. These radioactive particles emit three different types of waves: α emitters, β emitters, and γ emitters. There are different techniques to prepare such microspheres, and the process of preparation depends on the size of microspheres, route of administration, duration of drug crosslinking, duration of drug release, etc.

8.8 TYPES OF MICRO/NANOSPHERE BASED ON ORIGIN

Microspheres and nanospheres are polymer-based particles and can be classified based on the origin of the polymer. The polymers obtained through biological species or anthropological means are considered natural polymers while the engineered or synthetic polymers are produced by various methods including physical, biological, chemical, and hybrid of all. The major challenge in the use of polymers is their effect on biological species and the environment, which further classifies

TABLE 8.2
Polymers used in Micro/Nanospheres

Natural	Protein	Albumin, gelatin, collagen
	Carbohydrate	Agarose, starch, carrageenan, chitosan
	Chemically modified carbohydrate	Polydextran, polystarch
Synthetic	Biodegradable	Lactides, glycolides, co-polymer of lactides and glycolides, poly-alkyl-cyano acrylates, polyanhydrides
	Non-biodegradable	Polymethylmethacrylate, acrolein, epoxy polymer, glycidyl methacrylate

them into biodegradable and non-biodegradable polymers. The biodegradable synthetic and natural polymers that are usually consumed are given in Table 8.2.

The matrices used in nanospheres are natural and synthetic polymers or lipids that must meet certain requirements. They should be biodegradable and biocompatible. They cannot be toxic or carcinogenic, should not induce an immune response, and accumulate in the form of metabolic products. As matrices, mostly lactic acid polymers (PLA), glycol acid polymers (PGA), or mixtures of them (PLGA), as well as poly(methyl methacrylate) (PMMA) are used [66].

8.9 GENERAL METHODS FOR THE SYNTHESIS OF MICRO AND NANOSPHERES

8.9.1 ELECTROSPRAY METHOD

One of the most effective ways to create spherical nanoparticles is via the electrospray approach. To make a polymer solution emerge from the syringe as nanoparticles, the concept behind electro-spraying is to apply a high voltage to the polymer solution. The functional electrode in the experimental setup is a syringe pump filled with the polymer solution that is coupled to a high-voltage power source. The ground electrode is a metal foil collector that is positioned across from it. Depending on the type of solution used for electro-spraying, the flow rate and applied voltage were optimized. Because of surface tension, the liquid that emerges from the nozzle and enters the electric field forms a Taylor cone. The cone splits into highly charged droplets when the electric field is increased, and under the appropriate set of conditions, those droplets can attain the micro- or nanosize range [67]. This method offers consistent particle size distribution, effective encapsulation ability, minimal equipment cost, and a quick preparation cycle.

8.9.2 SOLVENT EVAPORATION METHOD

This method is based on the agitation-induced internal phase evaporation of an emulsion. Typically, a volatile organic solvent is used to dissolve the polymeric covering material. The aforesaid polymer solution is then used to dissolve or scatter the drug core, resulting in the formation of a suspension, emulsion, or solution. The organic phase is then emulsified while being stirred in a dispersion phase made up of a polymer diluent that is immiscible with the organic solvent and contains the proper emulsifying agent. After the emulsion has stabilized, the solvent diffuses through the continuous phase and evaporates, leaving behind solid, spherical particles that are recovered by filtration or centrifugation and then cleaned and dried. The systems of solvent evaporation method depend upon the external phase's nature organic or aqueous, the mode of incorporation of the core material that is dissolved, dispersed, or emulsified into the organic solution of the polymer, and the method used to get rid of the organic solvent either evaporation or extraction [68]. Due to its simplicity, scalability, and lower residual solvent potential compared to other procedures, the solvent evaporation method has garnered the most interest.

8.9.3 Sol-Gel Process

The sol-gel approach is one of the chemical processing techniques to develop promising drug-delivery formulations characterized by distinctive spherical nanoparticles. The initial homogeneous molecules (sol) undergo a series of steps and change into the endless, heavy, three-dimensional molecule known as a gel [69]. The process is distinguished by the first step, the development of stable colloidal solutions or sol, and the subsequent polycondensation stage, which creates the gel, a rigid 3D network made of polymeric molecules and encircled by the solvent. Acid-catalyzed acidic solutions produce a homogeneous, weakly crosslinked gel with a pH 6 value. Separate clusters make up the gel structure that is produced from basic or neutral solutions with pH > 6 (base catalyzed). The polymer condensation reactions continue to take place during the aging step, finishing the gel's creation. Additional crosslinks are added to the gel structure to strengthen it, which causes the gel matrix to contract and the solution to escape from the contracting pores. During this phase, the water and other liquids that have become trapped within the pores of the gel structure are removed by drying at a high temperature of roughly 400 °F (~200 °C) [70].

8.9.4 Emulsion Method

The emulsion method is frequently employed when creating nanoparticles to achieve high encapsulation effectiveness, high stability, and minimal toxicity. This method can be carried out by single or double emulsification. The single emulsification process [71] is suitable for hydrophobic drug encapsulation where oil in water emulsion contains a surfactant in the water phase while polymer and drug are in the oil phase. The double emulsification method [72] is appropriate for hydrophilic drugs where a surfactant is present in the external aqueous phase, the polymer is in the oil phase and another surfactant along with the drug is in the internal aqueous phase to obtain (water-in-oil)-in-water emulsion. It is necessary to conduct solvent evaporation in both instances to obtain nanospheres [73].

8.9.5 Nanoprecipitation Method

The method known as nanoprecipitation also referred to as solvent injection, spontaneous emulsification, solvent displacement, solvent diffusion, interfacial deposition, mixing-induced nanoprecipitation, or flash nanoprecipitation, is acknowledged as a practical and adaptable technique for encasing active molecules at the micro- and nanoscale range [74]. An organic polymer solution is emulsified in an aqueous solution using the nanoprecipitation process, either with or without the use of a surfactant. The organic solvent is then eliminated via stirring, either with or without a vacuum, which promotes the creation of nanoparticles. This method entails incorporating active molecules into colloidal drug-delivery systems, and the resulting particles allow for the optimization of the drug in vivo therapeutic performance by displaying traits like controlled release behaviors, target delivery, and improved stability in biological fluids. If the substance to be encapsulated is hydrophilic, this approach has a disadvantage in that the drug may leak out into the aqueous solution.

8.9.6 Coacervation Method

Coacervation is considered a commonly used method for the synthesis of nanoparticles. This process involves the separation of a polymeric solution into two immiscible liquids to generate two phases: a dilute equilibrium and a concentrated coacervate. It is mainly comprised of three steps initially oil-in-water emulsion is formed in which oil globules as a core material are disseminated into the aqueous phase and that phase was coated as a consistent film encircling suspended core particles. The coating is then solidified via heating, crosslinking, or desolvation methods.

Coacervation is broadly classified into simple and complex coacervation. A separation generates two phases in simple coacervation, one of which is saturated with the polymer in solution and the other of which is in equilibrium but depleted of the polymer [75]. A concentrated interface is created in polymers with an opposing charge in complex coacervation, which involves mixing two immiscible liquids. Weak electrostatic interaction creates an interface known as a coacervate [76]. Several advantages that have been noted with coacervation are enhanced resilience to mechanical stress or temperature, as well as providing regulated administration of therapeutic agents inside the particles [77].

8.9.7 Spray Drying Method

The transformation of liquid that is either in the form of a solution or, suspension into a powder can be accomplished in a single step using the spray technique. It is the most well-known and widely used method for creating spherical nanoparticles [78] due to its ability to embody delicate substances, use of mild conditions, accessibility to hardware, and ease of automation to produce drug and or excipients or a drug encapsulation method with the main benefit of obtaining free-flowing powders [79]. The basis of the spray-drying process is the removal of moisture while exposing the feed product to a hot environment. Pumping a solution into an atomizer causes it to disperse the liquid supply into a fine mist. After being discharged into a drying gas chamber, the droplets undergo moisture vaporization and produce dry particles. The dried particles are subsequently removed from the drying medium using the proper apparatus, and they are then collected in a tank.

8.9.8 Ion Gelation Method

Another technique for creating spherical nanoparticles is known as ion gelation. It is based on polymers that can crosslink and uses an electrostatic interaction with an oppositely charged ion to start the crosslinking process to create hydrogel beads, also known as gel spheres [80, 81]. These are sphere-shaped, crosslinked hydrophilic polymeric entities that can expand and congeal significantly in artificial biological fluids, with the release of drugs being regulated by polymer relaxation. Due to the ability to alter the degree of crosslinking and the polymer concentration, some factors might affect particle production that must be taken into consideration while using the ion gelation method these are the following:

- The concentration of polymer and electrolyte has a significant impact on how spheres are formed using the ion gelation process. Both should be concentrated in a ratio determined by the quantity of crosslinking units. The type of electrolytes and their concentration both affect the percent entrapment efficiency.
- The temperature has a significant impact on both the amount of time needed for crosslinking and the size of the sphere produced by ion gelation.
- The crosslinking solution's pH is a significant consideration in the formulation process because it has an impact on the reaction rate, shape, and size.
- The appropriate ratio of drug to polymer should be used to entrap the drug in the spheres since the drug concentration has a significant impact on how well it is captured. If the ratio of drug to polymer is out of range, bursting effects may be seen.

The ion gelation method has several benefits. Because of its simplicity, lack of use of organic solvents, minimal equipment requirements, and short processing times, it is, therefore, more efficient. To prevent potential reagent toxicity and other negative effects, it also uses reversible physical crosslinking by electrostatic contact rather than chemical crosslinking [82].

TABLE 8.3
Synthesis of Micro/Nanospheres of Anticancer Drugs using Different Methods

Method	Drug	Polymer Material	Size
Electrospray [86]	6-thioguanine	poly (d, l-lactide-co-glycolide) (PLGA)	Sustained release nanospheres of size 149.10 nm.
Emulsification [87]	Doxorubicin	alginate	Nanospheres of size 82.8 ± 3.6 nm, around ~ 83 nm.
Hydrothermal synthesis [88]	Docetaxel	poly (D, L-lactide-co-glycolic) acid (PLGA), Polyethylene glycol (PEG)	Iron oxide nanospheres of size range from 160–220 nm. With an average diameter of ~200 nm.
Ion gelation [89]	Cisplatin Rituximab	chitosan	Nanospheres loaded with cisplatin of size 308.10 nm and rituximab surface-linked nanospheres of size 349.40 ± 3.20 nm.
Nanoprecipitation [90]	Cytarabine	poly (ε-caprolactone) (PCL)	Nanospheres with an average diameter of ~150 nm and size range from 120±1.18 to 341± 3.0 nm. With the increase in polymer concentration, particle size was also increased.
Sol-gel [91]	Doxorubicin	polyethylene glycol PEG	TiO_2 nanospheres of size 25nm
Solvent evaporation [92]	Cisplatin	poly (lactic-co-glycolic acid) (PLGA), chitosan (CS), and sodium alginate (ALG)	Nanospheres of size range 228±72 nm (PLGA), 537±184 nm (PLGA/CS), and 895± 216 nm (PLGA/CS/ALG) size increases as the number of layers around the particles increases.
Spray drying [93]	Methotrexate/ doxorubicin	PEG	Hollow nanospheres of diameter < 50 nm, microspheres of range 3–5µm

8.9.9 HYDROTHERMAL SYNTHESIS

One of the most frequently employed alternative techniques for creating spherical nanoparticles is hydrothermal synthesis (Table 8.3). It primarily uses a solution reaction-based technique that entails hydrolysis and condensation in a medium (often water) under a variety of pressure and temperature conditions [83]. Using a unique apparatus known as a hydrothermal autoclave reactor consist of a strong vessel that can endure intense heat and pressure. An autoclave container is filled with a solution, and the opposite ends of the crystallizing compartment are kept at a constant thermal gradient. Wherever the solvent was dissolved was the end with the greater temperature. While the growth of the nanoparticles occurs at the opposite end, which is relatively cooler. This approach has several benefits, including the fact that it is affordable, requires just basic user-friendly equipment, and offers superb control over particle morphology, structure, and size [84, 85].

8.10 CONCLUSION

Traditional drug-delivery system is difficult to achieve precise control of drug release rate and release site [94, 95]. This situation leads to the development of advanced drug-delivery systems such as micro/nanomedicine which is designed to achieve slow and continuous release of the drug, maintain the drug at a constant release rate, and finally deliver it to the target tumor site in the body [96, 97]. Polymeric micro/nanocarriers particularly in the form of spheres have been used as a drug-loading system for a variety of anticancer therapeutic agents. The fluid intake ability of the polymeric matrix, the size of the sphere, and drug-loading efficiency are responsible for the release of the drug from the carrier system. This chapter has categorically discussed a wide range of micro/nanospheres, their methods of preparation for a targeted drug design, and factors that regularize the release of active drugs from the micro/nanospheres. The nanomaterials, which are both synthetic and natural, are elaborated in relation to their biocompatibility. Compared with traditional delivery methods, micro/nanocarrier drug delivery is preferred for producing prolonged therapeutic effect of drugs, reduce the number of drugs, improved patient compliance, and reduce systemic side effects of drugs.

REFERENCES

1. Dhadde, G.S., et al., *A review on microspheres: types, method of preparation, characterization and application. Asian Journal of Pharmacy and Technology*, 2021. **11**(2): pp. 149–155.
2. Jeevanandam, J., et al., *Review on nanoparticles and nanostructured materials: history, sources, toxicity and regulations. Beilstein Journal of Nanotechnology*, 2018. **9**(1): pp. 1050–1074.
3. Singh, A., G. Garg, and P. Sharma, *Nanospheres: a novel approach for targeted drug delivery system. International Journal of Pharmaceutical Sciences Review and Research*, 2010. **5**(3): pp. 84–88.
4. Sun, R., et al., *Nanomaterials and their composite scaffolds for photothermal therapy and tissue engineering applications. Science and Technology of Advanced Materials*, 2021. **22**(1): pp. 404–428.
5. Tang, L., et al., *Multifunctional inorganic nanomaterials for cancer photoimmunotherapy. Cancer Communications*, 2022. **42**(2): pp. 141–163.
6. Igaz, N., et al., *Modulating chromatin structure and DNA accessibility by deacetylase inhibition enhances the anti-cancer activity of silver nanoparticles. Colloids and Surfaces B: Biointerfaces*, 2016. **146**: pp. 670–677.
7. Liao, H., C.L. Nehl, and J.H. Hafner, *Biomedical applications of plasmon resonant metal nanoparticles. Nanomedicine*, 2006. **1**(2): pp. 201–208.
8. Liang, H., et al., *Controlled synthesis of uniform silver nanospheres. Journal of Physical Chemistry C*, 2010. **114**(16): pp. 7427–7431.
9. Pindiprolu, S.K.S., et al., *Formulation-optimization of solid lipid nanocarrier system of STAT3 inhibitor to improve its activity in triple negative breast cancer cells. Drug Development and Industrial Pharmacy*, 2019. **45**(2): pp. 304–313.
10. Chirio, D., et al., *Lipophilic prodrug of floxuridine loaded into solid lipid nanoparticles: In vitro cytotoxicity studies on different human cancer cell lines. Journal of Nanoscience and Nanotechnology*, 2018. **18**(1): pp. 556–563.
11. Rahiminejad, A., et al., *Preparation and investigation of indirubin-loaded SLN nanoparticles and their anti-cancer effects on human glioblastoma U87MG cells. Cell Biology International*, 2019. **43**(1): pp. 2–11.
12. Bhattacharya, S., M.M. Anjum, and K.K.J.D.D. Patel, *Gemcitabine cationic polymeric nanoparticles against ovarian cancer: Formulation, characterization, and targeted drug delivery. Drug Delivery*, 2022. **29**(1): pp. 1060–1074.
13. Yildiz, T., et al., *Doxorubicin-loaded protease-activated near-infrared fluorescent polymeric nanoparticles for imaging and therapy of cancer. International Journal of Nanomedicine*, 2018. **13**: pp. 6961.
14. Chen, J., et al., *Docetaxel loaded mPEG-PLA nanoparticles for sarcoma therapy: Preparation, characterization, pharmacokinetics, and anti-tumor efficacy. Drug Delivery*, 2021. **28**(1): pp. 1389–1396.
15. Hassani, S., N. Gharehaghaji, and B.J.M.T.C. Divband, *Chitosan-coated iron oxide/graphene quantum dots as a potential multifunctional nanohybrid for bimodal magnetic resonance/fluorescence imaging and 5-fluorouracil delivery. Materials Today Communications*, 2022. **31**: p. 103589.
16. Pandey, S., et al., *Inducing endoplasmic reticulum stress in cancer cells using graphene oxide-based nanoparticles. Nanoscale Advances*, 2020. **2**(10): pp. 4887–4894.
17. Muthoosamy, K., et al., *Exceedingly higher co-loading of curcumin and paclitaxel onto polymer-functionalized reduced graphene oxide for highly potent synergistic anticancer treatment. Scientific Reports*, 2016. **6**(1): pp. 1–14.

18. Sheth, R.A., et al., *Doxorubicin-loaded hollow gold nanospheres for dual photothermal ablation and chemoembolization therapy. Cancer Nanotechnology,* 2020. **11**(1): pp. 1–16.

19. Rozalen, M., et al., *Synthesis of controlled-size silver nanoparticles for the administration of methotrexate drug and its activity in colon and lung cancer cells. RSC Advances,* 2020. **10**(18): pp. 10646–10660.

20. Khafaji, M., M. Zamani, and M.J.I.J.o.N. Vossoughi, *Doxorubicin/cisplatin-loaded superparamagnetic nanoparticles as a stimuli-responsive co-delivery system for chemo-photothermal therapy. International Journal of Nanomedicine,* 2019. **14**: p. 8769.

21. Siminzar, P., et al., *Targeted delivery of doxorubicin by magnetic mesoporous silica nanoparticles armed with mucin-1 aptamer. Journal of Drug Targeting,* 2020. **28**(1): pp. 92–101.

22. Saini, K., et al., *Development of mesoporous silica nanoparticles of tunable pore diameter for superior gemcitabine drug delivery in pancreatic cancer cells. Journal of Nanscience and Nanotechnology,* 2020. **20**(5): pp. 3084–3096.

23. Yan, J., et al., *Fabrication of a pH/redox-triggered mesoporous silica-based nanoparticle with microfluidics for anticancer drugs doxorubicin and paclitaxel codelivery. ACS Applied Bio Materials,* 2020. **3**(2): pp. 1216–1225.

24. Whelehan, M. and I.W. Marison, *Microencapsulation using vibrating technology. Journal of Microencapsulation,* 2011. **28**(8): pp. 669–688.

25. Peanparkdee, M., S. Iwamoto, and R. Yamauchi, *Microencapsulation: A review of applications in the food and pharmaceutical industries. Reviews in Agricultural Science,* 2016. **4**: pp. 56–65.

26. Guterres, S.S., M.P. Alves, and A.R. Pohlmann, *Polymeric nanoparticles, nanospheres and nanocapsules, for cutaneous applications. Drug Target Insights,* 2007. **2**: p. 117739280700200002.

27. Zielińska, A., et al., *Polymeric nanoparticles: production, characterization, toxicology and ecotoxicology. Molecules,* 2020. **25**(16): p. 3731.

28. De Jong, W.H. and P.J. Borm, *Drug delivery and nanoparticles: applications and hazards. International Journal of Nanomedicine,* 2008. **3**(2): p. 133.

29. Patra, J.K., et al., *Nano based drug delivery systems: recent developments and future prospects. Journal of Nanobiotechnology,* 2018. **16**(1): pp. 1–33.

30. Kumar, S., et al., *Nanotechnology as emerging tool for enhancing solubility of poorly water-soluble drugs. Bionanoscience,* 2012. **2**(4): pp. 227–250.

31. Liechty, W.B., et al., *Polymers for drug delivery systems. Annual Review of Chemical and Biomolecular Engineering,* 2010. **1**: p. 149.

32. Kamaly, N., et al., *Degradable controlled-release polymers and polymeric nanoparticles: mechanisms of controlling drug release. Chemical Reviews,* 2016. **116**(4): pp. 2602–2663.

33. Jiang, H., et al., *Preparation of doxorubicin-loaded collagen-PAPBA nanoparticles and their anticancer efficacy in ovarian cancer. Annals of Translational Medicine,* 2020. **8**(14): p. 880

34. Gerami, S.E., et al., *Preparation of pH-sensitive chitosan/polyvinylpyrrolidone/α-Fe_2O_3 nanocomposite for drug delivery application: Emphasis on ameliorating restrictions. International Journal of Biological Macromolecules,* 2021. **173**: pp. 409–420.

35. Zavareh, H.S., et al., *Chitosan/carbon quantum dot/aptamer complex as a potential anticancer drug delivery system towards the release of 5-fluorouracil. International Journal of Biological Macromolecules,* 2020. **165**: pp. 1422–1430.

36. Khan, S., et al., *Lipid poly (ε-caprolactone) hybrid nanoparticles of 5-fluorouracil for sustained release and enhanced anticancer efficacy. Life Sciences,* 2021. **284**: p. 119909.

37. Khan, M.M., et al., *Lipid-chitosan hybrid nanoparticles for controlled delivery of cisplatin. Drug Delivery,* 2019. **26**(1): pp. 765–772.

38. Prabha, G. and V.J.J.o.B.M.R.P.B.A.B. Raj, *Preparation and characterization of chitosan—Polyethylene glycol-polyvinylpyrrolidone-coated superparamagnetic iron oxide nanoparticles as carrier system: Drug loading and in vitro drug release study. Journal of Biomedical Materials Research Part B: Applied Biomaterials* 2016. **104**(4): pp. 808–816.

39. Costa, P. and J.M.S.J.E.j.o.p.s. Lobo, *Modeling and comparison of dissolution profiles. European Journal of Pharmaceutical Sciences,* 2001. **13**(2): pp. 123–133.

40. Savjani, K.T., A.K. Gajjar, and J.K.J.I.S.R.N. Savjani, *Drug solubility: importance and enhancement techniques. ISRN Pharmacology,* 2012. **2012**: p. 195727.

41. Ahmad, N., et al., *Enhancement of oral bioavailability of doxorubicin through surface modified biodegradable polymeric nanoparticles. Chemistry Central Journal*, 2018. **12**(1): pp. 1–14.

42. Yu, H., et al., *pH- and NIR light-responsive micelles with hyperthermia-triggered tumor penetration and cytoplasm drug release to reverse doxorubicin resistance in breast cancer. Advanced Functyional Materials*, 2015. **25**(17): pp. 2489–2500.

43. Suzuki, H. and Y.H.J.B. Bae, *Evaluation of drug penetration with cationic micelles and their penetration mechanism using an in vitro tumor model. Biomaterials*, 2016. **98**: pp. 120–130.

44. Zhao, L. and S.-S. Feng, *-Enhanced oral bioavailability of paclitaxel formulated in vitamin E-TPGS emulsified nanoparticles of biodegradable polymers: in vitro and in vivo studies*, in *Chemotherapeutic Engineering*. 2014, New Delhi: Jenny Stanford. pp. 722–739.

45. Dabholkar, R.D., et al., *Polyethylene glycol–phosphatidylethanolamine conjugate (PEG–PE)-based mixed micelles: Some properties, loading with paclitaxel, and modulation of P-glycoprotein-mediated efflux. International Journal of Pharmaceutics*, 2006. **315**(1–2): pp. 148–157.

46. Kolluru, L.P., et al., *Development and evaluation of polycaprolactone based docetaxel nanoparticle formulation for targeted breast cancer therapy. Journal of Nanoparticle Research*, 2020. **22**(12): pp. 1–14.

47. Pornpitchanarong, C., et al., *Catechol-modified chitosan/hyaluronic acid nanoparticles as a new avenue for local delivery of doxorubicin to oral cancer cells. Colloids and Surfaces B: Biointerfaces*, 2020. **196**: p. 111279.

48. Alavi, S.E., et al., *Cisplatin-loaded polybutylcyanoacrylate nanoparticles with improved properties as an anticancer agent. International Journal of Molecular Sciences*, 2019. **20**(7): p. 1531.

49. Aftab, S., et al., *Nanomedicine: an effective tool in cancer therapy. International Journal of Pharmaceutics*, 2018. **540**(1–2): pp. 132–149.

50. Doppalapudi, S., et al., *Biodegradable polymers for targeted delivery of anti-cancer drugs. Expert Opinion on Drug Delivery*, 2016. **13**(6): pp. 891–909.

51. Florczak, A., et al., *Systemic and local silk-based drug delivery systems for cancer therapy. Cancers*, 2021. **13**(21): pp. 5389.

52. Mudshinge, S.R., et al., *Nanoparticles: emerging carriers for drug delivery. Saudi Pharmaceutical Journal*, 2011. **19**(3): pp. 129–141.

53. Mittal, P., et al., *Formulation, optimization, hemocompatibility and pharmacokinetic evaluation of PLGA nanoparticles containing paclitaxel. Drug Development and Industrial Pharmacy*, 2019. **45**(3): pp. 365–378.

54. Delrish, E., et al., *Efficacy of topotecan nanoparticles for intravitreal chemotherapy of retinoblastoma. Experimental Eye Research*, 2021. **204**: p. 108423.

55. Abdelfattah, A., et al., *Design and optimization of PEGylated silver nanoparticles for efficient delivery of doxorubicin to cancer cells. Journal of Drug Delivery Science and Technology*, 2022. **71**: pp. 103347.

56. Shaikh, R., et al., *Mucoadhesive drug delivery systems. Journal of pharmacy and Bioallied Sciences*, 2011. **3**(1): p. 89.

57. Sahatsapan, N., et al., *Doxorubicin-loaded chitosan-alginate nanoparticles with dual mucoadhesive functionalities for intravesical chemotherapy. Journal of Drug Delivery Science and Technology*, 2021. **63**: p. 102481.

58. Ak, G., *Covalently coupling doxorubicin to polymeric nanoparticles as potential inhaler therapy: In vitro studies. Pharmaceutical Development and Technology*, 2021. **26**(8): pp. 890–898.

59. Joshi, B. and A. Joshi, *Ultrasound-based drug delivery systems. Bioelectronics and Medical Devices*, 2019: pp. 241–260.

60. Yang, R.-M., et al., *Hyaluronan-modified superparamagnetic iron oxide nanoparticles for bimodal breast cancer imaging and photothermal therapy. International Journal of Nanomedicine*, 2017. **12**: p. 197.

61. Khafaji, M., M. Zamani, and M. Vossoughi, *Doxorubicin/cisplatin-loaded superparamagnetic nanoparticles as a stimuli-responsive co-delivery system for chemo-photothermal therapy. International Journal of Nanomedicine*, 2019. **14**: p. 8769.

62. Rauwel, E., et al., *Assessing cobalt metal nanoparticles uptake by cancer cells using live Raman spectroscopy. International Journal of Nanomedicine*, 2020. **15**: p. 7051.

63. Tian, J., et al., *CD271 antibody-functionalized HGNs for targeted photothermal therapy of osteosarcoma stem cells*. Nanotechnology, 2020. **31**(30): p. 305707.

64. Zhang, L., et al., *An optimized mesoporous silica nanosphere-based carrier system with chemically removable Au nanoparticle caps for redox-stimulated and targeted drug delivery*. Nanotechnology, 2020. **31**(47): p. 475102.

65. Banstola, A., et al., *Polydopamine-tailored paclitaxel-loaded polymeric microspheres with adhered NIR-controllable gold nanoparticles for chemo-phototherapy of pancreatic cancer*. Drug Delivery, 2019. **26**(1): pp. 629–640.

66. Rawat, M., et al., *Nanocarriers: promising vehicle for bioactive drugs*. Biological and Pharmaceutical Bulletin, 2006. **29**(9): pp. 1790–1798.

67. Bock, N., et al., *Electrospraying, a reproducible method for production of polymeric microspheres for biomedical applications*. Polymers, 2011. **3**(1): pp. 131–149.

68. Watts, P., M. Davies, and C.J.C.r.i.t.d.c.s. Melia, *Microencapsulation using emulsification/solvent evaporation: an overview of techniques and applications*. Critical Reviews in Therapeutic Drug Carrier Systems, 1990. **7**(3): pp. 235–259.

69. Verma, R., J. Gangwar, and A.K.J.R.a. Srivastava, *Multiphase TiO 2 nanostructures: A review of efficient synthesis, growth mechanism, probing capabilities, and applications in bio-safety and health*. RSC Advances, 2017. **7**(70): pp. 44199–44224.

70. Bokov, D., et al., *Nanomaterial by sol-gel method: synthesis and application*. Advances in Materials Science and Engineering, 2021. **2021:** p. 5102014

71. Wang, Y., et al., *Manufacturing techniques and surface engineering of polymer based nanoparticles for targeted drug delivery to cancer*. Nanomaterials, 2016. **6**(2): p. 26.

72. Liu, G., et al. *Porous PLGA microspheres effectively loaded with BSA protein by electrospraying combined with phase separation in liquid nitrogen*. Journal of Biomimetics, Biomaterials and Tissue Engineering. 2010. **6**: p. 1.

73. Panigrahi, D., et al., *Quality by design prospects of pharmaceuticals application of double emulsion method for PLGA loaded nanoparticles*. SN Applied Sciences, 2021. **3**(6): pp. 1–21.

74. Martínez-Muñoz, O.I., et al., *Nanoprecipitation: Applications for entrapping active molecules of interest in pharmaceutics*. Nano- and Microencapsulation 2020. London: InTechOpen.

75. Pak, C.W., et al., *Sequence determinants of intracellular phase separation by complex coacervation of a disordered protein*. Molecular Cell, 2016. **63**(1): pp. 72–85.

76. Pathak, J., et al., *Complex coacervation in charge complementary biopolymers: Electrostatic versus surface patch binding*. Advances in Colloid and Interface Science, 2017. **250**: pp. 40–53.

77. Aloys, H., et al., *Microencapsulation by complex coacervation: methods, techniques, benefits, and applications - A review*. American Journal of Food Science and Nutrition Research, 2016. **3**(6): pp. 188–192.

78. Sansone, F., et al., *Flavonoid microparticles by spray-drying: influence of enhancers of the dissolution rate on properties and stability*. Journal of Food Engineering, 2011. **103**(2): pp. 188–196.

79. Chandralekha, A., et al., *Encapsulation of yeast (Saccharomyces cereviciae) by spray drying for extension of shelf life*. Drying Technology, 2016. **34**(11): pp. 1307–1318.

80. Sacco, P., et al., *Insight into the ionotropic gelation of chitosan using tripolyphosphate and pyrophosphate as cross-linkers*. International Journal of Biological Macromolecules, 2016. **92**: pp. 476–483.

81. Patel, M.A., et al., *The effect of ionotropic gelation residence time on alginate cross-linking and properties*. Carbohydrate Polymers, 2017. **155**: pp. 362–371.

82. Debnath, S., R.S. Kumar, and M.N.J.R.J.P.T. Babu, *Ionotropic gelation – A novel method to prepare chitosan nanoparticles*. Reserach Journal of Pharmacy and Technology, 2011. **4**: p. 492–495.

83. Gan, Y.X., et al., *Hydrothermal synthesis of nanomaterials*. Journal of Nanomaterials, 2020. **2020**: p. 8917013.

84. Nadimpalli, N.K.V., R. Bandyopadhyaya, and V.J.F.P.E. Runkana, *Thermodynamic analysis of hydrothermal synthesis of nanoparticles*. Fluid Phase Equilibria, 2018. **456**: pp. 33–45.

85. Wasly, H., M. Abd El-Sadek, and M.J.A.P.A. Henini, *Influence of reaction time and synthesis temperature on the physical properties of ZnO nanoparticles synthesized by the hydrothermal method*. Applied Physics A, 2018. **124**(1): pp. 1–12.

86. Chatterjee, M., et al., *Development of 6-thioguanine conjugated PLGA nanoparticles through thioester bond formation: benefits of electrospray mediated drug encapsulation and sustained release in cancer therapeutic applications. Materials Science and Engineering: C* 2020. **114**: p. 111029.
87. Rosch, J.G., et al., *Nanoalginates via inverse-micelle synthesis: doxorubicin-encapsulation and breast cancer cytotoxicity. Nanoscale Research Letters,* 2018. **13**(1): pp. 1–10.
88. Panda, J., et al., *Engineered polymeric iron oxide nanoparticles as potential drug carrier for targeted delivery of docetaxel to breast cancer cells. Journal of Magnetism and Magnetic Materials,* 2019. **485**: pp. 165–173.
89. Sultan, M.H., et al., *Characterization of cisplatin-loaded chitosan nanoparticles and rituximab-linked surfaces as target-specific injectable nano-formulations for combating cancer. Scientific Reports,* 2022. **12**(1): pp. 1–16.
90. Jan, N., et al., *In vitro anti-leukemic assessment and sustained release behaviour of cytarabine loaded biodegradable polymer based nanoparticles. Life Sciences,* 2021. **267**: p. 118971.
91. Naghibi, S., et al., *Mortality response of folate receptor-activated, PEG–functionalized TiO$_2$ nanoparticles for doxorubicin loading with and without ultraviolet irradiation. Cermaics International* 2014. **40**(4): pp. 5481–5488.
92. Wang, F., et al., *PTX-loaded three-layer PLGA/CS/ALG nanoparticle based on layer-by-layer method for cancer therapy. Journal of Biomaterials Science,* 2018. **29**(13): pp. 1566–1578.
93. Nozohouri, S., et al., *A multilayer hollow nanocarrier for pulmonary co-drug delivery of methotrexate and doxorubicin in the form of dry powder inhalation formulation. Materials Science and Engineering: C,* 2019. **99**: pp. 752–761.
94. Li, C., et al., *Recent progress in drug delivery. Acta Pharmaceutica Sinica B,* 2019. **9**(6): pp. 1145–1162.
95. Li, D., et al., *Development of a redox/pH dual stimuli-responsive MSP@ P (MAA-Cy) drug delivery system for programmed release of anticancer drugs in tumour cells. Journal of Materials Chemistry B,* 2014. **2**(32): pp. 5187–5194.
96. Patil, P., S. Singh, and J. Sarvanan, *Preparation and evaluation of microspheres of flurbiprofen. International Journal of Pharmaceutical Sciences and Research,* 2018. **9**(12): pp. 5388–5393.
97. Zhou, X., et al., *Controlled released of drug from doubled-walled PVA hydrogel/PCL microspheres prepared by single needle electrospraying method. Colloids and Surfaces B: Biointerfaces,* 2020. **187**: p. 110645.

9 The Emergence of Liposomes in Cancer Therapy

Asia Naz Awan, Sabahat Abdullah, Ayesha Naseer, Muhammad Yasir Ali, and Daulat Haleem Khan

9.1 INTRODUCTION

The discipline of biomedicine is filled with enormous anticipation as a result of the rapid advancements in nanotechnology and nanoscience. Nanomaterials overcome various obstacles in a variety of medical sectors, including health, diagnostics, and therapy, because of their distinctive, versatile, and adaptable qualities.

One of the most often utilized nanoparticles in the field of medicine is liposomes. Its spherical lipid bilayer membranous structure offers both a hydrophilic and hydrophobic environment and is used to encapsulate a variety of therapeutic agents. In medicine, particularly drug delivery, liposomes are amazing structures because of their adaptability, flexibility, variety of components, simplicity of functionalization, tunability of the number of layers/sizes, biocompatibility, and biodegradability. In a wide range of biomedical and nanomedicine applications, liposomes serve as adaptable nanoplatforms for the enhancement of drug delivery and distribution in a specified manner at the target site. Furthermore, liposomes are the most significant category of clinically authorized therapeutic nanocarriers for the treatment of cancer due to their excellent biocompatibility and lack of toxicity.

9.2 LIPOSOMES

Liposomes are sphere shape nano- to micro-sized lipid-based vesicles ranging from 20 nm to 2.5 µm. They are made up of phospholipids, which include molecules with head and tail groups. The lengthy hydrocarbon chain that makes up the tail is orientated toward the lipid area away from water whereas the head is drawn to water when they are dispersed in an aqueous medium [1].

9.3 COMPOSITION OF LIPOSOMES

Phospholipids, a vital structural element of the bilayer membrane, are found in liposome vesicles, whereas cholesterol makes up the remaining portion and mostly stabilizes the membrane by increasing its rigidity. The nature and purpose of the phospholipids utilized in the construction of liposomes determine their properties [2].

9.3.1 PHOSPHOLIPIDS

The major constituents of liposomes are phospholipids. Furthermore, the formation of biological membranes mainly relies on these biomolecules [3]. Phospholipids comprise hydrophilic and hydrophobic regions therefore these are amphipathic molecules. The hydrophobic part contains two

DOI: 10.1201/9781003363958-12

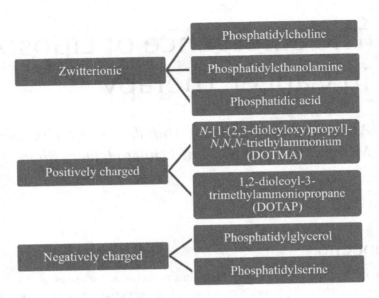

FIGURE 9.1   Classification of lipids used for liposomal preparation.

lipophilic tails that have lengthy hydrocarbon chains, while the hydrophilic region consists of a polar head that has a phosphorus molecule with a phosphoric acid group [4]. The polar head charge affects the surface characteristics of liposomes that it can be positively or negatively charged, zwitterionic, or neutral as described in Figure 9.1 [5].

9.3.2 CHOLESTEROL

Liposomes also contain cholesterol, which serves a purpose by modulating the lipid bilayer characteristics of the liposomes. The biological cell membrane's phospholipids' phosphate head group and cholesterol's OH group are joined, keeping the membrane flexible and firm [6] while simultaneously filling up the spacing between the phospholipid molecules [7] with strict regulation of sturdiness in liposomal structure [8] providing a more organized conformation. Cholesterol decreases the permeability of the bilayer for water-soluble molecules by enhancing its micro-viscosity [9, 10]. Additionally, the structural stability of liposomal membranes against environmental stress in the intestines depends on cholesterol [11]. The release of hydrophilic substances from liposomes was shown to be modulated by cholesterol, which was also found to affect liposome size because raising cholesterol content also causes a change in shape [12].

9.4   ADVANTAGES AND DISADVANTAGES OF LIPOSOMES

The advantages and disadvantages of liposomes can be summarized in Table 9.1, which includes some of the benefits and drawbacks of liposomes that both promote and restrict their potential uses [13, 14].

9.5   CLASSIFICATION OF LIPOSOMES

9.5.1 TYPES OF LIPOSOMES BASED ON SIZE

The circulation half-life of liposomes is significantly influenced by the size of the vesicles. Depending upon the size, liposomes are divided into different classes as mentioned in Table 9.2 [15, 16].

TABLE 9.1
Advantages and Disadvantages of Liposomes

Advantages	Disadvantages
• Non-poisonous and non-immunogenic, consistent, and amicable with the biological membrane.	• Expensive manufacturing materials for the creation of liposomes and the encapsulation of drugs.
• Can deliver hydrophilic, hydrophobic, and amphiphilic compounds because they have both lipophilic and hydrophilic moieties.	• May have an unexpected leakage that causes the enclosed molecules to fuse.
• Enhanced therapeutic potency and lowered toxicity of the enclosed substances.	• Unstable when structure degrades due to the possibility of phospholipids being subjected to oxidation and hydrolysis.
• Improved stability of entrapped molecules and function as a gradual release mechanism to safeguard them from the environment.	• Short half-life.
• Due to their adaptability in interacting with site-specific ligands, they facilitate active targeting.	• Low solubility in the aqueous medium.
• Exist in various forms including powder, emulsion, and suspension, and can be administered in a variety of ways.	• Required a nitrogen-sealed, dark environment for storage.

TABLE 9.2
Types of Liposomes Based on Size

Liposomes	Size	Marketed Products
Unilamellar vesicles (ULVs)		Doxil®
• Small Unilamellar vesicles (SUVs)	30–100 nm	
• Large Unilamellar vesicles (LUVs)	>100 nm	
• Giant Unilamellar vesicles (GUVs)	>1000 nm	
Oligolamellar vesicles (OLVs)	0.1–10 μm	Vyxeos™
Multilamellar vesicles (MLVs)	0.1–0.5 μm	Myocet® and Mepact®
Multivesicular liposomes/vesicles (MVLs or MVVs)	2–40 μm	Depocyt®, DepoDur® and Exparel®

9.5.2 Types of Liposomes Based on Structure and Lamellarity

The number of lipid bilayers in a liposome, or lamellarity (Figure 9.2), affects the effectiveness of encapsulation and the rate at which active pharmaceuticals are released. Additionally, the lamellarity of the liposome-drug combination influences how it behaves at the target site when taken up by the cells.

9.5.2.1 Unilamellar Vesicles (ULVs)

Vesicles with only a single lipid bilayer are unilamellar. They have a long circulation time and are not cleared from the bloodstream because of their small size. As a result, they stand a better chance of penetrating tissues and exerting therapeutic effects than LUVs, which have a lot of room to load substances, and GUVs, which are used for diagnostic and therapeutic purposes.

9.5.2.2 Oligolamellar Vesicles (OLVs)

This type of liposome has two–five concentric lipid bilayers and exhibits an onion-like structure [17].

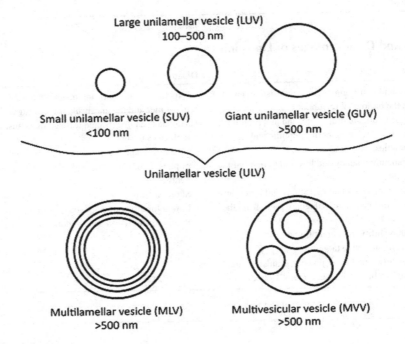

FIGURE 9.2 Types of different liposomes.

9.5.2.3 Multilamellar Vesicles (MLVs)

These vesicles have five or more concentric lipid bilayers, and their structure also looks like an onion. The simplicity of formation and stability of MLVs are their key advantages. The limited area for loading therapeutic molecules is the main drawback of these liposomes. The volume that can be loaded with the material is constrained by the number of concentric lipidic bilayers that surround more inner space, and the size of MLVs prevents them from being injected [13, 14].

9.5.2.4 Multivesicular Liposomes/Vesicles (MVLs or MVVs)

These are multipurpose liposomes and have a structure resembling a honeycomb and contain hundreds of non-concentric aqueous compartments enclosed by a single bilayer lipid membrane [18].

9.5.3 Types of Liposomes Based on Their Composition

9.5.3.1 Conventional Liposomes

These liposomes were created using phospholipids that were either natural or synthetic and may contain cholesterol or not [19]. Soy lecithin liposomes co-delivering letrozole/paclitaxel [20], and docetaxel/resveratrol [21] increase the effectiveness of dual therapy against breast and prostate cancer.

9.5.3.2 pH-Sensitive Liposomes

These liposomes can transport their contents into the interior of the cell through the fusion or destabilization of endosomes, which have a slightly acidic environment, due to their fusogenic characteristic, pH-sensitive liposomes are more effective than typical and long-circulating liposomes at conveying chemotherapeutic agents [22].

pH-sensitive liposomes were created and filled with doxorubicin [23] and daunorubicin [24]. It was discovered through an in vitro investigation that this system exhibits a rapid release profile of anticancer medicine at an acidic pH and is stable at the physiological pH. They showed a higher level of cytotoxicity and improved cellular uptake.

9.5.3.3　Thermos-Sensitive Liposomes

Targeted drug delivery is possible with thermosensitive liposomes, which liberate the enclosed drug when heated to a fever temperature of about 40–42 °C. These liposomes offer precise drug administration to a specific site when coupled with localized hyperthermia.

Liposomes coated with a polymer and adorned with gold encapsulating paclitaxel [25] and doxorubicin [26]. The designed thermosensitive liposomes have promising antineoplastic activity and have the potential for hyperthermia therapy since they can release the loaded medicine at a predetermined temperature with an accelerated release rate.

9.5.3.4　Cationic Liposomes

The term "cationic liposome" refers to liposomes that have a positive charge and are mostly made up of cationic lipids. They are well suited for delivering a variety of negatively charged drugs and macromolecules because their negative charge and relatively large size prevent passive diffusion into cells [27]. Additionally, angiogenic endothelium cells in malignancies are specifically targeted by cationic liposomes [28].

The positively charged methacrylate copolymer eudragit was used to modify doxorubicin-loaded liposomes. Compared to free doxorubicin or doxorubicin liposomes, the eudragit layering on the liposomal drug delivery system shows enhanced cellular absorption and anticancer activity. It was suggested that the cationic charge may have increased the interaction of the modified liposome with the partially negatively charged cell membranes, resulting in a higher liposome absorption rate and a more effective therapeutic outcome [29].

9.5.3.5　Immunoliposomes

Antibodies are coupled to the liposomal surface to create immunoliposomes, which enable active tissue targeting by attaching to receptors specific to tumor cells [30]. Paclitaxel and rapamycin co-loaded liposomes that were then coated with trastuzumab, an anti-HER-2 monoclonal antibody, to create immunoliposomes that were designed to aggressively target HER-2(+) breast cancer cells. When immunoliposomes were in vivo cytotoxically compared to medication solution, it was discovered that the immunoliposomes had greater cytotoxicity and were better able to suppress tumor growth [31].

9.5.3.6　PEG Liposomes

Wrapping the liposomes' surface with polyethylene glycol (PEG), shields against circulating proteins and increases the duration the medicine spends in the bloodstream while lowering immunological response (Table 9.3), thereby allowing drugs to be effectively absorbed and distributed throughout the body [32].

PEG-decorated thermosensitive liposomes were created utilizing the reverse-phase evaporation method for the targeted drug delivery of oxaliplatin against breast cancer. In vitro in vivo studies were conducted, which allowed researchers to assess the drug release pattern and cytotoxicity of the constructed liposomes. These investigations revealed that they are more target specific, increase cytotoxicity, and had longer circulation times of more than 24 hours, which improved their antitumor activity [33].

TABLE 9.3

Types of Liposomes Based on the Surface Modification

Types	Surface Modifiers
Polymeric liposomes	Docetaxel [34] and doxorubicin [35] encapsulated peg-stabilized liposomes for cancer treatment.
Metallic liposomes	Gold-decorated liposomes deliver doxorubicin [26] and paclitaxel [36] at the tumor site.
Carbon liposomes	For tumor Imaging and regression, doxorubicin-loaded graphene oxide-coated liposomes conjugated with poly (L-lysine) [37] and functionalized with folic acid [38] were developed.

9.5.4 Types of Liposomes Based on the Route of Administration

9.5.4.1 Oral Route of Administration

In addition to the usual benefits of nanocarriers for oral delivery, liposomes offer advantages derived from their lipidic bilayer structure. Liposomes are biocompatible carriers used to increase the oral bioavailability of drugs. They are good candidates for lymphatic uptake because they have improved biomembrane adhesion, can create mixed-micelle complexes with bile salts to boost the solubility of medicines with poor solubility, and can bind to biomembranes more effectively. The oral bioavailability of many different substances, including peptides, proteins, hydrophilic, and lipophilic medicines, has been successfully increased [39].

The thin film hydration approach was used to create multilamellar-type, cisplatin-loaded liposomes. To deliver cisplatin orally, liposomes were used, and the overall performance of the liposomal system was evaluated. It was found that these liposomes improved therapeutic effectiveness and reduced cisplatin toxicity to normal tissues thereby acting as a promising therapeutic approach for the management of colon cancer [40].

9.5.4.2 Local Route of Administration

Drugs that are administered locally may be thought of as a potential solution to the issues brought on by the numerous biological obstacles that are faced during drug delivery. Drug delivery through localized channels in conjunction with nanoformulations, like liposomes, may offer additional benefits. These benefits include greater protection of pharmaceuticals from potentially hostile conditions as well as prolonged retention of high drug loads at the target site and regulated drug release, ensuring sustained therapeutic impact [41].

Hybrid liposomes containing oxaliplatin and Cy5.5 dye were created using the magnetic property of Fe_3O_4. These liposomes were designed to assess their site-specific oxaliplatin delivery under magnetic field stimulation at high doses. The NIR radiation is used to monitor the cargo released by liposomes to confirm local distribution to the desired areas. This localized delivery system aims to improve survival rates in colorectal liver metastases by limiting exposure and toxicity to the drug elsewhere in the body and boosting local exposure to the drug, hence increasing antitumoral activity [42].

9.5.4.3 Systemic Route of Administration

Liposomes have undergone extensive clinical investigation and development as delivery vehicles for chemotherapeutic agents (Table 9.4). When taken systemically, medications encapsulated in liposomes are dispersed in the body in an extremely different manner unlike free drugs [43]. A significant portion of the parenteral delivery market now relies on liposomal formulations that are administered systemically.

TABLE 9.4
Examples of Marketed Brands of the Liposome

Trade Name	Encapsulated Agent	Indicated in
Depocyt® (1999) SkyPharma Inc.	Cytarabine	Acute Nonlymphocytic Leukemia, Meningeal Leukemia, Refractory Leukemia, and Lymphomatous Meningitis.
DaunoXome® (1996) NeXstar Pharmaceuticals	Daunorubicin	Kaposi's sarcoma, acute myeloid leukemia (AML)
Doxil® (1995) Sequus Pharmaceuticals	Doxorubicin	Kaposi's sarcoma, multiple myeloma, ovarian cancer, and breast cancer
Myocet® (2000) Elan Pharmaceuticals	Doxorubicin	Metastatic breast cancer
Mepact® (2009) Takeda Pharmaceutical Limited	Mifamurtide	Non-metastatic osteosarcoma
Marqibo® (2012) Talon Therapeutics, Inc.	Vincristine	Lymphoblastic leukemia
Onivyde™ (2015) Merrimack Pharmaceuticals Inc.	Irinotecan	Metastatic pancreatic cancer
ThermoDox® (2009) Zhejiang Hisun Pharmaceutical Company Ltd.	Doxorubicin	Liver cancer, recurrent chest wall breast cancer
Vyxeos™ (2017) Jazz Pharmaceuticals	Daunorubicin/ Cytarabine	Acute Myeloid Leukemia
Zolsketil (2022) Accord Healthcare Ltd.	Doxorubicin	Metastatic breast cancer, advanced ovarian cancer, progressive multiple myeloma, and Kaposi's sarcoma

9.6 METHODS OF PREPARATION OF LIPOSOMES

9.6.1 THIN FILM HYDRATION METHOD

The oldest, most popular, and easiest way for making MLV is the thin-film hydration process, also known as the bangham method. To create a homogenous mixture, the components of the phospholipid are first dissolved in an organic solvent, such as chloroform, ethanol, or dichloromethane, for the development of the lipid system. When a greater volume of organic solvent is added, the mixture is then exposed to rotary evaporation under a vacuum pump at a temperature of 45–60°C to remove the solvent from the mixture. In a fuming hood, a dry nitrogen or argon stream can be used to evaporate small volumes (less than 1 ml) of organic solvent until all traces are gone [44]. Following the repeated elimination of organic solvents, a uniform, dry, thin lipid film is created. The next step is hydration, which involves moistening the stacked lipid bilayers with a suitable aqueous medium such as distilled water or a phosphate buffer solution with a pH of 7.4 for 1–2 hours at a temperature of 60–70°C, which then causes phase transition because heating at a temperature will induce conformational changes in the lipid structure where the closely packed hydrocarbon chains are disordered to produce a liquid crystalline phase in which the particles are in random motion and become mobile. Now that the lipids are swelling, stirring may help to separate the lipid lamellae from the interior channel's surface. To aid in full lipid hydration, the resultant liposome suspension is subsequently left at 4°C overnight. Because of the lipid's swelling and hydration during the hydration stage, an MLV suspension with a very broad range of sizes and lamellarity is produced [45]. The main limitations of this process are its minimal production, low drug loading, and difficulty in extracting the organic solvent.

9.6.2 DETERGENT REMOVAL METHOD

As the name indicates this method involves the removal of detergent from the lipid that was initially added in the form of solution to the lipid and upon mixing the detergent will associate with the phospholipids shielding the hydrophobic portions from the direct interaction with the aqueous phase, as it hydrates and solubilized the lipids and thus formed mixed (detergent/lipids) micelles [13]. The formation of unilamellar vesicles occurs in the final stage of the progressive removal of the detergent when the total detergent concentration falls below the CMC of the detergent and the mixed micelles become more lipid-rich. Detergents with a high CMC, like sodium cholate, Triton X-100, sodium deoxycholate, and alkyl glycoside, are frequently used [46]. To get rid of the remaining detergent in the nanoformulation, various additional techniques need to be performed. The simplest and most common method is the dilution approach. When a detergent lipid mixture is diluted (by 10- to 100-fold) with an aqueous phase buffer, the initial micelles' size, and polydispersity increase. Finally, once the system is diluted beyond the equilibrium phase, a spontaneous change from elongated micelles to vesicles takes place [47]. The main downsides of this approach are the small number of liposomes obtained in the last phase and the low hydrophobic molecule entrapment effectiveness [2].

9.6.3 ETHANOL INJECTION METHOD

In this approach, the lipid is first thoroughly dissolved in ethanol while being constantly stirred, and then it is quickly injected into hot distilled water or buffer tris(hydroxymethyl)aminomethane hydrochloride is more commonly known as Tris-HCl. For 15 minutes, the solution is allowed to heat while being stirred [48]. When ethanol is diluted in an aqueous solution, the lipid components are more likely to spontaneously organize into an ordered structure. This spontaneous organization is then followed by interactions between the lipid components that cause the dissolved lipid to self-assemble in the aqueous medium. This precipitation causes bundles of bilayer fragments to form around the aqueous phase. The ethanol is evaporated in the final phase, which facilitates the fusion of lipid molecules and enables the subsequent creation of liposomes. Either rotary evaporation or centrifugation through a silica gel column can be used to remove the ethanol from the liposome suspension. SUVs are often prepared using the ethanol injection method, which produces liposomes with a size range of 30–170 nm. The size of the liposomes themselves is influenced by the volume and rate of the injection as well as the number of lipids. SUVs are homogeneous if the ethanol content is less than injection as well as the number of lipids. SUVs are homogeneous if the ethanol content is less than 7.5% of the total volume of the formulation. On the other hand, if ethanol is quickly introduced into an enormous quantity of buffer, a diverse population of MLVs is generated [49]. The key benefits of the ethanol injection technique are its ease of use, a significant level of reproducibility, use of ethanol as a non-harmful solvent, and ease of scaling up the procedure [50]. The two primary disadvantages are the difficulty in eliminating the remaining ethanol because it forms an azeotrope with water and the fact that the final liposome population is extremely diluted and diverse (30–110 nm). Moreover, to avoid liposome destabilization, the ethanol concentration should not go above 7.5%. Finally, even very small levels of ethanol carry the risk of inactivating physiologically active molecules [51].

9.6.4 ETHER INJECTION METHOD

With the significant exception that, unlike ethanol, the lipid solvent utilized in this case, ether, is not miscible with water, the ether injection method is remarkably similar to the ethanol injection method. As ether does not interfere with the development of liposomes, lipid prefers ether and opposes ethanol because of their great solubility in ether. This procedure involves slowly injecting lipid that has been dissolved in ether, diethyl ether, or a combination of diethyl ether and methanol into an aqueous phase or phosphate-buffered saline PBS while being continuously stirred. The mixture is heated to a temperature between 55 and 65°C to help the solvent evaporate from the liposomal product. LUVs are more likely to be produced when the organic solvent is gradually removed under decreasing pressure [52]. The ether injection method provides more effective elimination of the organic solvent from the finished product is a benefit of this strategy over the ethanol injection method. As a result, highly concentrated liposome solutions are more likely to form. Unlike the ethanol injection approach, LUVs rather than SUVs are created [53]. The main drawbacks of this approach are the active ingredient exposure to different chemical solvents and high temperatures, as well as the final liposomal population, showing high polydispersity (60–200 nm). This situation might jeopardize the liposome formulation's stability and safety parameters. This method has some shortcomings as well. During the injection process, both the phases ether and aqueous must be at different temperatures, the possibility that some therapeutic compounds may not be properly encapsulated by ether, and that will result in the creation of extremely uneven morphologies of the liposomes. It is recommended to inject the lipid mixture into the aqueous phase under a vacuum and at a slower rate than when using the ethanol injection method [2].

9.6.5   REVERSE-PHASE EVAPORATION METHOD

A mixture of organic solvents such as diethyl ether and chloroform (1:1v/v), diethyl ether/iso-propyl ether, or chloroform/methanol (2:1v/v), are used to dissolve lipids under constant stirring, and the resultant solution is then added to a PBS buffer or an aqueous phase containing citric-Na_2HPO_4 to promote the formation of inverted micelles enhance formulation characteristics [54]. Water-in-oil (W/O) microemulsion is produced when the lipids rearrange themselves at the water-oil interface. To aid in the creation of a homogenous dispersion, the W/O microemulsion can be emulsified using mechanical or sonication methods. The organic solvent can be eliminated by using a rotary evaporator under lower pressure, allowing for the development of a viscous gel. The breakdown of inverted micelles and the subsequent production of LUV-type liposomes are both favored by sluggish organic solvent removal. Many biologically active molecules can be enclosed inside the liposomes due to the microemulsions' extensive encapsulation of the aqueous phase. This technique allows for the encapsulation of 30–45% of the aqueous volume, with the potential for up to 65% entrapment under optimized conditions [55]. The primary downsides of this method are related to the existence of residual solvent, which can be eliminated using dialysis and centrifugation approach and the challenges of scaling up the procedure. The fact that the medicinal agents to be placed in the liposomes come into contact with an organic solvent makes this approach unsuitable for delicate molecules. Furthermore, the mechanical agitation and direct exposure to the organic solvent may also cause structural deformity in a variety of biomolecules [56].

9.6.6   MICROFLUIDIC METHOD

A unique method to create liposomal nanoparticles is developing recently called microfluidics. Dilution of a solvent in a microfluidic environment is a new and promising technique that is similar to the ethanol injection method. Through the use of microfluidics, homogeneous reaction conditions can be created by controlling liquid flows in channels with tens to hundreds of micrometers in width [57]. Lipids that have been dissolved in alcoholic solvents (ethanol or isopropanol) are successively injected into minuscule channels that have a cross-section area of 5–500 μm in the microfluidic procedure [58]. The microfluidic channel creates a hydrodynamically induced laminar flow and a diffusive mixing of the lipid alcoholic solution at the liquid interfaces that encourage the lipids to self-assemble into vesicles. This technique employs a low-toxicity solvent to produce liposomes. Besides this desirable sizes and size distributions can be obtained by carefully controlling the process parameters including mixing and flow rates [59]. The usage of organic solvents, delicate mechanical agitation, and the challenge of scaling up liposomal production are the main drawbacks of microfluidic technology, even though it offers high levels of diversity and flexibility in the development of liposomes. The finished product obtained from the microfluidic method does not need postproduction processing (i.e., extrusion, sonication, homogenization) in comparison to conventional processes [60].

9.6.7 Freeze Drying Method

The freeze-drying method is designed to improve development difficulties related to liposomes and overcome the challenges faced by hydrophilic molecules when they are encapsulated in liposomes. Liposomes being a lipid-based drug delivery system may cause leaking, precipitation, oxidation, or degradation of the water-soluble drugs using any chemical reaction making them devoid of their therapeutic activity all these serve as a limiting factor in the formation of liposomes [61]. The liposome formulation-containing water solution is frozen using the freeze-drying technique, and the ice is subsequently removed by sublimation. The freeze-drying approach is highly helpful for maintaining the stability of the liposomal drug delivery system. This technique favors the drying of thermos-liable liposomes where direct heating damages the structural integrity that results in the loss of its therapeutic response. Pharmaceuticals made of lipids have a longer shelf life when they are lyophilized, especially when they are carrying lipophilic agents that are unstable in an aqueous medium [62].

9.7 CHARACTERIZATION OF LIPOSOMES

At the molecular level, liposome behavior is governed by its geometric structure. Size, shape, morphology, lamellarity, and surface functionalization are a few of the controlling factors that have a big impact on liposome performance in biomedical and nanomedicine applications. It is important to characterize the structural properties of the conformation of the underlying bilayer vesicles to study the functionality of these nanocarrier systems, including their biodistribution and targeting capacities. To evaluate the physicochemical traits that affect the colloidal stability of liposome nanoformulation and their therapeutic and biological performances, the characterization of liposomes is performed after their production.

9.7.1 Atomic Force Microscopy (AFM)

Atomic force microscopy (AFM) is a crucial microscopic technique used to examine the shapes and sizes of liposomes. An example of a scanning probe microscope technique is also known as scanning-force microscopy (SFM). The fundamental principle of AFM is the relay on the cantilever/tip assembly that interacts with the sample and is also referred to as the probe. AFM can characterize surface modifications brought on by the presence of ligands, antibodies, or polymers conjugated at the liposomes' surface. It also has an exceptional resolution in the order of fractions of a nanometer and can provide a 3D image of liposomes along with information on morphology, size distribution, homogeneity, and stability [63, 64]. For the characterization of nanoparticles by AFM, they need to be adsorbed onto support surfaces like mica or silicon wafers of AFM so that they can function properly; this requirement is one of its limitations. There is a possibility of change in the vehicle's size, shape, and flatness as a result of liposome adhesion to a solid support [65].

9.7.2 Scattering Electron Microscopy (SEM)

The size, shape, and architecture of the liposomes are also shown using the SEM method. Since the sample must be dried or preserved before imaging, SEM is no longer frequently employed to study liposomes [66]. The concentric structure of the various lipid layers can be generally described by SEM, and it can also reveal specifics about the preparation's size and spherical morphology [67].

9.7.3 Transmission Electron Microscopy (TEM)

The imaging technique most frequently employed to assess the nanoparticles' structural integrity is transmission electron microscopy (TEM). TEM has the benefit of separating individual vesicles from aggregates and supplying details on lipid phase transitions, enabling a thorough evaluation of the structural characteristics of liposomes. Pre-treatment of the sample (drying) before characterizing with TEM arises several issues that cause swelling, shrinking, and deformation of the vesicles thereby changing the structural and morphological features of liposomes [66, 68].

The (cryo-)transmission electron microscopy (cryo-TEM) technology was created to address several of the drawbacks of the TEM method. To analyze the sample by cryo-TEM, there is no need to eliminate the solvent rather then the sample is treated with flash freezing to directly view the specimen in the solid state and prevent disturbance and damage to the liposomal structure. This quick freezing prevents the growth of ice crystals and maintains the integrity of the biological components. Before imaging, thin, vitrified liposome-hydrated films are employed, enabling the analysis to take place in its most natural state. Depending upon the film thickness cryo-TEM techniques provide resolutions in the range of 5–500 nm, besides shape and size it also offers precise insights into the interior of liposomes that includes lipid packing, phase behavior/transition, and drug inclusion features [69, 70].

9.7.4 Fluorescence Microscopy

A type of optical microscopy known as fluorescence microscopy focuses on the use of fluorophores that enables observation of the structure and provides crucial details regarding the composition and dynamics of membrane components [71]. To examine the structure of the liposome, fluorescent probes are employed and inserted into the sample. They can be positioned both within the lipid bilayer of liposomes and the aqueous compartment. The ability to identify the lamellarity of liposomes is made possible by rhodamine probes that were directly inserted into the lipid bilayer whereas rhodamine-labeled lipids were used to investigate various lipid packing confirmations. In addition to the probe, fluorescent molecules also include dye and proteins that are added to the lipid system, which may affect the liposomal delivery system's functionality. Low dye concentrations (1 mol%) have little effect on the physical characteristics of the liposomes, allowing for the avoidance of any modifications to the lipid phase [71]. Therefore, when utilizing fluorescence microscopy, the fluorescent dye selection and the creation of new membrane probes are crucial factors.

9.7.5 Confocal Microscopy

Confocal laser scanning microscopy is a promising approach developed as a result of advances in fluorescence microscopy. It is a method of choice since it offers a non-invasive means to look at the interior structure of liposomes and does structural analysis. Because it offers better image quality, the approach has grown increasingly appealing [66]. Using confocal microscopy, the structural features of lipid bilayers can be seen in the case of giant unilamellar vesicles, which is frequently not attainable with other imaging techniques. It also aids in the identification and visualization of the liposomal aqueous and lipid phase separation [72]. Additionally, it enables the localization and measurement of the degree of liposome distribution in cellular components throughout drug delivery procedures [73].

9.7.6 SMALL-ANGLE X-RAY SCATTERING (SAXS)

Small-angle x-ray scattering (SAXS) provides valuable information on the liposomal system including the size, distribution of particles in the lipid phase, lamellar thickness under variable conditions, and mainly the hydrophilic portion of a lipid bilayer and is sensitive to it [74].

9.7.7 WIDE-ANGLE X-RAY SCATTERING (WAXS)

Wide-angle x-ray scattering (WAXS) provides additional information on lipophilic chain packing and their lamellar features in the Å scale range when a kind of crystalline phase is a part of the liposome [74].

9.7.8 SMALL-ANGLE NEUTRON SCATTERING (SANS)

Small-angle neutron scattering (SANS) provides information on the hydrophobic tails section of the lipids and uses neutrons to provide a greater contrast for that region as compared to the hydrophilic part. Additionally, the assessment of the conformation of the lipid molecules at various conditions is made possible by neutron diffraction measurements and is selectively carried out on deuterated lipids. To describe the structure of liposome systems in detail, SAXS and SANS are complementing approaches [74, 75].

9.7.9 DYNAMIC LIGHT SCATTERING (DLS)

To analyze the liposome size distribution, dynamic light scattering (DLS), sometimes referred to as photon correlation spectroscopy, is performed. It assesses the variation in light reflected from particles moving in a Brownian manner. The basis for this method is the scattering phenomenon from the nanoparticles' surfaces. To detect the electron or light scattered by nanoparticles the sample usually a nanoformulation or dried nanoparticles is initially bombarded with light or electrons. The size is determined by the signal of these electrons or light scattering. This method allows for the determination of the polydispersity index (PDI) of a nanoformulation, a measure of particle size [76].

9.7.10 ZETA POTENTIAL

Zeta potential is the term used to describe the potential difference between the surface of the solid particles suspended in a dispersion medium. Zeta potential is a practical method for dealing with the electrostatic effects in charged nanoparticles. It is controlled by the makeup of the liposomes' surface charges and how well they are distributed, as well as by the charges present on the hydrophilic part of the lipids. The zeta potential is a significant element that tightly controls the drug uptake, its affinity towards the cell, biodistribution, pharmacokinetics, and colloidal stability of liposomes. When a liposome nanocarrier is disseminated in an aqueous solution, the ionization of surface endgroups or the adsorption of charged species on its surface causes the nanocarrier to develop a surface charge [77].

9.8 PASSIVE AND ACTIVE TARGETING OF LIPOSOMES

9.8.1 PASSIVE TARGETING

Passive drug targeting is a method of medication delivery that simply relies on the pathophysiological characteristics of cancerous tissues [78]. Nanodevices easily translocate through the capillary endothelium and reach the interstitial space because the vessels supplying blood to the tumor site are leaky. In contrast to the typical normal endothelium, which has gaps between endothelial cells of 5–10 nm, tumor capillaries have gaps between endothelial cells that range in size from 100–780 nm depending on the kind of malignancy. As a result, the extravasated molecules will only partially return to the bloodstream, causing macromolecules and nanoparticles to build up in the tumor microenvironment. Because more blood vessels that pass through the target amplify the EPR effect results in long-lasting systemic circulation and allows for longer liposome engagement with the target [79]. To prevent the reticuloendothelial system from absorbing the liposomes, the incorporation of a polymer such as PEG into liposomes is the main strategy to mask their identity, which increases their residence time in blood circulation. Liposomes typically have PEG added to the surface, which creates a protective hydrophilic barrier around the liposomes to stop them from aggregating and interacting with the blood constituents [80]. The liposomes' size is a crucial factor that affects passive targeting via the EPR effect. The size of the endothelial gaps in the capillary vasculature for a particular malignancy has a significant impact on how many liposomes accumulate in the tumor. The liposomes typically need to be smaller than 400 nm in size to take advantage of the EPR effect [81]. However, it has been demonstrated that numerous particles smaller than 200 nm can extravasate more effectively [82]. Other elements that affect passive targeting include the liposomes' composition and surface charge. The renal clearance is bypassed by anionic or neutral liposomes. Despite the cationic liposomes' propensity to localize in tumor vessels, their positive surface charge nonspecifically interacts with the anionic species in the blood, which leads to rapid clearance of liposomes from the bloodstream by the RES and lessens the EPR effect [83]. Nevertheless, when the number of cationic lipids in the liposomal membrane grows, the tendency for liposomes to aggregate rises. However, a suitable surface modification with cationic lipids could greatly improve tumor penetration.

The most popular method of clinical therapy has historically been passive targeting, although it has several drawbacks. According to the type and stage of tumors, neovascular porosity, and pore size change. As a result, not all cancers may respond to a passive targeting effect. The uniform targeting of the neoplastic cells within a tumor is not always an easy task and some chemotherapeutic medications cannot diffuse well across the cancerous region [84]. The increased interstitial fluid pressure might lead to multichemotherapeutic drug resistance [85] because it can also prevent nanocarriers from being distributed uniformly throughout the tissues of the majority of solid tumors [86].

9.9 ACTIVE TARGETING

Actively targeted liposomes are often made with a focus on minimizing astray effects. Targeting moieties, including small-molecule ligands, peptides, and monoclonal antibodies, are conjugated on the liposomal surface to create actively targeted liposomal systems [87]. To effectively target liposomes to cancer cells, the targeting moiety must be linked in large enough quantities to have a strong attraction for the cell surface receptors that are overexpressed in many malignancies [88].

To investigate the binding potential in cells overexpressing HER-2, PEGylated liposomal doxorubicin that is targeted against HER-2 was synthesized. This targeted drug delivery system showed greater accumulation in the tumor site when compared to numerous other ligands, demonstrating its efficacy as an anticancer therapeutic [89].

A liposomal delivery method that targets integrins to administer doxorubicin. The liposomes had a cyclic RGD (peptide) covalently attached to them. Doxorubicin was taken up by the glioma cells 2.5 times more readily by the RGD-coupled liposomal system than by the unaltered liposomes. An endocytic route regulated by an integrin receptor internalized the liposomes, according to competitive binding testing, indicating preferential targeting and extended circulating characteristics [90].

Long circulating liposomes with an exterior adorned with a thiolated oligonucleotide aptamer were produced to assess the target efficacy for breast cancer and pharmacokinetic aspects. The conjugated liposomes are efficiently and quickly absorbed, according to in vitro targeting tests. When administered intravenously, in vivo studies reveal liposomal buildup at the tumor vasculature with a longer circulatory half-life [91].

9.10 CONCLUSION

Due to their high biocompatibility and versatility, liposomes are the most used lipid-based nanoparticles. They are used as drug delivery systems due to their low toxicity and flexibility, which can be tailored for a variety of desirable purposes. Despite the wide range of physicochemical characteristics and administration routes, practically any medicine can be delivered using this incomparable method. This system exemplifies desirable liposomal preparation qualities, such as stability, sustained drug release over time, enhanced viscosity, and improved half-life for both the active ingredient and the liposomes. The system's polymeric component, on the other hand, aids in preserving and maintaining the bioactivity and efficacy of the encapsulated drugs. Apart from the significant advancements made with this system, they continue to face difficulties with synthesis, stability and targeting, such as the destruction of the drug during production due to hazardous organic solvents or high temperatures. The rapid polymer degradation results in overdose and its lack of degradation does not allow the loaded drug to liberate from the liposomes as it was intended to be. This changes the release pattern, thereby affecting pharmacokinetic parameters and encountering various biological mechanisms such as RES, opsonization, and vesicle destabilization to reach their target site and exert drug action at the cellular level. Despite this, liposomes act as a remarkable tool that creates new opportunities for customized chemotherapy for patients unresponsive or resistant to conventional forms of treatment. Therefore, they have the potential to revolutionize cancer treatment.

REFERENCES

1. Papahadjopoulos, D., *Liposomes and their uses in biology and medicine. Annuals of the New York Academy of Sciences*, 1978: pp. 308–324.
2. Torchilin, P.V., et al., *Liposomes: A practical approach.* 2003. Oxford: Oxford University Press.
3. Fahr, A., et al., *Transfer of lipophilic drugs between liposomal membranes and biological interfaces: consequences for drug delivery. European Journal of Pharmaceutical Sciences*, 2005. **26**(3–4): pp. 251–265.
4. Chowdhury, D., *Pharmaceutical nanosystems: Manufacture, characterization, and safety. Pharmaceutical Sciences Encyclopedia: Drug Discovery, Development, and Manufacturing*, 2010. **14**: pp. 1–38.
5. Munye, M.M., et al., *Role of liposome and peptide in the synergistic enhancement of transfection with a lipopolyplex vector. Scientific Reports*, 2015. **5**(1): pp. 1–9.
6. Alberts, B., et al., *Molecular biology of the cell. Scandinavian Journal of Rheumatology*, 2003. **32**(2): pp. 125–125.
7. Demel, R.A. and B. De Kruyff, *The function of sterols in membranes. Biochimica et Biophysica Acta (BBA)-Reviews on Biomembranes*, 1976. **457**(2): pp. 109–132.
8. Briuglia, M.-L., et al., *Influence of cholesterol on liposome stability and on in vitro drug release. Drug Delivery and Translational Research*, 2015. **5**(3): pp. 231–242.
9. Garg, T. and A. K Goyal, *Liposomes: Targeted and controlled delivery system. Drug Delivery Letters*, 2014. **4**(1): pp. 62–71.
10. Cogan, U., et al., *Microviscosity and order in the hydrocarbon region of phospholipid and phospholipid-cholesterol dispersions determined with fluorescent probes. Biochemistry*, 1973. **12**(3): pp. 521–528.
11. Liu, W., et al., *Kinetic stability and membrane structure of liposomes during in vitro infant intestinal digestion: Effect of cholesterol and lactoferrin. Food Chemistry*, 2017. **230**: pp. 6–13.
12. Kaddah, S., et al., *Cholesterol modulates the liposome membrane fluidity and permeability for a hydrophilic molecule. Food and Chemical Toxicology*, 2018. **113**: pp. 40–48.

13. Akbarzadeh, A., et al., *Liposome: classification, preparation, and applications. Nanoscale Research Letters*, 2013. **8**(1): pp. 1–9.

14. Dua, J., A. Rana, and A. Bhandari, *Liposome: Methods of preparation and applications. International Journal of Pharmaceutical Studies and Research*, 2012. **3**(2): pp. 14–20.

15. Fan, Y., M. Marioli, and K. Zhang, *Analytical characterization of liposomes and other lipid nanoparticles for drug delivery. Journal of Pharmaceutical Biomedical Analysis*, 2021. **192**: p. 113642.

16. Salimi, A., *Liposomes as a novel drug delivery system: Fundamental and pharmaceutical application. Asian Journal of Pharmaceutics (AJP)*, 2018. **12**(01): p. S31–S41.

17. Pattni, B.S., V.V. Chupin, and V.P. Torchilin, *New developments in liposomal drug delivery. Chemical Reviews*, 2015. **115**(19): pp. 10938–10966.

18. Kim, T., J. Kim, and S. Kim, *Extended-release formulation of morphine for subcutaneous administration. Cancer Chemotherapy and Pharmacology*, 1993. **33**(3): pp. 187–190.

19. Bangham, A., *A correlation between surface charge and coagulant action of phospholipids. Nature*, 1961. **192**(4808): pp. 1197–1198.

20. Vu, M.T., et al., *Development and characterization of soy lecithin liposome as potential drug carrier systems for codelivery of letrozole and paclitaxel. Journal of Nanomaterials*, 2020. **2020**: p. 8896455.

21. Zhang, L., et al., *Co-delivery of docetaxel and resveratrol by liposomes synergistically boosts antitumor efficiency against prostate cancer. European Journal of Pharmaceutical Sciences*, 2022. **174**: p. 106199.

22. Karanth, H. and R. Murthy, *pH-sensitive liposomes - principle and application in cancer therapy. Journal of Pharmacy and Pharmacology*, 2007. **59**(4): pp. 469–483.

23. Li, Y., et al., *Ultrasmall nanostructured drug based pH-sensitive liposome for effective treatment of drug-resistant tumor. Journal of Nanobiotechnology*, 2019. **17**(1): pp. 1–13.

24. Alrbyawi, H., et al., *pH-sensitive liposomes for enhanced cellular uptake and cytotoxicity of daunorubicin in melanoma (B16-BL6) cell lines. Pharmaceutics*, 2022. **14**(6): pp. 1128.

25. Xi, L., et al., *Novel thermosensitive polymer-modified liposomes as nano-carrier of hydrophobic antitumor drugs. Journal of Pharmaceutical Sciences*, 2020. **109**(8): pp. 2544–2552.

26. García, M.C., et al., *Cholesterol levels affect the performance of AuNPs-decorated thermo-sensitive liposomes as nanocarriers for controlled doxorubicin delivery. Pharmaceutics*, 2021. **13**(7): p. 973.

27. Majzoub, R.N., K.K. Ewert, and C.R. Safinya, *Cationic liposome–nucleic acid nanoparticle assemblies with applications in gene delivery and gene silencing. Philosophical Transactions of the Royal Society A: Mathematical, Physical and Engineering Sciences*, 2016. **374**(2072): p. 20150129.

28. Dass, C.R., *Improving anti-angiogenic therapy via selective delivery of cationic liposomes to tumour vasculature. International Journal of Pharmaceutics*, 2003. **267**(1–2): pp. 1–12.

29. Wang, W., et al., *Cationic polymethacrylate-modified liposomes significantly enhanced doxorubicin delivery and antitumor activity. Scientific Reports*, 2017. **7**(1): pp. 1–10.

30. Paszko, E. and M. Senge, *Immunoliposomes. Current Medicinal Chemistry*, 2012. **19**(31): pp. 5239–5277.

31. Eloy, J.O., et al., *Anti-HER2 immunoliposomes for co-delivery of paclitaxel and rapamycin for breast cancer therapy. European Journal of Pharmaceutics and Biopharmaceutics*, 2017. **115**: pp. 159–167.

32. Suk, J.S., et al., *PEGylation as a strategy for improving nanoparticle-based drug and gene delivery. Advanced Drug Delivery Reviews*, 2016. **99**: pp. 28–51.

33. Li, Y., et al., *Long-circulating thermosensitive liposomes for the targeted drug delivery of oxaliplatin. International Journal of Nanomedicine*, 2020. **15**: p. 6721.

34. Zawilska, P., et al., *Novel pegylated liposomal formulation of docetaxel with 3-n-pentadecylphenol derivative for cancer therapy. European Journal of Pharmaceutical Sciences*, 2021. **163**: p. 105838.

35. Grabarnick, E., et al., *PEGylated liposomes remotely loaded with the combination of doxorubicin, quinine, and indocyanine green enable successful treatment of multidrug-resistant tumors. Pharmaceutics*, 2021. **13**(12): p. 2181.

36. Zhang, N., et al., *Gold conjugate-based liposomes with hybrid cluster bomb structure for liver cancer therapy. Biomaterials*, 2016. **74**: pp. 280–291.

37. Hashemi, M., et al., *Layer-by-layer assembly of graphene oxide on thermosensitive liposomes for photo-chemotherapy. Acta Biomaterialia*, 2018. **65**: pp. 376–392.

38. Prasad, R., et al., *Graphene oxide supported liposomes as red emissive theranostics for phototriggered tissue visualization and tumor regression. ACS Applied Bio Materials*, 2019. **2**(8): pp. 3312–3320.

39. Daeihamed, M., et al., *Potential of liposomes for enhancement of oral drug absorption. Current Drug Delivery*, 2017. **14**(2): pp. 289–303.
40. Yucel, C., Z. De Gim, and S. Yilmaz, *Development of Cisplatin-loaded liposome and evaluation of transport properties through Caco-2 cell line. Turkish Journal of Pharmaceutical Sciences*, 2016. **13**: pp. 95–108.
41. Antimisiaris, S., et al., *Overcoming barriers by local drug delivery with liposomes. Advanced Drug Delivery Reviews*, 2021. **174**: pp. 53–86.
42. Gogineni, V.R., et al., *Localized and triggered release of oxaliplatin for the treatment of colorectal liver metastasis. Journal of Cancer*, 2020. **11**(23): p. 6982.
43. Ostro, M.J. and P.R. Cullis, *Use of liposomes as injectable-drug delivery systems. American Journal of Health-System Pharmacy*, 1989. **46**(8): pp. 1576–1588.
44. Zhang, H., *Thin-film hydration followed by extrusion method for liposome preparation*, in *Liposomes*. 2017, New York: Springer. pp. 17–22.
45. Xiang, B. and D.-Y. Cao, *Preparation of drug liposomes by thin-film hydration and homogenization*, in *Liposome-Based Drug Delivery Systems*, 2021. Berlin: Springer. pp. 25–35.
46. Jiskoot, W., et al., *Preparation of liposomes via detergent removal from mixed micelles by dilution. Pharmaceutisch Weekblad*, 1986. **8**(5): pp. 259–265.
47. Ollivon, M., et al., *Vesicle reconstitution from lipid–detergent mixed micelles. Biochimica et Biophysica Acta (BBA)-Biomembranes*, 2000. **1508**(1–2): pp. 34–50.
48. Pons, M., M. Foradada, and J. Estelrich, *Liposomes obtained by the ethanol injection method. International Journal of Pharmaceutics*, 1993. **95**(1–3): pp. 51–56.
49. Gouda, A., et al., *Ethanol injection technique for liposomes formulation: An insight into development, influencing factors, challenges and applications. Journal of Drug Delivery Science and Technology*, 2021. **61**: p. 102174.
50. Charcosset, C., et al., *Preparation of liposomes at large scale using the ethanol injection method: effect of scale-up and injection devices. Chemical Engineering Research and Design*, 2015. **94**: pp. 508–515.
51. Jaafar-Maalej, C., et al., *Ethanol injection method for hydrophilic and lipophilic drug-loaded liposome preparation. Journal of Liposome Research*, 2010. **20**(3): pp. 228–243.
52. Kanda, H., T. Katsube, and M. Goto, *Preparation of liposomes from soy lecithin using liquefied dimethyl ether. Foods*, 2021. **10**(8): p. 1789.
53. Deamer, D.W., *Preparation and properties of ether-injection liposomes. Annals of the New York Academy of Sciences*, 1978. **308**(1): pp. 250–258.
54. Shi, N.-Q. and X.-R. Qi, *Preparation of drug liposomes by reverse-phase evaporation. Liposome-Based Drug Delivery Systems*, 2021: pp. 37–46.
55. Szoka Jr, F. and D. Papahadjopoulos, *Procedure for preparation of liposomes with large internal aqueous space and high capture by reverse-phase evaporation. Proceedings of the National Academy of Sciences*, 1978. **75**(9): pp. 4194–4198.
56. Pidgeon, C., et al., *Multilayered vesicles prepared by reverse-phase evaporation: liposome structure and optimum solute entrapment. Biochemistry*, 1987. **26**(1): pp. 17–29.
57. Whitesides, G.M., *The origins and the future of microfluidics. Nature*, 2006. **442**(7101): pp. 368–373.
58. van Swaay, D. and A. DeMello, *Microfluidic methods for forming liposomes. Lab on a Chip*, 2013. **13**(5): pp. 752–767.
59. Jahn, A., et al., *Microfluidic directed formation of liposomes of controlled size. Langmuir*, 2007. **23**(11): pp. 6289–6293.
60. Carugo, D., et al., *Liposome production by microfluidics: potential and limiting factors. Scientific Reports*, 2016. **6**(1): pp. 1–15.
61. Li, C. and Y. Deng, *A novel method for the preparation of liposomes: freeze drying of monophase solutions. Journal of Pharmaceutical Sciences*, 2004. **93**(6): pp. 1403–1414.
62. Franzé, S., et al., *Lyophilization of liposomal formulations: still necessary, still challenging. Pharmaceutics*, 2018. **10**(3): p. 139.
63. Spyratou, E., et al., *Atomic force microscopy: a tool to study the structure, dynamics and stability of liposomal drug delivery systems. Expert Opinion on Drug Delivery*, 2009. **6**(3): pp. 305–317.

64. Robson, A.-L., et al., *Advantages and limitations of current imaging techniques for characterizing liposome morphology. Frontiers in Pharmacology*, 2018. **9**: p. 80.

65. Ruozi, B., et al., *Application of atomic force microscopy to characterize liposomes as drug and gene carriers. Talanta*, 2007. **73**(1): pp. 12–22.

66. Ruozi, B., et al., *AFM, ESEM, TEM, and CLSM in liposomal characterization: a comparative study. International Journal of Nanomedicine*, 2011. **6**: p. 557.

67. Nirale, N., R. Vidhate, and M. Nagarsenker, *Fluticasone propionate liposomes for pulmonary delivery. Indian Journal of Pharmaceutical Sciences*, 2009. **71**(6): p. 709.

68. Bibi, S., et al., *Microscopy imaging of liposomes: from coverslips to environmental SEM. International Journal of Pharmaceutics*, 2011. **417**(1–2): pp. 138–150.

69. Helvig, S., et al., *Recent advances in cryo-TEM imaging of soft lipid nanoparticles. Aims Biophysics*, 2015. **2**(2): pp. 116–130.

70. Almgren, M., K. Edwards, and G. Karlsson, *Cryo transmission electron microscopy of liposomes and related structures. Colloids and Surfaces A: Physicochemical and Engineering Aspects*, 2000. **174**(1–2): pp. 3–21.

71. Bouvrais, H., et al., *Impact of membrane-anchored fluorescent probes on the mechanical properties of lipid bilayers. Biochimica et Biophysica Acta (BBA)-Biomembranes*, 2010. **1798**(7): pp. 1333–1337.

72. Mertins, O. and R. Dimova, *Insights on the interactions of chitosan with phospholipid vesicles. Part II: Membrane stiffening and pore formation. Langmuir*, 2013. **29**(47): pp. 14552–14559.

73. Solomon, M.A., *Determination of the subcellular distribution of liposomes using confocal microscopy*, in *Liposomes*. 2017, New York: Springer. pp. 119–130.

74. Lombardo, D., P. Calandra, and M.A. Kiselev, *Structural characterization of biomaterials by means of small angle x-rays and neutron scattering (SAXS and SANS), and light scattering experiments. Molecules*, 2020. **25**(23): p. 5624.

75. Kinnun, J.J., et al., *Biomembrane structure and material properties studied with neutron scattering. Frontiers in Chemistry*, 2021. **9**: p. 203.

76. Surianarayanan, R., et al., *Effect of sample concentration on the characterization of liposomes using dynamic light scattering technique. Pharmaceutical Methods*, 2016. **7**(1): pp. 70–74.

77. Hunter, R.J., *Foundations of colloid science*. 2001. Oxford: Oxford University Press.

78. Lammers, T., et al., *Drug targeting to tumors: principles, pitfalls and (pre-) clinical progress. Journal of Controlled Release*, 2012. **161**(2): pp. 175–187.

79. Haley, B. and E. Frenkel. *Nanoparticles for drug delivery in cancer treatment.* in *Urologic oncology: seminars and original investigations*. 2008. Amsterdam: Elsevier.

80. Wang, M. and M. Thanou, *Targeting nanoparticles to cancer. Pharmacological Research*, 2010. **62**(2): pp. 90–99.

81. Danhier, F., O. Feron, and V. Préat, *To exploit the tumor microenvironment: passive and active tumor targeting of nanocarriers for anti-cancer drug delivery. Journal of Controlled Release*, 2010. **148**(2): pp. 135–146.

82. Torchilin, V.P., *Recent advances with liposomes as pharmaceutical carriers. Nature Reviews Drug discovery*, 2005. **4**(2): pp. 145–160.

83. Zhao, W., S. Zhuang, and X.-R. Qi, *Comparative study of the in vitro and in vivo characteristics of cationic and neutral liposomes. International Journal of Nanomedicine*, 2011. **6**: p. 3087.

84. Bae, Y.H., *Drug targeting and tumor heterogeneity. Journal of Controlled Release: Official Journal of the Controlled Release Society*, 2009. **133**(1): p. 2.

85. Ferrari, M., *Cancer nanotechnology: opportunities and challenges. Nature Reviews Cancer*, 2005. **5**(3): pp. 161–171.

86. Heldin, C.-H., et al., *High interstitial fluid pressure—an obstacle in cancer therapy. Nature Reviews Cancer*, 2004. **4**(10): pp. 806–813.

87. Byrne, J.D., T. Betancourt, and L. Brannon-Peppas, *Active targeting schemes for nanoparticle systems in cancer therapeutics. Advanced Drug Delivery Reviews*, 2008. **60**(15): pp. 1615–1626.

88. Egusquiaguirre, S.P., et al., *Nanoparticle delivery systems for cancer therapy: advances in clinical and preclinical research. Clinical and Translational Oncology*, 2012. **14**(2): pp. 83–93.

89. Shmeeda, H., et al., *Her2-targeted pegylated liposomal doxorubicin: retention of target-specific binding and cytotoxicity after in vivo passage. Journal of Controlled Release*, 2009. **136**(2): pp. 155–160.

90. Chen, Z., et al., *Cyclic RGD peptide-modified liposomal drug delivery system: enhanced cellular uptake in vitro and improved pharmacokinetics in rats. International Journal of Nanomedicine*, 2012. **7**: p. 3803.

91. Mann, A.P., et al., *Thioaptamer conjugated liposomes for tumor vasculature targeting. Oncotarget*, 2011. **2**(4): p. 298.

10 Niosome-Based Anticancer Therapies

Daulat Haleem Khan, Muhammad Yasir Ali,
Muhammad Asim Farooq, Muhammad Ali Syed,
Azhar Rasul, Shazia Anwer Bukhari, Sevki Adem,
and Maria Manan

10.1 INTRODUCTION

Niosomes are self-organizing vesicles prepared with the help of non-ionic surfactants and are stabilized with cholesterol with or without charge-imparting agents [1]. Niosomes are manufactured in the same way as liposomes and are similar in physical characterizations. They can be unilamellar or multilamellar. They have more benefits when compared with liposomes. The preparation of niosomes is easy with cost effectiveness, preservation, and versatility [2].

The conspicuous characteristics of niosomes, which lead to their massive applications in the development of pharmaceutical products and cosmetics are as follows:

- Niosomes can encapsulate hydrophilic and lipophilic drugs in the same way as liposomes.
- They are osmotically stable and active.
- Due to the presence of lipophilic and lipophobic constituents in the basic structure, they can load a wide variety of drugs depending on their solubility.
- They can be designed to the desired size and fluidity.
- They can transport the drug to the target site with improved bioavailability.
- Niosomes can allow the attachment of functional ligands for targeted delivery [3].
- They are produced to improve the bioavailability of less soluble drugs [4].

10.2 STRUCTURAL COMPONENTS OF NIOSOMES

Niosomes are prepared of non-ionic surfactants, cholesterol and sometimes charging agents is indicated in Figure 10.1 [5].

10.2.1 CLASSIFICATION OF NON-IONIC SURFACTANTS (GENERAL)

The non-ionic surfactants are neutral entities without charge (Table 10.1). When non-ionic surfactants are dispersed in the aqueous phase the lipophilic tails arrange themselves towards each other and lipophobic heads become oriented away from each other [6, 7]. Non-ionic surfactants are classified as follows:

10.2.1.1 Alkyl Ether

Alkyl ethers are divided into two sub-classes depending upon their hydrophilic heads, which are described as follows:

DOI: 10.1201/9781003363958-13

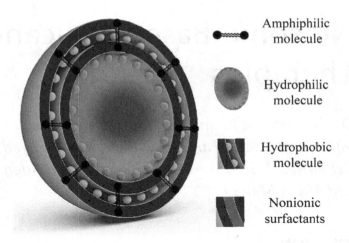

FIGURE 10.1   Structure of a typical noisome.

TABLE 10.1
Class of Non-Ionic Surfactant, Characteristic, and Application in Niosomal Preparations [8, 9]

Class of Non-Ionic Surfactants	Encapsulated Therapeutic Moiety	Distinct Characteristic and Applications
Alkyl ethers & alkyl glyceryl ether (Brij 30, 52, 56, 58, 72, 76, and 92)	Proteins and peptides	No skin allergy, a wide rangeof HLB allows the formation of inverse vesicles (Brij58) and multilamellar vesicles (Brij72 & 92)
Sorbitan fatty acid esters (Span 20, 40, 60, 80, and 85)	Acyclovir, colchicine, 5-Fluorouracil, Estradiol,	Lowest transition temperature (Span20 and Span80), act as a gelator (Span40 and Span 60)
Polyoxyethylene fatty acid esters (Tween 20, 40, 60, and 80) (synonyms: scattics, alkest & canarcel)	Methotrexate, Ciprofloxacin, and Curcumin, etc.	Stable formulations for a poorly soluble drug, Stabilize protein derivative
Block copolymer (pluronic L64, P105 etc.)	Doxorubicin, Curcumin, Paclitaxel, Calcein, Quarecetein, Rifampicin etc.	Biodegradable, pH-sensitive, helps in delivery of proteins and peptide through oral route

10.2.1.2   Alkyl Glycerol Ethers

These non-ionic surfactants have glycerol subunits or larger sugar molecules. These surfactants have been used to load cytotoxic drugs. They alter the pharmacokinetics of the drugs [10–12].

10.2.1.3   Alkyl Oxyethylene Ethers (Brij®)

The alkyl oxyethylene ethers are the non-ionic surfactants containing the oxyethylene repeated units. These non-ionic surfactants have been utilized for the oral delivery of the encapsulated drugs to prevent degradation of the drug by gastric acid. These non-ionic surfactants have been used for the oral delivery of insulin [3].

10.2.1.4 Alkyl Esters

These surfactants are fatty acid esters of poloxyethylene (tween®) and sorbitans (span®). They are used in the orally driven delivery system, parenteral, cosmeceuticals, topical, and foodstuffs [13, 14]. These surfactants are superior due to their non-toxic and non-irritant nature [15].

10.2.1.5 Pluronics

Pluronics are the surfactant types having different numbers of tri-block copolymers of poly (ethylene oxide) and poly (propylene oxide) units. They have been extensively used for the delivery of anticancer drugs. They can modify make the drug targeted and modify its response with increased efficacy [16]. Pluronics have the capacity to internalize cytotoxic drugs for a prolonged time by the nullification of the effect of P-glycoproteins and diminish anticancer drug resistance [17]. Pluronics increase the solubility of poorly water-soluble drugs [16].

10.2.2 CHOLESTEROL

The impact of cholesterol on the niosome preparation is also important. It affects the physical characterization of the niosomes, including shape and stability due to the interaction between the non-ionic surfactants and cholesterol. The content of cholesterol is needed between 30% and 50% for the vesicular formation. The quantity of the cholesterol depends on the HLB value of the surfactant. An HLB value greater than 10 needs more cholesterol for the preparation of niosomes [18]. Some studies proposed that the entrapment efficiency (%EE) of the drug is also dependent on the concentration of cholesterol. The mechanical and hydrodynamic stability to the niosomes is dependent on the concentration of cholesterol [19]. The quantity of cholesterol in the formulation must be assessed case by case, depending upon the type of the non-ionic surfactant and the model drug used [20].

10.2.3 CHARGE AIDING MOLECULES

The stabilized niosomes can be produced by the addition of a charging agent. The negative charge can be induced by dicetylphosphate (DCP) and phosphatidic acid. In the same way, positive charge can be induced by cetylpyridinium oxide and stearylamine (SA). The produced niosomes do not aggregate due to the repulsive forces [21].

The positively charged niosomes were used to encapsulate polynucleotide, which resulted in efficient cellular penetration [22]. Also, charge-aiding molecules increase niosomal aggregation and result in a prolonged plasma half-life ($t\frac{1}{2}$) of the loaded niosomes [22]. The concentration of charge imparting agent is a very important factor for the development of stable and least aggregating niosomes if the concentration is between 2.5–5 mol% and higher concentrations resulted in inhibition of niosomal vesicle formation [23, 24]. The zeta (ζ)-potentials over 30 mV resulted in niosomes in the stabilized form due to less niosomal aggregation with high entrapment efficiency and skin penetration [25–27].

10.3 GENERAL METHODS OF PREPARATION

Niosomes are generally prepared by the following methods.

10.3.1 THIN FILM HYDRATION TECHNIQUE

This is the widely used method of preparation of niosomes. In this method, non-ionic surfactant and cholesterol are dissolved in an organic solvent in a round bottom flask. The solvent is evaporated under a vacuum and a thin film is prepared on the walls of the round bottom flask. The thin film is hydrated with the addition of buffer, containing the drug. The solution is then heated above glass transition temperature and resulted in vesicular formation [28]. The schematic flow diagram of the thin-film hydration technique is shown in Figure 10.2 [29]. This method is used to encapsulate different types of drugs, i.e., anticancer, anti-inflammatory, and antibiotics.

10.3.2 REVERSE PHASE EVAPORATION TECHNIQUE (REV)

In the reverse phase evaporation method, surfactant and cholesterol are dissolved in an organic solvent and the aqueous solution of the drug is added. The solution is heated at 40–60°C and sonicated until the formation of an emulsion. The evaporation will continue until complete hydration is achieved and results in niosome formation [30]. The schematic flow chart of the REV technique is shown in Figure 10.3 [7].

10.3.3 ETHER INJECTION METHOD

In the ether injection method, the organic solvent used was ether mixed with a charge imparting agent and non-ionic surfactant. This organic solvent solution was injected into the aqueous solution of the drug at 60°C to remove the ether. After the evaporation of the ether resulted in niosome formation [31]. This technique has been adopted for the loading of naproxen [32], 5-fluorouracil, and azithromycin for ocular infections [33,34]. The schematic representation of the ether injection method is shown in Figure 10.4 [9].

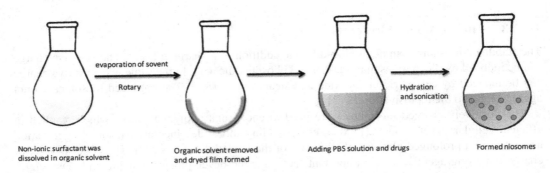

FIGURE 10.2   Schematic representation of the thin-film hydration technique.

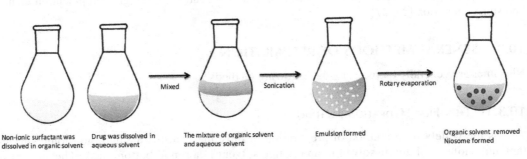

FIGURE 10.3   Schematic representation of reverse phase evaporation technique.

10.3.4 MICROFLUIDIZATION TECHNIQUE

In the microfluidization technique, the solutions of non-ionic surfactant and drug interacted in a chamber and after the collision they passed through a cooling loop to reduce the temperature [35].

10.3.5 TRANS-MEMBRANE TECHNIQUE

In this technique, non-ionic surfactants and cholesterol are dissolved in a relevant solvent and made into a thin film under reduced pressure. The hydration of the film is done with an acidic medium made of citric acid with subsequent vortex. The solution is then freeze-thawed and then the drug solution is added. The pH is adjusted at 7.4 with the addition of disodium hydrogen phosphate [10].

10.3.6 SUPERCRITICAL FLUID TECHNIQUE

In this technique, non-ionic surfactant, cholesterol along with organic solvent are subjected to a pressure cell under 200 bar pressure at 60°C temperature. The mixture is stirred with a magnet for 30 min. After mixing a niosome dispersion is obtained after the release of pressure [36].

10.3.7 BUBBLE METHOD

In the bubble method, phosphate buffer saline was mixed with non-ionic surfactant and cholesterol in a three-neck glass reactor. The temperature was monitored from one neck with the assistance of a thermometer. The nitrogen gas was introduced from the second neck and third neck used for cooled water. The ingredients for niosomes were mixed, heated at 70°C and homogenized for 15 min. due to the introduction of nitrogen gas, bubbling resulted in niosomes production [37].

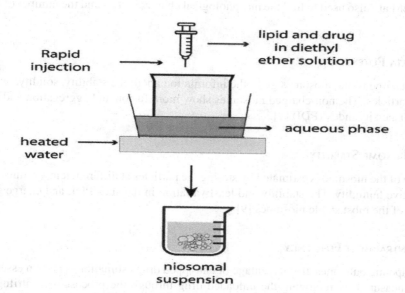

FIGURE 10.4 Schematic representation of ether injection method.

10.3.8 MEMBRANE CONTACTOR

In this method, the Shirasu membrane of porous glass is used in a two-chamber equipment. The dissolved non-ionic surfactant in organic solvent is introduced from one chamber and the aqueous dissolved drug from another chamber and is subjected to pressure and passed [38].

10.3.9 MICROFLUIDIC HYDRODYNAMIC FOCUSING

In this method, a scintillation vial is used for the organic solvent containing non-ionic surfactant, cholesterol, and charging agent. The solvent is removed to produce a thin film of the drug-dissolved in phosphate buffer saline and isopropyl alcohol for rehydration of the thin film in the microfluidic device. This resulted in the production of the niosomes [39].

10.3.10 PRONIOSOMAL TECHNOLOGY

In this technique, the precursor niosomes generated previously rehydrated with water and resulted in niosomes production [9]. The niosomes produced by this technique have been used to load a variety of drugs and are also used for transdermal and ophthalmic drug delivery [40]. A different method of preparation has advantages and disadvantages, which are tabulated in the following Table 10.2 [41].

10.4 NIOSOMES' CHARACTERIZATION

10.4.1 SIZE AND SIZE DISTRIBUTION

The size of the niosome is an important factor in reference to particle stability and physical characteristics. The size of the niosomes is needed to be small enough for cellular penetration. The size of the niosome ranges from 10 nm to 50 µm. The size of the niosome is carried out with the differential light scattering (DLS) technique. Transmission electron microscopy (TEM), scanning electron microscopy (SEM), and light microscopy can be done for particle size estimation. The TEM and SEM are also used to find the morphological characteristics and the number of the bilayer [1, 9].

10.4.2 ZETA POTENTIAL

The surface charge of the niosomes gives the information about the stability, solidity, and aggregation of the particles. The non-charged niosomes show more fusion and aggregation and resulted in a high polydispersity index (PDI) [9].

10.4.3 NIOSOME STABILITY

The stability of the niosome is estimated by storing the particles at different temperatures (4, 25, and 40°C at relative humidity. The stability and least variation in the size, PDI, and charge provide the information of the most stable niosomes [9].

10.4.4 ENTRAPMENT EFFICIENCY

For the therapeutic outcomes, the percentage of entrapped drug estimation is also an essential factor. The EE is measured by removing the unloaded drug through the process of centrifugation. The removal of the drug from niosomes is carried out by using 50% of n-propanol or 0.1% of Triton

TABLE 10.2

Advantages and Disadvantages of Niosomal Methods of Manufacturing

Preparation Method	Advantages	Disadvantages
Thin-film hydration	An easy technique for laboratory research	Involves the use of organic solvents
Reverse phase evaporation	High drug EE	Involves the use of organic solvents
Ether injection	An easy technique for laboratory researches	Cannot be used for heat labile drugs
Microfluidization	No organic solvents involved	Cannot be used for heat labile drugs
Trans-membrane	High drug EE	Involves the use of organic solvents
Bubble method	No organic solvents involved	Cannot be used for heat labile drugs
Emulsion method	An easy technique for laboratory research	Involves the use of organic solvents
Lipid injection method	No organic solvents involved	Cannot be used for heat labile drugs
Proniosomes	No organic solvents involved Better physical stability	Complex process Complete drug entrapment may not be possible during hydration
Supercritical reverse phase evaporation method	No organic solvents involved	Special equipment required for this method

X-100. This resulted in rupturing of niosomes after the incubation of 1 h. After incubation, particles are centrifuged and the drug solution is separated from the supernatant, and concentration is measured by diving the amount of drug entrapped with total amount of the drug used [9].

10.4.5 IN VITRO DRUG RELEASE

The release behavior of the drug from the particles is measured to assess the behavior of the particles inside the body. Therefore, the particles are loaded in a dialysis bag (pre-washed) or even without the dialysis bag directly to the dissolution media. After different time intervals, the samples of the dissolution media are withdrawn and the drug is estimated by using UV-Vis spectrophotometer or HPLC [42]. Different kinds of drugs encapsulated in niosomes and their obtained results are indicated in Table 10.3 [9].

10.5 ANTICANCER APPLICATION OF NIOSOMES

Several treatment strategies have been developed to reduce the mortality rate, including pain management with better life quality. The cancer treatments are flawed due to the inadequacy of treatments. The efficacy and adequacy of the treatment could be possible with the timely diagnosis of cancer with very specific drug administration for that cancer type. Due to the severe toxicity of the drug, poor diagnosis, and poor therapeutic outcomes, several strategies have been made to overcome these problems. Nanotechnologies have been developed to reduce toxicities with better diagnosis. The nanotechnological immunotherapeutic agents have been developed to reduce the toxicity of the drug with site-specific and targeted drug delivery and preservation of normal cells [43].

The poor bioavailability of the drug is caused by the poor solubility of the drug. To solve this problem, S. Agarwal et al. used non-ionic surfactant span 60 and cholesterol to prepare niosomal system to improve the solubility of the drug. The size of the niosomes was 479 nm with smooth and

TABLE 10.3
Different Drug-Loaded Niosomes and Their Characterization

Drug	Method of Preparation	The Highest EE (%)	Size (nm)	Zeta Potential (mV)
Methotrexate	Ether injection method	94.8±4.6	115.2±7.0	-
Paclitaxel	Thin-film hydration method	98.7±0.8	134±3	−81.1±2.2
Curcumin	Thin-film hydration,	ND	80-200	ND
Rifampicin	Probe sonication (5 min)	75.37	190-893	−27.5±0.9
Acetazolamide	REV, TFH	65.71±1.09	3.46	-
Sodium Stibo-gluconate	Ether injection method	77.0±0.3	146±15	−40.3±0.2
Vinblastine	Thin-film hydration method	99.92±1.6	234.3±11.4	−34.6±4.2
siRNA	Micro-fluidization method	93.18±2.10	46.30±0.18	51.48±2.99
Tetanus toxoid	Reverse-phase evaporation method	42.1±2.1	2.9±0.5	-
Tenofovir	Proniosome-derived niosome method	33.68	50	7.7
Embelin	Thin-film hydration method	85.20	500	-
Ganciclovir	Reverse-phase evaporation method	89±2.13	144±3.47	−9.5±0.9
Minoxidil	Thin-film hydration method	69.526±2.9	200-1300	−44.71±1.3
Nystatin	Thin-film hydration method	97.88±1.58	164.8±22.3	-
Letrozole	Reverse-phase evaporation method	66.60	231.4	−8.71
Diallyl disulfide	Sonication method	68.6±3.3	140±30	−30.67±0.45
Morin hydrate (MH)	Thin-film hydration method	98.62±0.01	109±0.35	−27.48±3.02
Ellagic acid (EA)	Reverse-phase evaporation method	38.73±1.58	312–402	-
Topotecan	Micro-fluidization method	37.50–39.30	128.47	−27.00
Hydroxychloroquine	Hand shaking method	26.3±3.98	4.16±0.03	-
Glucocorticoid	Thin-film hydration	77.0±0.3	186±24	−25.1±0.1
Gemifloxacin	Solvent injection	64.9±0.66	213.2±1.5	−34.7±2.2
Doxorubicin	Thin-film hydration	75±1.22	338±3.14	−23.7±0.39

spherical morphology. The high entrapment efficiency of morusin (97%) was estimated with free dispersion in the aqueous medium as compared to the free morusin. The controlled and sustained drug release profile of the morusin was observed, which resulted in improved therapeutic efficacy against four different cancerous cell lines. The morusin niosomes showed targeted and more effective anticancer [44].

Another study was carried out that facilitates penetration through the skin. Hyaluronic acid niosomes were considered effective antitumor nanoparticles, which were endocytosed through the skin. Due to the presence of hyaluronic acid it enhances dermal penetration and more anticancer activity [45]. In another study, Ru (III)-complex was loaded in niosomes for targeted delivery against HeLa cells [45].

Poloxamers are block-copolymers and are less utilized non-ionic surfactants. They have the capacity to enclose drugs with the characteristic of a more solubilizing effect and result in increased bioavailability. For this purpose, pluronic L121 was used to prepare the cytotoxic drugs paclitaxel and doxorubicin-loaded niosomes. The anticancer activity of the niosomes was evaluated by using breast cancer cell line (MCF7) and prostatic cancer cell lines (PC3). The niosomes showed high entrapment efficiency (99%), small size (137–893 nm), and increased antiproliferative effect [46].

Niosomes with plant extracts have also been designed to enhance their activity. *withania somnifera* is a plant with an active constituent withaferin-A and anticancer activity. Niosomes loaded with withaferin-A were designed by using span 60 as a non-ionic surfactant and showed small-sized niosomes (278 nm) and high entrapment efficiency (87%). Niosomes were tested against HeLa cancer cells. They showed a threefold increase in anticancer activity [47].

Niosomes loaded with green tea extract and cholesterol hemisuccinate were used as pH-responsive polymer and these niosomes were PEGylated. The results indicated a small particle size (240 nm) and high entrapment efficiency (81%). These niosomes were evaluated for anticancer activity against MCF-7, HepG2, and HL-60 cancer cell lines. Niosomes showed the least cell toxicity and high targeted anticancer with antiproliferation activity [48].

In another study, niosomes were prepared to encapsulate letrozole and ascorbic acid and then folate-PEG was used to target the cancer cell. The niosomes were evaluated against the breast cancer cell and the results indicated that the niosomes were targeted to the breast cancer and not being destroyed by the macrophages [49].

One group of researchers prepared niosomes to target colon cancer. They were loaded with oxaliplatin and paclitaxel as hydrophilic and hydrophobic anticancer drugs, respectively. Different molar ratios of surfactants and cholesterol were used to prepare the niosomes. The surfactant d-α-tocopheryl polyethylene glycol 1000 succinate (TPGS) (4 molar ratios) and cholesterol (2 molar ratios) were used. The particle size (278.5±19.7 nm and 251.6±18.1 nm) and zeta-potential were (32.7±1.01 mV and 31.69±0.98 mV) with a high EE of more than 90%. The anticancer activity against colon cancer cell line HT-29 was evaluated. The niosomes showed high cytotoxicity and apoptosis activity with reduced toxicity [50].

Using $Fe_3O_4@SiO_2$ magnetic niosomes were fabricated, and then PEGylation was used to change their surface. Niosomes were magnetized to enable them to target particular tissues, and PEGylation was employed to increase their bioavailability. There was a huge difference in vitro drug release with these modified niosomes as compared to naked niosomes. Surprisingly, PEGylation of these magnetized niosomes led to a more prolonged drug release, despite the fact that loading naked niosomes with magnetic particles increased the rate of drug release. PEGylation of magnetic niosomes led to a slower, more sustained release of the medication over time in addition to increasing their bioavailability. Finally, research on the in vitro effects of niosomal formulations on MCF-7, a breast cancer cell line, revealed that these cells were sufficiently toxic to PEGylated magnetic niosomes in the presence of an external magnetic field [51].

PEGylated niosome containing siRNA, doxorubicin, quercetin, or both anticancer drugs were also prepared as cationic moiety. The goal of this study was to assess the antitumor effects of a combination therapy that targeted the genes and proteins responsible for the growth of gastric cancer. Oncogene CDC20 is a promising option for the treatment of gastric cancer. The research group adjusted the cationic PEGylated niosome in terms of cationic lipid content in order to maximize the loading capacity of siRNA and achieve the desired physical qualities. The co-delivery system was loaded with drugs (doxorubicin and quercetin) and CDC20siRNA, and its physical properties, thermos-sensitive controlled-release, gene silencing effectiveness, and apoptosis rate were assessed. The findings demonstrated that, when compared to siRNA or drug delivery made separately, the co-delivery system for the drugs and gene silencer had an appropriate size, a high positive charge for loading siRNA, and also displayed a thermos-sensitive drug release behavior that effectively silenced the CDC20 expression. Moreover, CDC20 siRNA and medication administration had shown a significantly inhibitive property for the proliferation of gastric cancer cells. The novel cationic PEGylated niosomes appeared to have promise for the treatment of gastric cancer when combined with an anticancer medication and CDC20siRNA [52].

In another study, niosomes were prepared with the loading of curcumin and methotrexate individually and in combination. The prepared niosomes were evaluated against a colorectal cell line HCT-116 and also with pure drugs. The resultant niosomes were evaluated against a cell line of colorectal cancer and showed significant antiproliferative activity and the least toxicity [53].

In another study, Artemether loaded niosomes were prepared and further evaluated for morphology, size, drug release entrapment efficiency, and anticancer activity. Cell proliferation, necrosis, and angiogenesis of the tumor were calculated by immunostaining with Ki-67, H&E, and CD-34. The results indicated that angiogenesis and proliferation is decreased with increased activity of necrosis against breast cancer cell [54].

In a study, pH-responsive niosomes modified with ergosterol and loaded with paclitaxel (PTX) were created. MCF7, Hela, and HUVEC cell lines were used to evaluate the in vitro effectiveness of free PTX and niosome/PTX. Rats were given intraperitoneal doses of 2.5 mg/kg and 5 mg/kg of niosomal PTX for 2 weeks in order to compare in vivo effectiveness to that of free PTX. The pH-responsive niosomes, according to the findings, were nanometric in size, spherical in shape, 77% EE, and released at pH 5.2 and 7.4. It was noticed that in the presence of PTX IC50 was reduced after treatment for 48 h [55].

PEGylated niosomes were also loaded with brucine and composed of non-ionic surfactants, i.e., Brigj-52, span 60, and poloxamer-184. The size of the niosomes was less than 311 nm and EE was between 53%–64%. The niosomes prepared with span 60 showed significant anticancer activity when compared with niosomes prepared with other surfactants against MDA-MB-231 cancer cell line [56].

To improve transfection efficacy and stability, cationic niosomal formulations were formulated using tween 80, tween 60, cholesterol, and dioleoyl-3-trimethylammonium propane (DOTAP). High-efficiency entrapment of the anticancer medication curcumin inside stable, spherical niosomes with positive charges of around +27 mV was achieved. When niosomal curcumins were loaded with miR-34a, the surface charge was reduced to +15 mV and the diameter was increased to almost 68 nm. According to the findings, co-delivery affected cancer cells more than the other groups in terms of cytotoxicity, uptake, and anticancer activity. The toxicity of curcumin and miR-34a to healthy human cells was significantly reduced in both niosomal and free forms. Also, the 4T1 xenografted Balb/C mouse tumor model was used to study the effects of these anticancer drugs. Tumor inhibition rates were higher than in other groups when curcumin and miR-34a were delivered together to cancer model organisms. As a result, it was possible to recognize the combined therapy of curcumin and miR-34a using the novel cationic niosomal delivery as a key tactic for more successful cancer treatments [57].

Due to the antihepatocarcinoma and hepatoprotective effects, ursolic acid was encapsulated in niosomes manufactured with span 60 by thin-film hydration method and chitosan was added. The size of niosome was between 255 to 439 nm with zeta-potential from –46 to –21 mV. The in vivo studies showed that the niosomes were having high anticancer activity when compared with the niosomes loaded with ursolic acid without chitosan. The chitsan also improved the stability and drug release profile of the drug [58].

A promising contender for cancer treatment is melittin, a peptide found in honey bee venom. Melittin-loaded and empty niosomes were optimized, and the anticancer impact was tested in vivo on BALB/C mice as well as in vitro on the breast cancer cell lines 4T1 and SKBR3. Moreover, in another experiment, the melittin-loaded niosome impacts the expression of the genes in the examined cells; it up-regulates the expression of the genes Bax, caspase3, and caspase9 while down-regulating the expression of the genes Bcl2, MMP2, and MMP9. According to this study, melittin-loaded niosomes had more anticancer effects than free melittin [59].

In another study, gold nanoparticles were prepared through a green synthesis process by using *artemisia annua* extract, within the niosomes. Different molar ratios of span 60 and cholesterol were used for the manufacturing of niosomes. By using the MTT assay, the cytotoxicity of free and noisy encapsulated AuNPs was assessed against the human ovarian cancer cell line (A2780). The outcomes demonstrated that the optimized niosomal formulation's entrapment effectiveness and particle size of AuNPs were 34.49%±0.84 nm and 153.6±4.62 nm, respectively, with a regular spherical shape. After 8 h, the AuNPs release profile from the niosomal formulation was 59%±1.0, indicating a controlled release profile. Via the stimulation of apoptosis and a large increase in the mRNA expression of the Bax gene, this formulation significantly reduced the expression of the antiapoptotic gene Bcl-2, causing dose-dependent cytotoxicity against the A2780 cells. The results imply that AuNP-loaded niosomal formulation is a potentially effective and targeted method for enhancing antitumor activity against A2780 cells [60].

Similarly, for the manufacture of tamoxifen-loaded niosomes, a water-in-oil emulsion was used as a template for a reverse-phase evaporation process employing span 120 as a non-ionic surfactant. To construct niosomes for prolonged drug release over 12 h and better surface shape, dicetyl phosphate and span 120 were utilized. The spherical niosomes had a −34.6mV zeta potential and ranged in size from 260 to 300 nm. The surface of niosomes had a rough roughness, according to scanning electron microscopy. The medication was released by niosomes in a first-order, continuous release pattern for up to 12 h. The cellular uptake of tamoxifen was enhanced by niosomes, which also made apoptosis (29%) the predominant mode of cell death as opposed to necrosis (17%). Tamoxifen's anticancer activity was increased by up to five times with an IC50 against MCF-7 cells that was decreased from 1 to 0.2 µM [61].

Dual character baring niosomes loaded with acemetacin were prepared for anticancer activity and radio-kinetic evaluation. By using the ether injection method, niosomes were fabricated and evaluated for in vitro drug release, entrapment efficiency, zeta potential, polydispersity index, and particle size (PS). The optimum formula had an average droplet size, zeta potential, and in vitro release after 24 h of 315.23±5.37 nm, −9.16±2.91 nm, and 76%, respectively. The highest ^{131}I-ACM labeling yield was 93.1±1.1%. After 60 minutes after intravenous administration, radio-kinetic analysis revealed a maximum tumor absorption of 5.431%ID/g for ^{131}I-ACM niosomal formula and 2.601% ID/g for ^{131}I-ACM solution. By passively targeting the nanosized niosomes, niosomal formula improved tumor absorption of ACM. Also, employing ^{131}I-ACM niosomes, the chemotherapeutic effects of ACM and the radio-therapeutic effects of ^{131}I were successfully coupled in one treatment plan [62].

A brand-new poly (lactic-co-glycolic acid)-polyethylene glycol (PEG) nano-niosome was created using folic acid (FA). Curcumin (Cur) was loaded into the niosome as a model medication and fluorescent probe for cervical cancer therapy and cell imaging. The results of the MTT experiment showed that the blank niosomes had high biocompatibility. The nanoniosome demonstrated extremely high efficacy as a drug carrier in an in vitro study of drug loading and release behavior. Cur-loaded Fe_3O_4@PLGA-PEG@FA niosomes achieved considerably high targeting efficiency for cervical cancer, as shown by the confocal laser scanning microscopy (CLSM) and flow cytometry (FCM) tests. By damaging the mitochondrion of cervical tumorvff cells, curcumin-loaded niosomes caused HeLa229 cells to undergo apoptosis, while simultaneously altering the nuclear shape and preventing tumor cell growth [63].

By using the thin-film hydration process, a PEGylated niosomal formulation of vinblastine (Pn-VB) was prepared and physicochemically characterized. Pn-cytotoxicity of VB towards murine lung cancer TC-1 cells was examined using the MTT test, and its tumor-inhibitory impact was assessed in C57BL/6 mice carrying lung tumors. The average niosome particle size, zeta potential, entrapment, and loading efficiency were found to be around 234.3±11.4 nm, -34.6±4.2 mV, 99.92±1.6%, and 2.673±0.30%, respectively. A prolonged release behavior was visible in the drug's in vitro release pattern from niosomes. In comparison to free VB, Pn-VB showed a much higher level of toxicity against TC-1 cells. Pn-VB had a longer lifespan and a better tumor-inhibitory impact in the animal model than free VB [64].

In another investigation, niosome structure (NISM) and bovine serum albumin (BSA), which was created to BSA coat NISM (NISM-B). Furthermore, selenium nanoparticles (SeNPs) were separately prepared using BSA-mediated biosynthesis. Eventually, the NISM-B was hybridized with SeNPs and created as NISM-B@SeNPs for drug delivery applications. The anticancer activity of the niosomes was assessed against A549 cell line. Against the A549 cell line, the niosomes had a substantial cytotoxic impact. Although the Bax/Bcl-2 expression ratio was considerably higher in cancer cells treated with NISM-B@SeNPs, the expression of MDR1 was non-significantly reduced [65].

In a study, selenium-nanoparticles (SeNPs) were encapsulated in niosomes. The antibacterial and anticancer activity of SeNPs and niosomes containing SeNPs were evaluated. The findings showed that the ideal formulation had a spherical shape, an average size of 177.9 nm, and an encapsulation effectiveness of 37.58%. The findings also showed that the release rates of free SeNPs and SeNPs loaded on niosomes were 100% and 61.26%, respectively, in 72 h. Moreover, niosome-loaded SeNPs may drastically down-regulate the expression of the Bcl2 gene while considerably up-regulated the expression of the apoptotic genes Bax, cas3, and cas9. Also, according to the results of the MTT test, free niosomes had no discernible harmful effects on the HFF cell line, demonstrating the biocompatibility of the generated niosomes [66].

The herbal extract of *carum carvil* seeds contains thymoquinne, which has a lot of pharmaceutical applications including anticancer activity. Thymoquinone (TQ) is a hydrophobic drug with low permeability and solubility. Niosomes were used to encapsulate two distinct mixtures of TQ and carum (designated Nio/tQ and Nio/Carum, respectively), and their characteristics were contrasted. According to the findings, both loaded formulations exhibit a negative zeta potential, a nanometric size, and a spherical shape. Around 92.32%±2.32 and 86.25%±1.85 of TQ and carum-loaded niosomes had EE%, respectively. The MTT experiment demonstrated that loaded niosomes have more anticancer activity against the MCF-7 cancer cell line compared to free TQ and free Carum, and these findings were supported by a flow cytometric study [67].

In photodynamic treatment (PDT), light and photosensitizers (PS) are used to create reactive oxygen species (ROS), which are capable of destroying tumor cells and dangerous bacteria. The outstanding PS zinc phthalocyanine (ZnPc) has a water solubility issue that can be fixed by encapsulating it in niosomes. One of the research intended to create niosomes containing ZnPc to support PDT for melanoma, the most dangerous form of skin cancer, and skin diseases brought on by harmful bacteria. The fabricated niosomes were having an average size of 233±5.6 nm, PDI of 0.22±0.07 nm, a charge of 36.73±0.65 mV, and exhibited spherical and regular form. The surface of vesicles was also modified to form cationic niosomes, which had improved photobiological activity. After being exposed to light, niosomes (anionic and cationic) containing ZnPc showed high photobiological activity and minimal dark cytotoxicity. The optimized formulations showed excellent anticancer activity [68].

A few examples of body organs treated with cytotoxic drug-loaded niosomes are listed in Table 10.4.

10.6 CONCLUSION

Niosomes are non-ionic surfactant-based vesicles that are stabilized with the help of cholesterol and with or without charge-inducing agents. They are small-sized vesicles enclosing hydrophilic and hydrophobic drugs with high entrapment capacity. The drugs that are least water-soluble and have poor bioavailability can be enclosed in niosomes. The anticancer drugs having the least water-solubility can be loaded in niosomes and showed improved bioavailability and solubility. The niosomes that are having surface moieties showed targeted delivery of the anticancer drugs with the least toxicity and more antiproliferative characteristics.

TABLE 10.4
A Few Examples of Cytotoxic Drug-Loaded Niosomes and Their Composition

Types of Cancers	Drug Used	Ingredients for Niosome Formulation	In Vitro Release Profile (pH 7.4)	Method of Preparation	Encapsulation Efficiency
Breast and Lung	Doxorubicin	Monoalkyl triglycerol ether & cholesterol	-	Ether injection method	70%
Lung and leukemia	vincristine sulfate	Cholesterol and surfactant	-	Thin-film hydration	90%
Breast, Lung and adenocarcinoma	Doxorubicin	Pluronic L64, Tween60, cholesterol	50%	Thin-film hydration	55-65%
Breast and ovarian cancer	Paclitaxel	Brij 72/76/78, Span 20/40/ 60, Tween 20/60	33.10%	Thin-film hydration	96.60%
Human colon adenocarcinoma	Imatinib mesylate	Span60, cholesterol, DCP, STR	89.45%	Thin-film hydration	82.96%
Breast	Silibinin	Span20, PEG 2000, cholesterol	22.05%	Reverse phase evaporation	70.61%
Skin	5-fluorouracil	Tween 20, cholesteryl hemisuccinate	-	Thin-film hydration and probe	45.10%
Breast and ovary	Mitoxantrone	Hemisuccinate Poly (monomethylitaconate) (PMMI)	91.50%	Modified ethanol injection method	70.9- 73.2%
Antioxidant and antitumor activity	Morine hydrate	Tween 60, Span 60/80, Cholesterol, Dicetyl phosphate	98.3-100%	Modified thin-film hydration	71-93.3%
Breast, ovary, nonsmall cell lung cancer	Paclitaxel and curcumin	Tween60 and cholesterol	29.93%	Thin-film hydration	100%
Leukemia	Cytarabine hydrochloride	Span 60, 80, Tween 20, 80, and cholesterol	70%	Thin-film hydration	88.20%
Breast	Cisplatine	Span60 and cholesterol	32%	Thin-film hydration	41.20%
Liver and colon	Hydroxy-camptothecin	Span60 and cholesterol	95%	Thin-film hydration	93%

REFERENCES

1. D.H. Khan, S. Bashir, M.I. Khan, P. Figueiredo, H.A. Santos, L. Peltonen, *Formulation optimization and in vitro characterization of rifampicin and ceftriaxone dual drug loaded niosomes with high energy probe sonication technique. J. Drug Deliv. Sci. Technol.* **58** (2020): p. 101763.

2. I.F. Uchegbu, A.T. Florence, *Non-ionic surfactant vesicles (niosomes): Physical and pharmaceutical chemistry. Adv. Colloid Interface Sci.* **58** (1995): pp. 1–55.

3. A. Pardakhty, E. Moazeni, *Nano-niosomes in drug, vaccine and gene delivery: a rapid overview. Nanomedicine J.* **1** (2013): pp. 1–12.

4. N. Puvvada, S. Rajput, B.N.P. Kumar, M. Mandal, A. Pathak, *Exploring the fluorescence switching phenomenon of curcumin encapsulated niosomes: In vitro real time monitoring of curcumin release to cancer cells. RSC Adv.* **33** (2013): pp. 2553–2557.

5. S.M. Mawazi, T.J. Ann, R.T. Widodo, *Application of niosomes in cosmetics: A systematic review. Cosmetics.* **9** (2022): pp. 1–16.

6. H. Abdelkader, A.W.G. Alani, R.G. Alany, Recent advances in non-ionic surfactant vesicles (niosomes): self-assembly, fabrication, characterization, drug delivery applications and limitations, *Drug Deliv.* **21** (2014): pp. 87–100.

7. S. Moghassemi, A. Hadjizadeh, *Nano-niosomes as nanoscale drug delivery systems: An illustrated review. J. Control. Release.* **185** (2014): pp. 22–36.

8. P. Aparajay, A. Dev, *Functionalized niosomes as a smart delivery device in cancer and fungal infection. Eur. J. Pharm. Sci.* 168 (2022): p. 106052.

9. M. Moghtaderi, K. Sedaghatnia, M. Bourbour, M. Fatemizadeh, Z. Salehi Moghaddam, F. Hejabi, F. Heidari, S. Quazi, B. Farasati Far, *Niosomes: A novel targeted drug delivery system for cancer. Med. Oncol.* **39** (2022): p. 240.

10. A.J. Baillie, A.T. Florence, L.R. Hume, G.T. Muirhead, A. Rogerson, *The preparation and properties of niosomes-non-ionic surfactant vesicles. J. Pharm. Pharmacol.* **37** (1985): pp. 863–868.

11. K. Kuotsu, K. Karim, A. Mandal, N. Biswas, A. Guha, S. Chatterjee, M. Behera, *Niosome: A future of targeted drug delivery systems. J. Adv. Pharm. Technol. Res.* **1** (2010): p. 374.

12. I.F. Uchegbu, J.A. Double, J.A. Turton, A.T. Florence, *Distribution, metabolism and tumoricidal activity of doxorubicin administered in sorbitan monostearate (Span 60) niosomes in the mouse, Pharm. Res.* **12** (1995): pp. 1019–1024.

13. J. Varshosaz, A. Pardakhty, V.I. Hajhashemi, A.R. Najafabadi, *Development and physical characterization of sorbitan monoester niosomes for insulin oral delivery. Drug Deliv. J. Deliv. Target. Ther. Agents.* **10** (2003): pp. 251–262.

14. R. Muzzalupo, L. Tavano, R. Cassano, S. Trombino, T. Ferrarelli, N. Picci, *A new approach for the evaluation of niosomes as effective transdermal drug delivery systems. Eur. J. Pharm. Biopharm.* **79** (2011): pp. 28–35.

15. M.J. Lawrence, *Sorbitan esters (sorbitan fatty acid esters).* In *Handbook of Pharmaceutical Excipients*, 4th ed., London: Pharmaceutical Press, 2003: pp. 591–595.

16. V.Y.A. Alexander, V. Kabanova, E.V. Batrakova, *Pluronic block copolymers as novel polymer therapeutics for drug and gene delivery. J. Control. Release.* **82** (2002): pp. 189–212.

17. A. Batrakova, E., Lee, S., Li, S., Venne, A., Alakhov, V. Kabanov, *Fundamental relationships between the composition of pluronic block copolymers and their hypersensitization effect in MDR cancer cells. Pharm. Res.* **16** (1999): pp. 1373–1379.

18. P. Bandyopadhyay, M. Johnson, *Fatty alcohols or fatty acids as niosomal hybrid carrier: Effect on vesicle size, encapsulation efficiency and in vitro dye release. Colloids Surfaces B Biointerfaces.* **58** (2007): pp. 68–71.

19. T. Liu, R. Guo, W. Hua, J. Qiu, *Structure behaviors of hemoglobin in PEG 6000/Tween 80/Span 80/ H2O niosome system. Colloids Surfaces A Physicochem. Eng. Asp.* 293 (2007): pp. 255–261.

20. C. Marianecci, L. Di Marzio, F. Rinaldi, C. Celia, D. Paolino, F. Alhaique, S. Esposito, M. Carafa, *Niosomes from 80s to present: The state of the art. Adv. Colloid Interface Sci.* **205** (2014): pp. 187–206.

21. I.F. Uchegbu, S.P. Vyas, *Non-ionic surfactant based vesicles (niosomes) in drug delivery. Int. J. Pharm.* **172** (1998): pp. 33–70.

22. P.R. Maurer, N., Zhigaltsev, I., & Csullis, *Encapsulation of nucleic acid–based therapeutics. In Liposome Technol. Entrapment Drugs Other Mater. into Liposomes.* 3rd ed., New York: Informa Healthcare, 2007: pp. 149–68.

23. D.G.R. Hu, Chengjiu., *Proniosomes: A novel drug carrier system, Int. J. Pharm.* 185 (1999) pp. 23–35.

24. V.B. Junyaprasert, V. Teeranachaideekul, T. Supaperm, *Effect of charged and non-ionic membrane additives on physicochemical properties and stability of niosomes. AAPS PharmSciTech.* **9** (2008): pp. 851–859.

25. A. Pardakhty, M. Shakibaie, H. Daneshvar, A. Khamesipour, T. Mohammadi-Khorsand, H. Forootanfar, *Preparation and evaluation of niosomes containing autoclaved Leishmania major: A preliminary study. J. Microencapsul.* **29** (2012): pp. 219–224.

26. Y.-K. Oh, M.Y. Kim, J.-Y. Shin, T.W. Kim, M.-O. Yun, S.J. Yang, S.S. Choi, W.-W. Jung, J.A. Kim, H.-G. Choi, *Skin permeation of retinol in Tween 20-based deformable liposomes: In-vitro evaluation in human skin and keratinocyte models. J. Pharm. Pharmacol.* **58** (2006): pp. 161–166.

27. C. Cametti, *Polyion-induced aggregation of oppositely charged liposomes and charged colloidal particles: The many facets of complex formation in low-density colloidal systems. Chem. Phys. Lipids.* **155** (2008): pp. 63–73.

28. M.I. Khan, A. Madni, L. Peltonen, *Development and in-vitro characterization of sorbitan monolaurate and poloxamer 184 based niosomes for oral delivery of diacerein. Eur. J. Pharm. Sci.* **95** (2016): pp. 88–95.

29. X. Ge, M. Wei, S. He, W.E. Yuan, *Advances of non-ionic surfactant vesicles (niosomes) and their application in drug delivery. Pharmaceutics.* **11** (2019): p. 55.

30. S. Moghassemi, E. Parnian, A. Hakamivala, M. Darzianiazizi, M.M. Vardanjani, S. Kashanian, B. Larijani, K. Omidfar, *Uptake and transport of insulin across intestinal membrane model using trimethyl chitosan coated insulin niosomes. Mater. Sci. Eng. C.* **46** (2015): pp. 333–340.

31. V. Ravalika, A.K. Sailaja, *Formulation and evaluation of etoricoxib niosomes by thin film hydration technique and ether injection method. Nano Biomed. Eng.* **9** (2017): pp. 242–248.

32. A.K. Sailaja, M. Shreya, *Preparation and characterization of naproxen loaded niosomes by ether injection method. Nano Biomed. Eng.* **10** (2018): pp. 174–180.

33. N. Akhtar, R.K. Singh, K. Pathak, *Exploring the potential of complex-vesicle based niosomal ocular system loaded with azithromycin: Development of in situ gel and ex vivo characterization. Pharm. Biomed. Res.* 3 (2017): pp. 22–33.

34. V.S. Shukla, V. Mastiholimath, *Effect of tween 20 and tween 40 surfactants on 5-fluorouracil niosomes, Int. J. Sci. Res.* **7** (2018): pp. 34–35.

35. F. Duncan, R. Florence, A. Uchegbu, I. Cociacinch, *Drug Polymer conjugates encapsulated within niosomes*, (1997).

36. A. Manosroi, P. Jantrawut, J. Manosroi, *Anti-inflammatory activity of gel containing novel elastic niosomes entrapped with diclofenac diethylammonium. Int. J. Pharm.* 360 (2008): pp. 156–163.

37. V. Verma, S. Singh, S.K. Syan, N. Mathur, P. Valecha, *Nanoparticle vesicular systems: A versatile tool for drug delivery. J. Chem. Pharm. Res.* **2** (2010): pp. 496–509.

38. T.T. Pham, C. Jaafar-Maalej, C. Charcosset, H. Fessi, *Liposome and niosome preparation using a membrane contactor for scale-up. Coll. Surf. B Biointer.* **94** (2012): pp. 15–21.

39. C.T. Lo, A. Jahn, L.E. Locascio, W.N. Vreeland, *Controlled self-assembly of monodisperse niosomes by microfluidic hydrodynamic focusing. Langmuir.* **26** (2010): pp. 8559–8566.

40. R.M. Khalil, G.A. Abdelbary, M. Basha, G.E.A. Awad, H.A. El-Hashemy, *Design and evaluation of proniosomes as a carrier for ocular delivery of lomefloxacin HCl. J. Liposome Res.* **27** (2017): pp. 118–129.

41. J.W. Shuo Chen, S. Hanning, J. Falconer, M. Locke, *Recent advances in non-ionic surfactant vesicles (niosomes): Fabrication, characterization, pharmaceutical and cosmetic applications. Eur. J. Pharm. Biopharm.* **144** (2019): pp. 19–39.

42. D. Haleem Khan, S. Bashir, A. Correia, M. Imran Khan, P. Figueiredo, H.A. Santos, L. Peltonen, *Utilization of green formulation technique and efficacy estimation on cell line studies for dual anticancer drug therapy with niosomes. Int. J. Pharm.* **572** (2019): p. 118764.

43. C. Jin, K. Wang, A. Oppong-Gyebi, J. Hu, *Application of nanotechnology in cancer diagnosis and therapy-a mini-review. Int. J. Med. Sci.* **2020** (2020): pp. 2964–2973.

44. S. Agarwal, M.S. Mohamed, S. Raveendran, A.K. Rochani, T. Maekawa, D.S. Kumar, *Formulation, characterization and evaluation of morusin loaded niosomes for potentiation of anticancer therapy.* RSC Adv. **8** (2018): pp. 32621–32636.

45. R. Muzzalupo, L. Tavano, *Niosomal drug delivery for transdermal targeting: recent advances.* Res. Rep. Transdermal Drug Deliv. **4** (2015): pp. 23–33.

46. K. Haleem, Daulat, S. Bashir, A. Correia, M. Imran, *Utilization of green formulation technique and efficacy estimation on cell line studies for dual anticancer drug therapy with niosomes.* Int. J. Pharm. **572** (2019): p. 118764.

47. H.S. Shah, F. Usman, M. Ashfaq-Khan, R. Khalil, Z. Ul-Haq, A. Mushtaq, R. Qaiser, J. Iqbal, *Preparation and characterization of anticancer niosomal withaferin – A formulation for improved delivery to cancer cells: In vitro, in vivo, and in silico evaluation.* J. Drug Deliv. Sci. Technol. **59** (2020): p. 101863.

48. M. Baranei, R.A. Taheri, M. Tirgar, A. Saeidi, F. Oroojalian, L. Uzun, A. Asefnejad, F.R. Wurm, V. Goodarzi, *Anticancer effect of green tea extract (GTE)-loaded pH-responsive niosome coated with PEG against different cell lines.* Mater. Today Commun. **26** (2021): p. 101751.

49. M. Bourbour, N. Khayam, … H.N.-… S.D. & undefined 2022, Evaluation of anti-cancer and anti-metastatic effects of folate-PEGylated niosomes for co-delivery of letrozole and ascorbic acid on breast cancer cells, *Pubs.Rsc.Org.* (n.d.). https://pubs.rsc.org/en/content/articlehtml/2022/me/d2m e00024e (accessed February 21, 2023).

50. S.W. El-Far, H.A.A. El-Enin, E.M. Abdou, O.E. Nafea, R. Abdelmonem, *Targeting colorectal cancer cells with niosomes systems loaded with two anticancer drugs models; comparative in vitro and anticancer studies.* Pharmaceuticals. **15** (2022): pp. 2–18.

51. F. Davarpanah, A.K. Yazdi, M. Barani, M. Mirzaei, *Magnetic delivery of antitumor carboplatin by using PEGylated-Niosomes.* DARU J. Pharm. Sci. **26** (2018): pp. 57–64.

52. M. Hemati, F. Haghiralsadat, F. Jafary, S. Moosavizadeh, A. Moradi, *Targeting cell cycle protein in gastric cancer with CDC20siRNA and anticancer drugs (Doxorubicin and quercetin) co-loaded cationic PEGylated nanoniosomes.* Int. J. Nanomedicine. **14** (2019): pp. 6575–6585.

53. N. Mousazadeh, M. Gharbavi, H. Rashidzadeh, H. Nosrati, H. Danafar, B. Johari, *Anticancer evaluation of methotrexate and curcumin-coencapsulated niosomes against colorectal cancer cell lines.* Nanomedicine. **17** (2022): pp. 201–217.

54. M.J. Mirzaei-Parsa, M.R.H. Najafabadi, A. Haeri, M. Zahmatkeshan, S.A. Ebrahimi, H. Pazoki-Toroudi, M. Adel, *Preparation, characterization, and evaluation of the anticancer activity of artemether-loaded nano-niosomes against breast cancer.* Breast Cancer. **27** (2020): pp. 243–251.

55. M. Barani, M.R. Hajinezhad, S. Sargazi, A. Rahdar, S. Shahraki, A. Lohrasbi-Nejad, F. Baino, *In vitro and in vivo anticancer effect of pH-responsive paclitaxel-loaded niosomes.* J. Mater. Sci. Mater. Med. **32** (2021): pp. 1–13.

56. H.M.E. Michelyne Haroun, H.S. Elsewedy, T.M. Shehata, C. Tratrat, B.E. Al Dhubiab, K.N. Venugopala, M.M. Almostafa, H. Kochkar, *Significant of injectable brucine PEGylated niosomes in treatment of MDA cancer cells.* J. Drug Deliv. Sci. Technol. **71** (2022): p. 103322.

57. B.Z.D. Najmeh, A. Abtahi, S.M. Naghib, S.J. Ghalekohneh, Z. Mohammadpour, H. Nazari, S.M. Mosavi, S.M. Gheibihayat, F. Haghiralsadat, J.Z. Reza, *Multifunctional stimuli-responsive niosomal nanoparticles for co-delivery and co-administration of gene and bioactive compound: In vitro and in vivo studies.* Chem. Eng. J. **429** (2022): p. 132090.

58. A. Miatmoko, S. Safitri, F. Aquila, D. Cahyani, B. Hariawan, E. Hendrianto, E. Hendradi, R. Sari, *Characterization and distribution of niosomes containing ursolic acid coated with chitosan layer.* Res. Pharm. Sci. **16** (2021): pp. 660–673.

59. F. Dabbagh Moghaddam, I. Akbarzadeh, E. Marzbankia, M. Farid, L. Khaledi, A.H. Reihani, M. Javidfar, P. Mortazavi, *Delivery of melittin-loaded niosomes for breast cancer treatment: an in vitro and in vivo evaluation of anti-cancer effect.* Cancer Nanotechnol. **12** (2021): pp. 1–35.

60. F. Rezaie Amale, S. Ferdowsian, S. Hajrasouliha, R. Kazempoor, A. Mirzaie, M. Sedigh Dakkali, I. Akbarzadeh, S. Mohammadmahdi Meybodi, M. Mirghafouri, *Gold nanoparticles loaded into niosomes: A novel approach for enhanced antitumor activity against human ovarian cancer.* Adv. Powder Technol. **32** (2021): pp. 4711–4722.

61. G.N. Devaraj, S.R. Parakh, R. Devraj, S.S. Apte, B.R. Rao, D. Rambhau, *Release studies on niosomes containing fatty alcohols as bilayer stabilizers instead of cholesterol. J. Colloid Interface Sci.* **251** (2002): pp. 360–365.

62. H.M. Shewaiter, M.A. Selim, A.A. Moustafa, Y.M. Gad, S. Rashed, *Radioiodinated acemetacin loaded niosomes as a dual anticancer therapy. Int. J. Pharm.* **628** (2022): p. 122345.

63. L. You, X. Liu, Z. Fang, Q. Xu, Q. Zhang, *Synthesis of multifunctional Fe_3O_4@PLGA-PEG nano-niosomes as a targeting carrier for treatment of cervical cancer. Mater. Sci. Eng. C.* **94** (2019): pp. 291–302.

64. B. Amiri, H. Ahmadvand, A. Farhadi, A. Najmafshar, M. Chiani, D. Norouzian, *Delivery of vinblastine-containing niosomes results in potent in vitro/in vivo cytotoxicity on tumor cells. Drug Dev. Ind. Pharm.* **44** (2018): pp. 1371–1376.

65. M. Gharbavi, B. Johari, N. Mousazadeh, B. Rahimi, M.P. Leilan, S.S. Eslami, A. Sharafi, *Hybrid of niosomes and bio-synthesized selenium nanoparticles as a novel approach in drug delivery for cancer treatment. Mol. Biol. Rep.* **47** (2020): pp. 6517–6529.

66. A. Haddadian, F.F. Robattorki, H. Dibah, A. Soheili, E. Ghanbarzadeh, N. Sartipnia, S. Hajrasouliha, K. Pasban, R. Andalibi, M.H. Ch, A. Azari, A. Chitgarzadeh, A.B. Kashtali, F. Mastali, H. Noorbazargan, A. Mirzaie, *Niosomes-loaded selenium nanoparticles as a new approach for enhanced antibacterial, anti-biofilm, and anticancer activities. Sci. Rep.* 12 (2022): pp. 1–16.

67. M. Barani, M. Mirzaei, M. Torkzadeh-Mahani, M. Adeli-sardou, *Evaluation of carum-loaded niosomes on breast cancer cells: physicochemical properties, in vitro cytotoxicity, flow cytometric, DNA fragmentation and cell migration assay. Sci. Rep.* **9** (2019): pp. 1–10.

68. E.R.-J. Luciana, B. de Oliveira de Siqueira, A. Paula dos Santos Matos, P.E. Feuser, R.A. Machado-de-Ávila, R. Santos-Oliveira, *Encapsulation of photosensitizer in niosomes for promotion of antitumor and antimicrobial photodynamic therapy. J. Drug Deliv. Sci. Technol.* **68** (2022): p. 103031.

11 Solid Lipid Nanoparticle-Based Anticancer Therapies

*Mulazim Hussain Asim, Muhammad Yasir Ali,
Shumaila Arshad, Ummaima Shahzad,
Arshad Mahmood, Syed Atif Raza, Alia Erum,
and Ali Moghadam*

11.1 INTRODUCTION

Cancer usually begins by dividing and spreading abnormal body cells without control. Nowadays, different surgical, radiation, and chemotherapeutic treatments are being used for cancer. I.v. route of administration is the most commonly used route for chemotherapeutic treatment in cancer, as this route provides better drug bioavailability. But this route also causes serious side effects, including nephrotoxicity, myelosuppression, and hair loss [1–3]. I.v. chemotherapy is very uncomfortable and hurtful for patients, depending upon the nature, dose, and frequency of the chemotherapeutic agent used [4]. In contrast, oral chemotherapy is a more convenient route due to patient compliance. However, most anticancer drugs possess low bioavailability due to limited drug-water solubility and poor drug diffusion [5]. New drug delivery systems are being developed to overcome these limitations. Drug encapsulation into nanoparticles, mucoadhesive thiomers, liposomes, dendrimers, polymeric micelles, carbon nanotubes, nanocrystals, polymeric microparticles, and nanoparticles such as lipid nanoparticles are some examples of the newly developed drug delivery systems [6–8]. Presently, solid lipid nanoparticles (SLNs) are getting attention for their prominent use in oral cancer drug delivery. SLNs were first developed as an alternative carrier system in 1991 to combine the advantages of existing colloidal carriers while avoiding their disadvantages. They have gained prominence in recent years [9].

Lipid nanoparticles are usually less toxic and biocompatible as compared to other polymeric nanoparticles [10]. SLNs are made up of a lipid matrix solid at physiological temperature, surfactants, and co-surfactants. They work as a specific drug carrier system that can increase therapeutic effectiveness and enhance the safety of different chemotherapeutic agents used for cancer treatment. These nanoparticles have the benefits of controlled drug release and protection of active pharmaceutical compounds. Moreover, the small size of nanoparticles is one of the key factors resulting in the close contact of SLNs with the stratum corneum for better diffusion [11].

11.2 PREPARATION OF SOLID LIPID NANOPARTICLES

High-pressure homogenization (HPH) was the predominant production method until recently. However, two further SLN production techniques seemed to have been dropped by the researchers [12]. The usage of organic solvents, a significant quantity of surfactants, and other additions make several obvious shortcomings of this process clear. While both high shear homogenization and ultrasound were initially employed for the manufacture of SLNs, they did not involve organic solvents, significant amounts of surfactants, or other additives, in contrast to HPH [13]. The two approaches previously stated were both popular and easy to utilize. However, one

DOI: 10.1201/9781003363958-14

drawback of these conventional methods was their poor dispersion quality. The conventional dispersing methods were altered to create high-quality solid lipid nanodispersion utilizing these straightforward, commonplace tools that were virtually always accessible in every laboratory. SLNs are prepared from lipids, emulsifiers, and water/solvent by using different methods and are discussed below.

11.2.1 HOMOGENIZATION BY HIGH SHEAR (HSH)

This process is trustworthy and was first utilized to make solid lipid nanoemulsions. It entails high-pressure homogenization by forcing a liquid through a small gap of a few microns under high pressure (100–2000 bar). The fluid accelerates to a very small distance with a viscosity of over 1000 km/h. The particles, as small as a submicron, are dispersed by shear stress and cavitation forces. A 5–40% range in the use of lipid content has been studied for this method. Two general methods for attaining HSH are hot homogenization and cold homogenization.

11.2.1.1 Hot Homogenization

Usually, hot homogenization takes place at temperatures higher than the lipid's melting point. The drug-loaded lipid melt and the aqueous emulsifier phase are mixed vigorously to form a pre-emulsion (both at the same temperature). The result is a heated o/w emulsion that, when cooled, crystallizes lipids and produces SLNs. Smaller particle sizes are produced by this technique because higher processing temperatures diminish the viscosity of the lipid phase. On the other hand, high temperatures hasten the deterioration of the medicine and the carrier. The high kinetic energy of the particles causes an increase in the particle size when the homogenization temperature or cycle counts are increased. This method usually takes 3–5 homogenization cycles at 500–1500 bar [14].

11.2.1.2 Cold Homogenization

Cold homogenization was created to address the problems with the hot homogenization method like partitioning and then loss of the drug in the aqueous phase and temperature-related degradation difficulties. Due to the intricate nature of the nanoemulsion's crystallization phase, lipid polymeric transitions occur, leading to several modifications, and/or supercooled melts. The active pharmaceutical ingredient (API) is blended with melted fat and quickly cooled by using liquid nitrogen or dry ice. The obtained solid substance is ground using a mortar mill. Then, a cold emulsifier solution that is at or below room temperature is used to disperse the lipid microparticles. This method is economical and easy to handle at a laboratory scale. However, the drawbacks of this method include intensive use of energy, biomolecule damage at the laboratory scale, polydisperse distributions, and unproven scalability [15].

11.2.2 ULTRASONICATION

High-speed homogenization or ultrasonication is another technique for the preparation of SLNs (Figure 11.1). An advantage of this method is that the equipment is frequently accessible at the laboratory scale. The broader size dispersion of this approach, which extends into the micrometer range, is one of its disadvantages. Potential metal contamination and physical instability, such as particle development during storage, are the drawbacks of this approach [16, 17].

11.2.3 SOLVENT EVAPORATION

The procedure of solvent evaporation can also be utilized to make SLNs (Figure 11.2). The lipophilic material (such as cyclohexane) is dissolved in the water-immiscible organic solvent dispersed

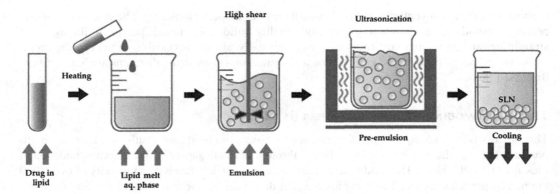

FIGURE 11.1   The method of preparation of SLNs including high shear or high speed and ultrasonication homogenization [18].

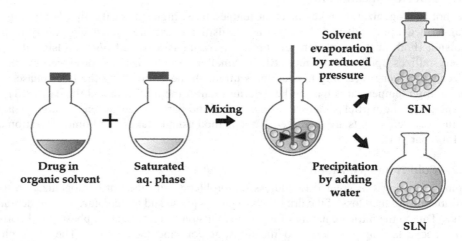

FIGURE 11.2   The method of synthesis including emulsification solvent diffusion or evaporation [18].

in the aqueous phase, generating an o/w emulsion. The emulsion's organic solvent is evaporated at lowered pressure (40–60 mbar). Lipid precipitates as nanoparticles with a mean size of 25 nm after solvent evaporation, resulting in a dispersion of nanoparticles. The advantages of this method include that it is easily scalable, uses advanced technology, continual procedure, and is commercially displayed. The drawbacks of this method include the consumption of a lot of energy, polydisperse distributions, and harm to biomolecules [19, 20].

11.2.4   Solvent Emulsification-Diffusion Method

This technique enables the production of particles with typical diameters between 30 and 100 nm. No involvement of heat during preparation is the key advantage of this method [20].

11.2.5   Supercritical Fluid Method

This is a different way to make SLNs by using particles from gas-saturated fluids (PGSS). This technique is performed at moderate temperature and pressure conditions and gets particles as a dry powder rather than a suspension because it avoids the use of solvents [21–23].

11.2.6 Microemulsion-Based Method

In this method, microemulsions are diluted to attain the SLNs. The microemulsions (like o/w microemulsions) are two-phase systems composed of an inner and an outer phase (Figure 11.3). They are formed by stirring an optically transparent liquid and typically contain water, an emulsifier (like polysorbate 20), a low melting fatty acid (like stearic acid), and co-emulsifiers (like butanol). The hot microemulsion is dispersed in cold water (2–3°C) while being stirred. When the particle content is low, too much water must be removed to turn the SLN dispersion into solid goods (tablets, pellets) through the granulation process. High-temperature gradients promote rapid lipid crystalliza-tion and inhibit aggregation. In this method, minimal mechanical energy is required, and SLNs are theoretically stable. However, this process is extremely susceptible to change and requires a lot of work for formulation design [24].

11.2.7 Spray Drying Method

It acts as a replacement for the lyophilization process and manipulates the combining of lipids with melting points greater than 70°C. The best results of this technique were obtained using 20% tre-halose in an ethanol-water mixture or water with a 1% SLNs content [25].

11.2.8 Double Emulsion Method

Here, a stabilizer has been added to the medicine to avoid partitioning into the external water phase of the w/o/w double emulsion when the solvent evaporates [26].

11.2.9 Precipitation Method

In this method, the glycerides are dissolved in an organic solvent (such as chloroform), and the mix-ture is then emulsified in an aqueous phase. Lipids then precipitate out and form nanoparticles after the evaporation of the organic solvent.

11.2.10 Dispersion of Film Ultrasonic

After adding the lipid and active ingredient to the appropriate organic solutions, they are then rotated, decompressed, and evaporated to create a lipid film. The aqueous solution containing the

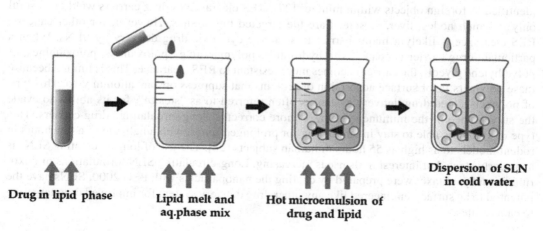

Drug in lipid phase   Lipid melt and aq.phase mix   Hot microemulsion of drug and lipid   Dispersion of SLN in cold water

FIGURE 11.3 The microemulsion method for SLNs synthesis [18].

emulsifiers is then introduced. Finally, the SLNs with small and uniform particle sizes are generated using ultrasound with the probe/bath diffuser.

11.2.11 Secondary Production Steps

11.2.11.1 Freeze Drying

A strategy for improving the chemical and physical stability of SLNs over extended periods is lyophilization. To obtain long-term stability for a product comprising hydrolyzable pharmaceuticals or a product suited for oral administration, lyophilization is necessary. Oswald's ripening would be stopped and hydrolytic processes would be avoided by transformation into a solid state. The entire lipid matrices utilized create bigger solid lipids when the product is freeze-dried. They have a greater size distribution because there are aggregates between the nanoparticles. SLN aggregation is facilitated by the freeze-drying conditions and the elimination of water. The conglomeration of solid lipid nanoparticles during the freezing drying process can be avoided with the use of enough cryoprotectants.

11.2.11.2 Sterilization

Sterilization of the nanoparticles is desirable for parenteral delivery and is done by autoclaving. Investigations into how sterilization affects particle size have conclusively shown that it does so.

11.2.11.3 Spray-Drying

Spray-drying is a possible substitute for freeze-drying, for turning the aqueous SLN dispersions into dry goods. Even though spray-drying is less expensive than freeze-drying, the SLN formulations rarely employ this technique. Spray-drying is suggested for lipids with melting points greater than 70°C.

11.2.12 Development of an SLN System to Avoid Clearance by the Reticuloendothelial System (RES)

Following intravenous administration, drug delivery systems, such as polymeric nanoparticles and liposomes, are rapidly cleared from the systemic circulation by the RES. The RES is part of the immune system consisting of phagocytic cells, which usually reside in the spleen, lymph nodes, and also in liver in the form of kupffer cells. These phagocytic cells can remove drug carriers identified as foreign objects within minutes [27]. RES clearance of drug carriers would be useful only if lymph nodes, liver, or spleen are the targeted tumor sites. However, for other cancers, RES clearance is likely a major barrier to systemic cytotoxic drug delivery by SLNs. When a particulate drug carrier is coated with hydrophilic polymers (e.g., poloxamers, poloxamines, or polyethylene glycol), the carrier becomes more resistant to RES clearance. This is limited because these polymers favor surface adsorption of proteins that suppress opsonization in vivo. This type of polymer-coated drug delivery system is often referred to as "stealth", for its ability to evade the surveillance of the immune system, or more correctly "long-circulating" drug carriers. This type of system is able to stay in circulation for prolonged times, with a half-life of a few hours in rodent models to as high as 55 hours in human subjects [28]. The use of long-circulating SLNs is at an early stage, but interest in its use is increasing. Long-circulating SLN formulations of doxorubicin and paclitaxel were prepared by coating the nanoparticles with PEG 2000. SLNs have the potential to be surface-engineered like any other drug delivery system for improved drug targeting to cancer sites.

11.3 EXPERIMENTAL VARIABLES

11.3.1 FORMULATION VARIABLES IN THE PRODUCT QUALITY

The physical stability of lipid particles, the loaded drug's bio-status, and its release kinetics are all greatly impacted by size changes. As a result, it is important to keep the SLN size within safe limits. The concept of colloidal particles states that well-formulated systems, such as liposomes, nanospheres, and nanoparticles, should have a narrow submicron particle size distribution (μm in size) [29].

11.3.2 IMPACT OF THE INGREDIENTS ON PRODUCT QUALITY

The makeup of the formulation (such as the surfactant/co-surfactant combination, lipid characteristics, and the API being evaluated) as well as other factors might affect the particle size of lipid nanoparticles, techniques, and manufacturing circumstances (such as time, temperature, pressure, number of cycles, equipment, sterilization, and freeze-drying). Low processing temperatures result in large particle sizes. In comparison to cold homogenization, the hot homogenization approach produces particles with narrower size dispersion, often less than 500 nm. According to reports, the average particle size and the polydispersity index (PDI) value decreased when the homogenization pressure was increased up to 1500 bar, and the number of cycles was (3–7 cycles) [30].

11.3.2.1 Effects of Lipids

It was discovered by hot homogenization that the average particle size of the SLN dispersion increased when the lipids' melting temperature rose. However, various lipids will have varied effects on other crucial factors in the production of nanoparticles. Examples include the rate of lipid crystallization and the hydrophilicity of lipids, which influences the crystal structure and self-emulsifying capabilities of lipids (and thus the surface). Additionally, when the lipid content is increased by 5–10%, bigger particles, including microparticles, and a broader particle size distribution usually follow [31].

11.3.2.2 Emulsifier Effect

The particle size of the lipid nanoparticle is significantly influenced by the surfactant mixture/surfactant concentration. Higher surfactant-to-lipid ratios were often associated with lower particle sizes. Particle size increased during storage as a result of the drop in surfactant content. The surfactant causes the particles to break apart and so increases the surface area by lowering the surface tension between the contacts.

11.3.2.3 Drug Delivery Through SLNs

Drug delivery to the site of action predicts enhancement in their efficiency, as well as a decrease in side effects [32]. There are different mechanisms by which SLNs improve their delivery.

11.3.2.3.1 Passive Drug Delivery

SLNs can concentrate anticancer drugs at the tumor site to achieve the desired antitumor effect. However, in the case of complex treatment, it is impossible to identify cancerous cells sometimes [32]. To overcome this problem, SLNs target cancer cells because of the enhanced permeability and retention effect (EPR) [33]. This effect is primarily based on the fast angiogenesis carried out by solid tumors to maintain sufficient oxygen supply and nutrients [34]. Recently, it was reported that EPR is not providing desired results although it has a valuable mechanism to increase drug delivery. This effect shows a huge variation in results and depends on many factors including the type and size of the tumor [35].

11.3.2.3.2 Active Drug Delivery

This mechanism of drug delivery is dependent upon target receptors or transporters on the tumor surface. In tumor tissues, nutrient demand is higher due to the enhanced proliferation of tumor cells, and therefore for entry into cells selective transporters are required for nutrient transport. Therefore, enhanced transporters serve an additional benefit in contrast to surface receptors [36]. In contrast, it is also important that surface modification does not change the biodistribution of SLNs.

For SLNs, different types of ligands can be used for active drug delivery for instance hyaluronic acid. A group of researchers proved that paclitaxel-loaded SLNs functionalized with hyaluronic can overcome drug resistance and decrease the viability of HeLa and MCF-7 cell lines. SLNs also showed increased drug concentration at the tumor site in comparison to free drugs and SLNs without hyaluronic acid [37]. Another modification of docetaxel-loaded SLNs having more than one ligand showed an enhanced active drug delivery with hyaluronic acid and tetraiodothyroacetic acid [38]. Moreover, sugar addition (galactose) to SLNs is useful for the effective cellular uptake of anticancer drugs due to the presence of lectin receptors [39].

11.3.2.4 Co-Drug Delivery

Another approach to overcoming drug resistance in tumor cells is the co-administration of anticancer drugs in SLNs. In a study, it was shown that when different preventive agents were co-administered with cytotoxic drugs, efficacy was enhanced against chemotherapy. For instance, dexrazoxane is capable of decreasing the P-glycoprotein expression that drugs can induce, thus preventing the development of multidrug resistance [40]. Similarly, the efficacy of combined paclitaxel and tanespimycin was enhanced as co-delivery results in an enhanced antitumor effect [41].

11.3.2.5 SLN Drug Incorporation Models

Factors affecting a drug's ability to load in lipids are as follows [42]:

- Its solubility in molten lipids.
- Lipid melt and drug melt are miscible.
- The solid matrix lipid's chemical and structural makeup.
- Lipid substance in a polymorphic condition.

11.3.2.6 Capacity for Loading and Drug Incorporation

It has been demonstrated that the manufacturing process, the type of emulsifier (anionic, cationic, non-ionic), the type of lipid (triglycerides, fatty acids, steroids, waxes, etc.), and the size distribution of SLNs all have an impact on the particle size, loading capacity, and size distribution of SLNs [26, 42].

11.4 PHYSICOCHEMICAL EVALUATION

11.4.1 CALCULATION OF THE DRUG INCORPORATED

Numerous drugs have been developed, some of which contain compounds that are very hydrophilic [43, 44].

The in vitro release of the medication is investigated using the following methods:

- Reverse dialysis bag technique.
- Dialysis bag diffusion technique.
- Parallel diffusion cells using a biological or artificial membrane.
- Agitation followed by centrifugal ultra-filtration or ultra-centrifugal separation.

11.4.1 Efficiency of Entrapment

This is extremely important in SLNs because it determines how a drug molecule is released. The quantity of drug per unit weight of nanoparticles is determined after isolating the entrapped drug from the SLN formulation. This separation can be accomplished using methods such as gel permeation chromatography, centrifugation filtration, and ultracentrifugation [42, 45, 46].

11.4.1.2 Filtration by Centrifugation

Ultra-free MC and ultra-sort 10 filters are employed in addition to traditional centrifugation techniques. The quantity of API remaining after centrifuging, filtering, or ultra-centrifuging the SLNs suspension, or by dissolving the sediment in a suitable solvent and then analyzing the results, can be used to infer the level of encapsulation [43].

11.4.1.3 In Vitro Drug Release

11.4.1.3.1 Dialysis Tubing

In vitro drug release may be accomplished using dialysis tubing. In pre-washed, hermetically sealable dialysis tubing, solid lipid nanoparticle dispersion is placed. The dialysis sac is then dialyzed against a suitable dissolving solution at ambient temperature. The drug content of the samples is then determined using a suitable analytical method after they are centrifuged and removed from the dissolving fluid at the proper intervals [47].

11.4.1.3.2 Reverse Dialysis

In this procedure, small dialysis sacs holding 1 ml of the dissolving medium are held in place by SLN dispersion. The SLNs are then moved into the medium after that.

11.4.2 SLN Storage Stability

It is possible to determine the physical properties of SLNs over prolonged storage by keeping track of changes in zeta potential, particle size, drug content, appearance, and viscosity as a function of time. External variables, like temperature and light, appear to be most important for long-term stability. In general, for dispersion to remain physically stable, the zeta potential must be larger than -60 mV [43].

- The best storage temperature is $4°C$.
- Long-term storage at $20°C$ did not cause drug-loaded SLNs to aggregate or lose drug.
- A rapid increase in particle size was seen at $50°C$.

11.4.3 Characteristics of SLNs

SLNs must be correctly identified for the purpose of maintaining product quality. The following variables that directly impact the stability and release kinetics must be taken into account:

- Particle size and zeta potential.
- The degree of crystallization and variation of lipids.
- The existence of additional structures and dynamic phenomena.

11.4.3.1 Particle Size Measurement and Zeta Potential

For typical particle size measurements, photon-correlated spectroscopy (PCS) and laser diffraction (LD) are the most effective methods. PCS, often referred to as dynamic light scattering, examines variations in the brightness of scattered light brought on by particle motion. This technique can handle sizes ranging from a few nanometers to around three microns. Although, PCS is a useful technique for analyzing nanoparticles, it is unable to pick much bigger microparticles. Unlike PCS and LD electron microscopy, which directly discloses the shape of the particles? Distributed optimized SLN is often more physically stable than 12 months. ZP measurements aid in predicting the stability of colloidal dispersions during storage [48].

11.4.3.1.1 Dynamic Light Scattering (DLS)
DLS also known as PCS records the change in intensity of scattered light over a time scale of microseconds [49].

11.4.3.1.2 Static Light Scattering (SLS)/Fraunhofer Diffraction
In the SLS synthetic approach, light that has been dispersed by a particle solution is collected and fitted to the fundamental variable.

11.4.3.1.3 Acoustic Method
By fitting the pertinent physical equations, it evaluates the attenuation of dispersed sound waves as a way of sizing.

11.4.3.1.4 Nuclear Magnetic Resonance (NMR)
Nanoparticles' size and qualitative makeup can both be determined via NMR.

11.4.3.1.5 Infrared Imaging
The two direct methods for calculating nanoparticle quantities and describing their physical characteristics are scanning electron microscopy (SEM) and transmission electron microscopy (TEM), with the former method being employed for morphological research. The detection size limit for TEM is smaller [50].

11.4.3.1.6 Atomic Force Microscopy (AFM)
It creates a topological map of the sample based on forces acting between the probe tip and the surface as it is rastered over the sample.

11.4.3.2 Powder X-Ray Diffraction and Differential Scanning Calorimetry (DSC)
The geometric scattering of radiation from crystal planes inside a solid is used to ascertain the presence or absence of the original solid and consequently the degree of crystallinity. By measuring glassware and melting point temperatures, DSC can be used to characterize the nature of crystallinity in nanoparticles [51].

11.5 STERILIZATION OF SLNS

The SLNs need to be sterile for delivery via intravenous and ophthalmic routes. The production of hot microemulsions and changes in hot nanoparticle size can both be attributed to the temperature attained during autoclave sterilization. After a slow cooling period, the SLNs reassemble, but some nanodroplets are able to unite once again to generate a bigger SLN than the original droplet. The nanodroplets might not be stable enough, since the SLNs are rinsed before sterilization and there is less surfactant and co-surfactant in the heating system [52].

11.6 FATE OF SLNS AFTER ORAL INTAKE

It remains challenging and alluring to give drugs orally because of their evident commercial potential. The bioavailability of drugs contained within lipid nanoparticles may be enhanced and/or less variable, and their plasma levels may last longer. While these technologies could provide the greatest degree of versatility in terms of adjusting the medicine release profile inside the GIT and providing labile drug molecules with protection against chemical degradation (peptide drugs) [53].

11.7   ROUTES OF USE AND THEIR BIOLOGICAL DISTRIBUTION

Interactions of SLNs with biological media include processes of biomaterial distribution on the surface of particles and desorption of SLNs components in biological media along with enzymatic processes. The different routes of administration are as follows [54, 55].

11.7.1   PARENTERAL ADMINISTRATION

Parenteral medicines containing peptides and proteins are often sold. Because of the digestive tract's enzymatic degradation, they cannot be consumed as normal. The potential negative effects of SLN caused by its higher bioavailability are lessened when administered parentally.

11.7.2   ORAL ADMINISTRATION

According to reports, the controlled release characteristic of SLNs enables bypassing the intestinal and gastric degradation of encapsulated medications as well as their capacity to absorb and transport across the mucosa. For ensuring their appropriateness for oral administration, colloidal carriers' stability in the digestive fluids must first be assessed.

11.7.3   RECTAL USE

In some circumstances, parenteral or rectal usage is recommended when a quick pharmacological effect is desired. Due to its simplicity of usage, this method is used for treating pediatric patients.

11.7.4   INTRANASAL ADMINISTRATION

The nasal route is recommended because of its quick absorption and quick commencement of the action, which also prevents the unstable medication from being degraded in the GIT and from being transported insufficiently through epithelial cell layers.

11.8   ADVANTAGES OF SLNS

The following are a few advantages of SLNs [56, 57]:

- Avoiding chemical solvents and using biodegradable physiological lipids in production procedures reduces the risk of acute and chronic toxicity.
- Increased bioavailability of compounds with weak water solubility.
- The ability to scale up.
- Site-specific drug delivery; improved drug penetration into the skin by dermal application.
- Enhance the bioavailability of entrapped bioactive and chemical synthesis of labile integrated substance.
- Protect chemically labile agents from degradation in the gut and sensitive molecules from the environment.
- SLNs are more stable than liposomes.
- Achieved high concentration of a functional chemical.
- Possibility of lyophilization.

11.9 DISADVANTAGES OF SLNS

The following are a few disadvantages of SLNs [58]:

- Drug repulsion during storage following polymeric change.
- Insufficient drug loading capacity.
- Relatively high-water content of the dispersions (70–99.9%).

11.10 SPECIFIC ROLE OF SLNS IN ANTICANCER DRUG DELIVERY

For cancer therapy, chemotherapy is widely used through the conventional route of drug administration. However, chemotherapy has many problems including low drug solubility, less specificity,
enhanced toxicity, and drug resistance [33, 34]. Patient compliance is another concern due to the
discomfort of needles while injecting drugs [59].

SLNs have the potential to overcome these limitations and overcome drug resistance. The size
of SLNs in the nanometer range makes them suitable to diffuse through barriers and deliver drugs
at the site of action with fewer chances of toxicity [60]. SLNs enhance the contact time of cancer to
drugs in comparison to the different ways of administration [59]. Therefore, SLNs are considered
promising drug delivery systems for the development of cancer treatment.

11.10.1 ENCAPSULATION OF WATER-SOLUBLE ANTICANCER COMPOUNDS

Regardless of the choice of the SLNs' preparation process, at some point in the SLNs' fabrication,
the lipid must be melted and dispersed into submicron-sized lipid droplets in an aqueous medium,
either by mechanical or thermodynamic means to enable the formation of nanoparticles. The drug
to be encapsulated must be effectively partitioned into these melt lipid droplets to attain better drug
loading in SLNs [29]. Thus hydrophobic anticancer compounds (taxanes and camptothecin-based
drugs) can be proficiently encapsulated in SLNs as they are anticipated to partition well in lipids but
cytotoxic drugs are physicochemically different. Several anticancer drugs are hydrophilic (FuDR,
5-fluorouracil (5-FU), or mi tomycin-C). Moreover, salt forms of many lipophilic drugs are more
commonly utilized as they can be easily diluted and administered using ordinarily available water-
based vehicles (for example, 0.9% saline). Examples are hydrochloride salts of doxorubicin and
vincristine, which are more often used compared to their parent drugs. Typically fabricated SLNs of
such hydrophilic or ionic anticancer drugs tend to possess low drug loading and drug encapsulation
efficiency (i.e., the relative amount of drug loaded compared to that in the feed). SLNs are appropriate carriers for such hydrophilic drugs, which are very potent [61], but this normally is not appropriate for anticancer drugs. Indeed, several milligrams of cytotoxic agents are required to attain the
desired anticancer effects. It is important to design a method that results in substantial encapsulation
of these hydrophilic drugs in SLNs.

Numerous approaches are developed to encapsulate the ionic salts of cytotoxic drugs. One
involves the addition of organic counter-ions to form ionic pairs with the charged drug molecules
reported by Gasco and co-workers. Decyl phosphates/hexadecyl phosphates were used to improve
the loading of the salt forms of doxorubicin and idarubicin into SLNs composed of stearic acid.
Other noteworthy advancements in drug partitioning into the lipid have been demonstrated to fabricate "lipid drug conjugate" (LDC) nanoparticles [62]. Firstly, an insoluble drug-lipid conjugate
mass is fabricated either by covalent linkage (e.g., ester linkage) or salt formation. Secondly, using
the standard method, an aqueous surfactant solution and this LDC mass are mixed for nanoparticle
fabrication (e.g., homogenization). Another approach employs the complexation of ionic polymers
and drugs, which was investigated earlier for the transport of ionic anticancer drugs and chemosensitizers to prepare "polymer-lipid hybrid nanoparticles" (PLN). In such preparation, the oppositely charged ions of polymer neutralize the charges on ionic drug molecules; the drug-polymer

complexes thus formed are then incorporated into lipids for nanoparticle fabrication. The drug encapsulation efficiencies of ionic drugs such as doxorubicin HCl and verapamil HCl are improved from 20–35% up to 80% by this method [63]. For particular nonionic hydrophilic anticancer drugs, all the above-mentioned approaches based on charge neutralization are not valid. A potential way out is to chemically synthesize lipophilic drug derivatives. For example, 5-FU is a nonionic, extremely hydrophilic antimetabolite of low molecular weight. To increase its loading capacity and encapsulation efficiency in SLNs, Wang et al. synthesized chemically a lipophilic derivative of 5-FU and assimilated it in SLNs. The encapsulation efficiency was reported to be more than 90% [64]. The key problem of this method is the involvement of monotonous techniques of chemical synthesis and purification. Careful evaluations of the stability, safety, and efficacy of the drug derivative are also required, which are not easy tasks in themselves.

11.10.2 ENCAPSULATION OF WATER-INSOLUBLE ANTICANCER COMPOUNDS

SLNs are distinguished by the incorporation of lipids that persist to be solid at normal body temperature. Various biocompatible and physiological lipids like fatty acids, triglycerides, steroids, and waxes are abundantly used in the formation of SLNs. The freedom of choosing a formulation method from a diversity of techniques including homogenization (hot or cold), makes these nanocarriers attractive from a pharmaceutical frame of reference. Such methods ensure high reproducibility and production free of toxic organic solvents, along with easy scale up [55, 65]. Looking from the perspective of drug delivery, the encapsulation of water-insoluble lipophilic compounds is more efficient in NLCs due to their high content of lipids [66]. The nanocarriers based on the solid lipids are shown to possess intrinsic capabilities to carry the anticancer substances into tumor cells, conveniently bypassing the efflux transporters like the P-glycoprotein via exhibiting enhanced endocytosis [67]. This indicates that formulating SLNs for the lipophilic anticancer compounds can be more effective for drug-resistant tumor treatment. Many researchers have already studied the SLNs for water-insoluble anticancer substances. Yang et al. demonstrated that the encapsulation efficiency of campothecin was enhanced following the oral administration when the drug was incorporated into SLNs [68]. These nanocarriers have also been used extensively for the incorporation of taxanes like docetaxel and paclitaxel [69, 70]. Yuan and his coworkers reported that the folate receptor targeted SLNs show a lesser IC50 value in comparison to free paclitaxel solution, in the A549 cells. SLNs of all-trans-retinoic acid (ATRA) show a reduced hemolytic potential and better delivery as compared to the free drug. One of the main disadvantages of SLNs is their high burst drug release and easier drug expulsion. But studies have shown that the use of a mixture of lipids having different lengths, can easily overcome this limitation by providing more capacity for the drug's encapsulation in lipid structure [71].

11.10.3 IMPROVED CONTROL OF THE RATE AND EXTENT OF DRUG RELEASE

The SLN systems established in the early 1990s frequently release drugs in an uneven, biphasic fashion. Initially, fast drug release was observed followed by slow and incomplete release [26]. The burst release that was initially observed, depicts a substantial difficulty in anticancer drug delivery because of the high potency of cytotoxic compounds [66]. A large dose of anticancer drug rapidly released into the systemic circulation (if administered systemically) or close to local injection locations (if injected in a specific region) can result in a considerable health hazard. The burst effect in SLNs is often accredited to the irregular dispersal of the drug within the particle. Several lipids such as tripalmitin may develop close to perfect crystal lattice in the solid state during SLNs' fabrication, with lipid molecules compact and orderly packed within. These crystals possess limited imperfections and have little room for a large number of drugs. It will therefore push the drug molecules to the outer portion of the nanoparticle. Moreover, polymorphic transitions in nanoparticles result in lipid crystallinity during long-term storage, which may also cause drug expulsion to the nanoparticle surface [72]. In both cases, the drug concentrated at or near the particle surface can rapidly diffuse away into the surrounding medium, and give rise to the burst effect. Conditions of fabrication of nanoparticles can be accustomed to overcome or diminish the above burst release effect, e.g., decreasing the surfactant concentration and/or cooling the lipid emulsion speedily to permit the formation of nanoparticles comprising primarily of solid drug solution [29]. As high lipid crystallinity is the major cause of the burst release of drugs from SLNs, this undesirable phenomenon may be lessened by choosing lipids that do not form good crystals, including mono- or di-glycerides, or triglycerides with chains of different lengths [73]. Drug release can be slow and incomplete from SLNs after the initial burst. For instance, the release was less than 0.1% in different systems delivering anticancer drugs including doxorubicin, idarubicin, and paclitaxel [74]. Extended drug release is usually considered to be a positive feature in most forms of therapy. However, in terms of cancer chemotherapy, its impact is difficult to predict. It has been shown that continuous exposure to sub-optimal levels of cytotoxic agents may induce the expression of membrane-associated drug transporters (P-glycoprotein) and thus renders cancer cells more drug-resistant [75]. A SLN system that may release anticancer drugs faster without a strong burst release may avoid this theoretical risk.

11.10.4   USE OF SLNs IN VARIOUS TUMORS

SLNs have been used for the treatment of tumors in various body parts due to their unique structure, good encapsulation efficiency, and the ability to even cross the blood–brain barrier (BBB). Over time, SLN formulations have been implied in the tumors of the breast, lungs, brain, liver, etc. Some of the examples are discussed below.

11.10.4.1   Breast Tumors

Breast cancer has become one of the most common cancers in women worldwide. Studies refer to it as the second most abundant cancer in women after skin cancer. Localized SLNs containing drugs for the treatment of breast cancer are a good treatment option for early-stage breast cancer. For example, drug-resistant anticancer cells have been treated with paclitaxel-loaded SLNs. The effectiveness of paclitaxel-SLNs was compared to the other formulations, including cremophor EL vehicles (commercial formulation) and dimethyl sulfoxide solubilization, against drug-sensitive and drug-resistant MCF-7 cells. The analysis of concentration-dependent cytotoxicity revealed that the IC50 concentration in drug-resistant cells was significantly increased by SLNs containing paclitaxel. Additionally, these nanocarriers offered improved cellular uptake compared to the other formulations, particularly in drug-resistant cells, demonstrating that SLNs are successful in preventing multidrug resistance mechanisms in breast cancer cells [70]. Other studies, such as one in which SLNs were used as curcumin carriers against the breast cancer cell line MDA-MB-231, have also supported the effectiveness of SLNs against breast cancer. Additionally, compared to curcumin diluted in dimethyl sulfoxide, curcumin-SLN promoted a greater reduction in cell viability and an increase in the apoptotic cells [76].

11.10.4.2   Brain Tumors

Brain tumors pose a serious hazard to the quality of life, along with their duration. Brain tumors are complicated because the BBB is a crucial barrier. SLNs have a good ability to cross the BBB, and hence they are proven to be an effective carrier. The surface of SLNs can be altered with molecules that target receptors that are highly expressed in the blood–brain barrier to improve drug delivery in these therapies. Apolipoprotein E (ApoE), for example, is a molecule that the receptors of low- or very low-density lipoproteins (LDL or VLDL) can specifically recognize. Since, these receptors are expressed in blood–brain barrier cells, aiming ApoE at them would enable active cellular uptake of ApoE-SLN. Therefore, using this method could result in more nanoparticles building up in the brain. Additionally, it has been demonstrated that SLNs modified with ApoE, promoted cellular transcytosis and incorporation across the blood–brain barrier. In a hCMEC/D3 cell monolayer simulating the properties of the BBB, SLNs were coated with ApoE using DSPE-PEG-avidin or palmitate-avidin as linkers. This increased cellular uptake [77, 78].

11.10.4.3 Lung Tumors

Lung tumors are another leading cause of death worldwide. They are of significant interest here because they can be treated by the SLNs via direct inhalation into the lungs. However, as a result of an uncontrolled drug release, this type of therapy is linked to some restrictions, including brief residence times and low tolerance. In this regard, paclitaxel-loaded SLNs coated with a polymer made up of folate-poly (ethylene glycol) and chitosan have been used to overcome some of these limitations. Some studies showed that SLNs decreased the in vitro IC50 value for M109HiFR lung cancer cells. Additionally, it was discovered that SLNs, when inhaled, could raise the drug concentration in vivo in the lungs of healthy and ill mice [79]. According to other researchers, the poorly soluble substance erlotinib could be added to SLNs and used as an inhalation drug to treat A549 cells. Furthermore, erlotinib-loaded SLNs demonstrated a sufficient aerosol dispersion performance, suggesting that this system may be appropriate for pulmonary delivery [80].

11.10.4.4 Hepatic Tumors

Hepatic tumors or liver tumors can be benign or malignant. Despite the vast number of research in this area, new treatment approaches are still needed due to their growth rate. In a research study, SLNs were created with various lipid compositions, and the substance linalool was added to those formulations. This drug's ability to treat tumors was confirmed in both the HepG2 human hepatocarcinoma cell line and the A549 lung adenocarcinoma cells. Linalool-containing SLNs demonstrated potent antiproliferative activity in HepG2 cells, which was dose- and time-dependent [81]. Another study revealed that to control drug delivery using an external magnetic field, superparamagnetic iron oxide nanoparticles (SPIONs) can be added to SLNs. As a result, sorafenib was loaded into SLNs, and SPIONs were added to HepG2 human hepatocarcinoma cells. Although this method of drug delivery demonstrated a sizable cytotoxic effect, it was still not as potent as the free drug. Despite this, experiments using magnetic targeting and cellular uptake from SLNs showed that these nanoparticles may improve the treatment of hepatocarcinoma [82].

Many successful studies have also been performed on the utilization of SLNs in colon cancer, leukemia, prostate cancer, etc.

11.11 CONCLUSION

SLNs are the most commonly used carrier systems for the treatment of different types of cancer due to their better compatibility. SLNs are made of a lipid matrix solid and surfactants at physiological temperature and these systems work as a specific drug carrier system that can increase therapeutic effectiveness and enhance the safety of different chemotherapeutic agents used for cancer treatment. In comparison with other vehicles such as suspension, creams, and emulsions, these nanoparticles have the benefits of controlled drug release and protection of active pharmaceutical compounds. Moreover, the small sizes of nanoparticles confirm close contact of SLNs with the stratum corneum for better diffusion. Mostly, SLNs are less toxic and biocompatible as compared to other polymeric nanoparticles.

REFERENCES

1. Kruijtzer, C., J. Beijnen, and J. Schellens, *Improvement of oral drug treatment by temporary inhibition of drug transporters and/or cytochrome P450 in the gastrointestinal tract and liver: an overview. The Oncologist*, 2002. **7**(6): pp. 516–530.

2. Kalyanaraman, B., et al., *Doxorubicin-induced apoptosis: implications in cardiotoxicity. Molecular and Cellular Biochemistry*, 2002. **234**(1): pp. 119–124.

3. Wheate, N.J., et al., *The status of platinum anticancer drugs in the clinic and in clinical trials. Dalton Transactions*, 2010. **39**(35): pp. 8113–8127.

4. Borner, M., et al., *Answering patients' needs: Oral alternatives to intravenous therapy. The Oncologist*, 2001. **6**(S4): pp. 12–16.

5. Thanki, K., et al., *Oral delivery of anticancer drugs: Challenges and opportunities. Journal of Controlled Release*, 2013. **170**(1): pp. 15–40.

6. Mazzaferro, S., K. Bouchemal, and G. Ponchel, *Oral delivery of anticancer drugs I: General considerations. Drug Discovery Today*, 2013. **18**(1–2): pp. 25–34.

7. C Silva, A., et al., *Lipid-based nanocarriers as an alternative for oral delivery of poorly water-soluble drugs: Peroral and mucosal routes. Current Medicinal Chemistry*, 2012. **19**(26): pp. 4495–4510.

8. Gaumet, M., R. Gurny, and F. Delie, *Localization and quantification of biodegradable particles in an intestinal cell model: The influence of particle size. European Journal of Pharmaceutical Sciences*, 2009. **36**(4–5): pp. 465–473.

9. Westesen, K. and B. Siekmann, *Particles with modified physicochemical properties, their preparation and uses*. 2001, Google Patents.

10. H Muller, R., R. Shegokar, and C. M Keck, *20 years of lipid nanoparticles (SLN & NLC): present state of development & industrial applications. Current Drug Discovery Technologies*, 2011. **8**(3): pp. 207–227.

11. Liu, J., et al., *Isotretinoin-loaded solid lipid nanoparticles with skin targeting for topical delivery. International Journal of Pharmaceutics*, 2007. **328**(2): pp. 191–195.

12. Lander, R., et al., *Gaulin homogenization: a mechanistic study. Biotechnology Progress*, 2000. **16**(1): pp. 80–85.

13. Speiser, P., *Lipidnanopellets als Trägersystem für Arzneimittel zur peroralen Anwendung. European Patent EP*, 1990. **167825**: p. 0167825.

14. Siekmann, B. and K. Westesen, *Investigations on solid lipid nanoparticles prepared by precipitation in o/w emulsions. European Journal of Pharmaceutics and Biopharmaceutics*, 1996. **42**(2): pp. 104–109.

15. Mukherjee, S., S. Ray, and R. Thakur, *Solid lipid nanoparticles: a modern formulation approach in drug delivery system. Indian Journal of Pharmaceutical Sciences*, 2009. **71**(4): p. 349.

16. Boltri, L., et al. *Lipid nanoparticles: evaluation of some critical formulation parameters. Proc Int Symp Control Release Bioact Mater*, 1993. **20**(20): pp. 346–347.

17. De Labouret, A., et al., *Application of an original process for obtaining colloidal dispersions of some coating polymers. Preparation, characterization, industrial scale-up. Drug Development and Industrial Pharmacy*, 1995. **21**(2): pp. 229–241.

18. Satapathy, M.K., et al., *Solid lipid nanoparticles (SLNs): an advanced drug delivery system targeting brain through BBB. Pharmaceutics*, 2021. **13**(8): p. 1183.

19. Cavalli, R., et al., *Effects of some experimental factors on the production process of solid lipid nanoparticles. European Journal of Pharmaceutics and Biopharmaceutics*, 1996. **42**(2): pp. 110–115.

20. Chen, Y., et al., *Preparation of solid lipid nanoparticles loaded with Xionggui powder-supercritical carbon dioxide fluid extraction and their evaluation in vitro release. China Journal of Chinese Materia Medica*, 2006. **31**(5): pp. 376–379.

21. Drake, B., et al., *Imaging crystals, polymers, and processes in water with the atomic force microscope. Science*, 1989. **243**(4898): pp. 1586–1589.

22. Jannin, V., J. Musakhanian, and D. Marchaud, *Approaches for the development of solid and semi-solid lipid-based formulations. Advanced Drug Delivery Reviews*, 2008. **60**(6): pp. 734–746.

23. Yang, S., et al., *Body distribution of camptothecin solid lipid nanoparticles after oral administration. Pharmaceutical Research*, 1999. **16**(5): pp. 751–757.

24. Cortesi, R., et al., *Production of lipospheres as carriers for bioactive compounds. Biomaterials*, 2002. **23**(11): pp. 2283–2294.

25. Yang, S.C., et al., *Body distribution in mice of intravenously injected camptothecin solid lipid nanoparticles and targeting effect on brain. Journal of Controlled Release*, 1999. **59**(3): pp. 299–307.

26. Zur Mühlen, A. and W. Mehnert, *Drug release and release mechanism of prednisolone loaded solid lipid nanoparticles. Pharmazie*, 1998. **53**(8): pp. 552–555.

27. Moghimi, S.M. and J. Szebeni, *Stealth liposomes and long circulating nanoparticles: Critical issues in pharmacokinetics, opsonization and protein-binding properties. Progress in Lipid Research*, 2003. **42**(6): pp. 463–478.

28. Park, J.W., *Liposome-based drug delivery in breast cancer treatment. Breast Cancer Research*, 2002. **4**(3): pp. 1–5.

29. Mehnert, W. and K. Mäder, *Solid lipid nanoparticles: production, characterization and applications. Advanced Drug Delivery Reviews*, 2012. **64**: pp. 83–101.

30. Kabra, R., et al., *Role of solid lipid nanoparticles in oral drug delivery: A review. International Journal of Current Pharmaceutical Sciences*, 2014. **1**: pp. 47–62.

31. Lee, C.H. and Y.W. Chien, *Drug delivery: Vaginal route*, in *Encyclopedia of Pharmaceutical Science and Technology, Fourth Edition*. 2013, Boca Raton: CRC Press. pp. 1236–1259.

32. Moon, J.H., et al., *Nanoparticle approaches to combating drug resistance. Future Medicinal Chemistry*, 2015. **7**(12): pp. 1503–1510.

33. Din, F.u., et al., *Effective use of nanocarriers as drug delivery systems for the treatment of selected tumors. International Journal of Nanomedicine*, 2017: pp. 7291–7309.

34. Sun, T., et al., *Engineered nanoparticles for drug delivery in cancer therapy. Angewandte Chemie International Edition*, 2014. **53**(46): pp. 12320–12364.

35. Natfji, A.A., et al., *Parameters affecting the enhanced permeability and retention effect: The need for patient selection. Journal of Pharmaceutical Sciences*, 2017. **106**(11): pp. 3179–3187.

36. Kou, L., et al., *Transporter-guided delivery of nanoparticles to improve drug permeation across cellular barriers and drug exposure to selective cell types. Frontiers in Pharmacology*, 2018. **9**: p. 27.

37. Wang, F., et al., *Hyaluronic acid decorated pluronic P85 solid lipid nanoparticles as a potential carrier to overcome multidrug resistance in cervical and breast cancer. Biomedicine & Pharmacotherapy*, 2017. **86**: pp. 595–604.

38. Shi, S., et al., *Synergistic active targeting of dually integrin $\alpha v\beta 3$/CD44-targeted nanoparticles to B16F10 tumors located at different sites of mouse bodies. Journal of Controlled Release*, 2016. **235**: pp. 1–13.

39. Jain, A., et al., *Galactose engineered solid lipid nanoparticles for targeted delivery of doxorubicin. Colloids and Surfaces B: Biointerfaces*, 2015. **134**: pp. 47–58.

40. Wang, J., et al., *Novel strategies to prevent the development of multidrug resistance (MDR) in cancer. Oncotarget*, 2017. **8**(48): p. 84559.

41. Ma, L., et al., *Co-delivery of paclitaxel and tanespimycin in lipid nanoparticles enhanced anti-gastric-tumor effect in vitro and in vivo. Artificial Cells, Nanomedicine, and Biotechnology*, 2018. **46**(sup2): pp. 904–911.

42. Üner, M. and G. Yener, *Importance of solid lipid nanoparticles (SLN) in various administration routes and future perspectives. International Journal of Nanomedicine*, 2007. **2**(3): p. 289.

43. Lv, Q., et al., *Development and evaluation of penciclovir-loaded solid lipid nanoparticles for topical delivery. International Journal of Pharmaceutics*, 2009. **372**(1–2): pp. 191–198.

44. Suresh, G., et al., *Preparation, characterization, and in vitro and in vivo evaluation of lovastatin solid lipid nanoparticles. Aaps Pharmscitech*, 2007. **8**(1): pp. E162–E170.

45. Stuchlík, M. and S. Zak, *Lipid-based vehicle for oral drug delivery. Biomedical Papers-Palacky University in Olomouc*, 2001. **145**(2): pp. 17–26.

46. Kuo, Y.-C. and H.-H. Chen, *Entrapment and release of saquinavir using novel cationic solid lipid nanoparticles. International Journal of Pharmaceutics*, 2009. **365**(1–2): pp. 206–213.

47. zur Mühlen, A., C. Schwarz, and W. Mehnert, *Solid lipid nanoparticles (SLN) for controlled drug delivery–drug release and release mechanism. European Journal of Pharmaceutics and Biopharmaceutics*, 1998. **45**(2): pp. 149–155.

48. Shah, R., et al., *Optimisation and stability assessment of solid lipid nanoparticles using particle size and zeta potential. Journal of Physical Science*, 2014. **25**(1): pp. 59–75.

49. Teja, V.C., et al., *A glimpse on solid lipid nanoparticles as drug delivery systems. Journal of Global Trends in Pharmaceutical Science*, 2014. **5**(2): pp. 1649–1657.

50. Üner, M., *Characterization and imaging of solid lipid nanoparticles and nanostructured lipid carriers*, in *Handbook of Nanoparticles*. 2016, Berlin: Springer. pp. 117–141.

51. Vivek, K., H. Reddy, and R.S. Murthy, *Investigations of the effect of the lipid matrix on drug entrapment, in vitro release, and physical stability of olanzapine-loaded solid lipid nanoparticles*. *Aaps Pharmscitech*, 2007. **8**(4): pp. 16–24.

52. Li, H., et al., *Enhancement of gastrointestinal absorption of quercetin by solid lipid nanoparticles*. *Journal of Controlled Release*, 2009. **133**(3): pp. 238–244.

53. Kaur, I.P., et al., *Potential of solid lipid nanoparticles in brain targeting*. *Journal of Controlled Release*, 2008. **127**(2): pp. 97–109.

54. Mozafari, M.R., *Nanocarrier Technologies: Frontiers of Nanotherapy*. 2006. Berlin: Springer.

55. Müller, R.H., K. Mäder, and S. Gohla, *Solid lipid nanoparticles (SLN) for controlled drug delivery—a review of the state of the art*. *European Journal of Pharmaceutics and Biopharmaceutics*, 2000. **50**(1): pp. 161–177.

56. Rupenagunta, A., et al., *Solid lipid nanoparticles-A versatile carrier system*. *Journal of Pharmaceutical Research*, 2011. **4**(7): pp. 2069–2075.

57. Fahr, A. and X. Liu, *Drug delivery strategies for poorly water-soluble drugs*. *Expert Opinion on Drug Delivery*, 2007. **4**(4): pp. 403–416.

58. Schwarz, C., et al., *Solid lipid nanoparticles (SLN) for controlled drug delivery. I. Production, characterization and sterilization*. *Journal of Controlled Release*, 1994. **30**(1): pp. 83–96.

59. Mei, L., et al., *Pharmaceutical nanotechnology for oral delivery of anticancer drugs*. *Advanced Drug Delivery Reviews*, 2013. **65**(6): pp. 880–890.

60. Geszke-Moritz, M. and M. Moritz, *Solid lipid nanoparticles as attractive drug vehicles: composition, properties and therapeutic strategies*. *Materials Science and Engineering: C*, 2016. **68**: pp. 982–994.

61. Morel, S., M.R. Gasco, and R. Cavalli, *Incorporation in lipospheres of [D-Trp-6] LHRH*. *International Journal of Pharmaceutics*, 1994. **105**(2): pp. R1–R3.

62. Olbrich, C., et al., *Lipid-drug-conjugate (LDC) nanoparticles as novel carrier system for the hydrophilic antitrypanosomal drug diminazenediaceturate*. *Journal of Drug Targeting*, 2002. **10**(5): pp. 387–396.

63. Wong, H.L., et al., *Development of solid lipid nanoparticles containing ionically complexed chemotherapeutic drugs and chemosensitizers*. *Journal of Pharmaceutical Sciences*, 2004. **93**(8): pp. 1993–2008.

64. Wang, J.-X., X. Sun, and Z.-R. Zhang, *Enhanced brain targeting by synthesis of 3', 5'-dioctanoyl-5-fluoro-2'-deoxyuridine and incorporation into solid lipid nanoparticles*. *European Journal of Pharmaceutics and Biopharmaceutics*, 2002. **54**(3): pp. 285–290.

65. Saupe, A. and T. Rades, *Solid lipid nanoparticles*, in *Nanocarrier Technologies: Frontiers of Nanotherapy*, 2006. Berlin: Springer. pp. 41–50.

66. Wong, H.L., et al., *Chemotherapy with anticancer drugs encapsulated in solid lipid nanoparticles*. *Advanced Drug Delivery Reviews*, 2007. **59**(6): pp. 491–504.

67. Wong, H.L., et al., *A new polymer–lipid hybrid nanoparticle system increases cytotoxicity of doxorubicin against multidrug-resistant human breast cancer cells*. *Pharmaceutical Research*, 2006. **23**: pp. 1574–1585.

68. Yang, S., et al., *Body distribution of camptothecin solid lipid nanoparticles after oral administration*. *Pharmaceutical Research*, 1999. **16**: pp. 751–757.

69. da Rocha, M.C.O., et al., *Docetaxel-loaded solid lipid nanoparticles prevent tumor growth and lung metastasis of 4T1 murine mammary carcinoma cells*. *Journal of Nanobiotechnology*, 2020. **18**: pp. 1–20.

70. Xu, W., E.J. Bae, and M.-K. Lee, *Enhanced anticancer activity and intracellular uptake of paclitaxel-containing solid lipid nanoparticles in multidrug-resistant breast cancer cells*. *International Journal of Nanomedicine*, 2018. **13**: p. 7549.

71. Narvekar, M., et al., *Nanocarrier for poorly water-soluble anticancer drugs—barriers of translation and solutions*. *Aaps Pharmscitech*, 2014. **15**: pp. 822–833.

72. Freitas, C. and R. Müller, *Correlation between long-term stability of solid lipid nanoparticles (SLN™) and crystallinity of the lipid phase*. *European Journal of Pharmaceutics and Biopharmaceutics*, 1999. **47**(2): pp. 125–132.

73. Wissing, S., O. Kayser, and R. Müller, *Solid lipid nanoparticles for parenteral drug delivery. Advanced Drug Delivery Reviews*, 2004. **56**(9): pp. 1257–1272.

74. Cavalli, R., O. Caputo, and M.R. Gasco, *Preparation and characterization of solid lipid nanospheres containing paclitaxel. European Journal of Pharmaceutical Sciences*, 2000. **10**(4): pp. 305–309.

75. Campone, M., et al., *Induction of chemoresistance in HL-60 cells concomitantly causes a resistance to apoptosis and the synthesis of P-glycoprotein. Leukemia*, 2001. **15**(9): pp. 1377–1387.

76. Rompicharla, S.V.K., et al., *Formulation optimization, characterization, and evaluation of in vitro cytotoxic potential of curcumin loaded solid lipid nanoparticles for improved anticancer activity. Chemistry and Physics of Lipids*, 2017. **208**: pp. 10–18.

77. Battaglia, L., et al., *Solid lipid nanoparticles by coacervation loaded with a methotrexate prodrug: Preliminary study for glioma treatment. Nanomedicine*, 2017. **12**(6): pp. 639–656.

78. Neves, A.R., et al., *Apo E-functionalization of solid lipid nanoparticles enhances brain drug delivery: uptake mechanism and transport pathways. Bioconjugate Chemistry*, 2017. **28**(4): pp. 995–1004.

79. Rosiere, R., et al., *New folate-grafted chitosan derivative to improve delivery of paclitaxel-loaded solid lipid nanoparticles for lung tumor therapy by inhalation. Molecular Pharmaceutics*, 2018. **15**(3): pp. 899–910.

80. Naseri, N., et al., *Development, in vitro characterization, antitumor and aerosol performance evaluation of respirable prepared by self-nanoemulsification method. Drug Research*, 2017. **67**(06): pp. 343–348.

81. Rodenak-Kladniew, B., et al., *Design, characterization and in vitro evaluation of linalool-loaded solid lipid nanoparticles as potent tool in cancer therapy. Colloids and Surfaces B: Biointerfaces*, 2017. **154**: pp. 123–132.

82. Grillone, A., et al., *Active targeting of sorafenib: preparation, characterization, and in vitro testing of drug-loaded magnetic solid lipid nanoparticles. Advanced Healthcare Materials*, 2015. **4**(11): pp. 1681–1690.

12 Mesoporous Nanoparticle-Based Anticancer Therapies

Tanzeela Awan, Uzma Saher, Muhammad Yasir Ali,
Muhammad Umair Amin, and Sajid Ali

12.1 INTRODUCTION

Nanocarriers have recently received a lot of attention due to their successful applications in disease diagnosis, monitoring, and treatment. Nanocarriers have been employed successfully for targeted drug delivery because of their high therapeutic efficacy and less side effects. A number of nanoparticles such as liposomes, micelles, carbon nanoparticles, metal oxides or metals (gold, silver), silica-based nanocarriers, and many others have been studied to obtain maximum drug delivery to the targeted site.

Inorganic nanoparticles have been extensively studied for their versatility of functions, their vast availability, and their functional biocompatibility. Among inorganic nanocarriers, mesoporous silica nanoparticles (MSNs) are one of the most effective types of nanocarriers that have been employed for theranostics (diagnosis and therapeutic use). MSNs are materials made of silica with pores that are in the nanometer range. The pore size of MSNs is classified by IUPAC as being between 2–50 nm [1]. Its initial discovery was made by Mobil Oil Research Group, and it was called M41S [2]. These have a high surface area, flexible pore size, adaptable particle size and shape, and surfaces with double function, which make them appealing for use as nanoparticles. These particles are suitable for controlled drug delivery systems (DDS) as they prevent the premature release of loaded drugs.

12.2 PROPERTIES OF MSNS

MSNPs have developed as novel inorganic materials for therapeutic uses because of their distinctive characteristics [3]. Due to their big surface area (up to 1000 m^2/g), increased pore volume (>0.9 cm^3/g), and good biocompatibility, MSNs having a particle size of 30–200 nm, are suitable to be loaded with many therapeutic/diagnostic compounds [4]. They are able to prevent the premature release of a drug, which prevents unintended degradation of particles in the stomach and intestines before reaching the target sites [5]. They are inexpensive, flexible in pore size, barely harmful, and easy to synthesize [6, 7]. MSNPs have optically transparent characteristics, are resistant to chemicals, and are stable at high temperatures [8, 9]. Additionally, they have fixed-diameter pores with regular arrangements that range in size from 2–50 nm, and their surfaces are easily functionalizable [10–12] to increase their cellular transportation [13]. MSNPs possess greater loading capacity than organic carriers, like micelle, gel, and liposome [14], and due to this property, they have considerably affected nanobiotechnology research. They are successfully employed as a carrier for the oral administration of hydrophobic drugs, thus their dissolution rate and bioavailability are enhanced significantly in comparison to the conventional drugs [15].

DOI: 10.1201/9781003363958-15

12.3 SYNTHESIS OF MSNS

In addition to the silica source, MSNs can be produced by adjusting a number of synthesis factors, such as reagent concentration, the type of structure-directing agent, for example, with the help of surfactants and copolymers, and by the help of controlling some physical factors, for example, temperature and pH of the reaction mixture [16]. Three main elements are required for the synthesis of MSNs: the template, often a surfactant, which acts as the agent to produce the pores; the silica source, which creates the walls around the pores; and an acid or base, which aids in the particle formation. Some supplementary compounds and/or settings, such as diluents, temperature, stirring rate, additives, and others are also part of these particles. These supplementary components will change the characteristics of developed MSNs. Sol-gel, hydrothermal, and a more contemporary green method can be used as the three different types of synthesis processes for the production of MSNs.

12.3.1 SOL-GEL METHOD

Stöber discovered that monodispersed sphere-shaped silica particles of very small size (microns) are the precursors to MSN production. The four main elements of the Stöber synthesis are water, alcohol, base, and silica source. The improved Stöber process generally involves the following four steps for synthesizing MSNs:

Step 1: In the first step, water is mixed with the template and the base.
Step 2: Afterward, the silica is mixed in it by stirring. During this step, the hydrolysis and condensation reactions occur resulting in the formation of silica sol.
Step 3: Subsequently, the sol is passed by the process of aging procedure that leads to the gel formation.
Step 4: At the end, MSNs are obtained in the form of powder, and then the template is separated by a calcination or acidic-solvent extraction procedure [17].

Many researchers emphasize the sol-gel approach for the development of MSNs since the reaction took place over a short period of time (2 h), and the amount of the solution was very small, making the production and collection procedure straightforward. This approach generates MSNs using sodium silicate as the silica source and polyethylene glycol (PEG) having a molecular mass of 3000 g/mol as the template. MSNs obtained by this method are of spherical shape with MCM-41 properties [18]. In another study, a chain of MSNs was prepared by consuming cetyltrimethylammonium chloride (CTAC) as the template and tetraethylorthosilicate (TEOS) as the silica source [19].

12.3.2 HYDROTHERMAL METHOD

The hydrothermal method involves hot water solutions coming from cooled magma to produce minerals. This process involves a chemical reaction that happens at high pressure and temperature inside a sealed container. Different steps in the hydrogel approach for creating MSNs include the following:

Step 1: Mixing of catalyst, water, and template together is the first step, which is the same as for the sol-gel method.
Step 2: In step 2, a silica source is added.

Step 3: Sometimes, the mixture underwent aging, while in others, it is agitated briefly before being transferred to an autoclave lined with teflon.

Step 4: The autoclave is heated for a specific amount of time at a specific temperature.

Step 5: After obtaining MSN's powder, a template removal procedure is carried out.

In some studies MSNs' production was done by using CTAB as a template and TEOS as a silica source, ammonia was used to enhance the reaction rate and ethanol is used to regulate the hydrolysis rate. Hydrothermal treatment was done by providing 100°C temperature for 12 h resulting in MSNs of sphere morphology. In another study, hydrothermal synthesis was successful in producing MSNs with fibrous dendritic or KCC-1 structures. This study revealed that a mixture of CTAB, TEOS, cyclohexane, and urea was used in the production process. This combination underwent a hydrothermal reaction at 120°C and 60 rpm for 4 h. The MSNs had a spherical form, and their centers were filled with organized fibers [20]. Successful hydrothermal production of MSNs with SBA-15 was characterized using pluronic F-127 and TEOS as templates and sources of silica, respectively. The procedure was carried out for 30 h under acidic hydrothermal conditions. The MSNs obtained have an impressive surface area of 1098 m^2/g [21].

MSNs produced by the hydrothermal approach have increased mesoscopic regularity, enhanced hydrothermal stability, and larger pore sizes. Although this process can yield MSNs, it also has a number of drawbacks, including the need for specialized equipment and extreme temperatures that translate to expensive costs over extended periods of time. Therefore, the sol-gel approach has been chosen for the majority of contemporary research.

12.3.3 GREEN METHOD

The "green technique" has recently been put forth as an alternative way for the creation of MSNs. The process is supposed to be environmentally benign and use waste materials as the source of silica, as suggested by the moniker "green." In the lack of a template, Abburi et al. were able to produce MSNs by employing hexafluorosilicic acid, a byproduct of the fertilizer industry, as the silica source. According to the XRD data, the produced MSNs have a hexagonal, structured mesoporous structure [22]. Another study used CTAB as a template and banana peel ash as a source of silica. [23]. Li and colleagues created MSNs using TEOS as a source of silica and a modified amino acid as a template. The MSNs appear to have pores with a "wormhole" layout, according to the TEM pictures. The MSNs produced have particle sizes between 130 nm and 270 nm and surface areas between 239 m^2/g and 678 m^2/g [24].

12.4 HYBRID MESOPOROUS SILICA NANOPARTICLES (MSNS)

Hybrid MSNs are formed after the functionalization of MSNs with organic or inorganic functional groups [25]. The silanol group present on the surface of silica can be changed into various compounds to enhance the use of MSNs in the biomedical field [26, 27]. Functionalization of MSNs can be done by three methods; co-condensation, a post-synthetic process by grafting, and the surfactant displacement method. In the co-condensation process, the functional group is combined with the surfactant and silica group during the synthesis of MSNs, which resulted in the homogenous attachment of the desired functional group to the MSNs' surface. The disadvantage of this method is that the MSNs cannot be calcined for template elimination because the functional group can also be calcined. However, with the grafting procedure, the functional group is added to MSNs after they have formed, either before or after the template has been removed. The active/functional sites like the external surface, pore surface, and pore entrance are very specific in the grafting method [28]. The surfactant displacement method is an extension of the grafting process in which direct surface silylation is done without prior calcination. Acidic alcohol is used as a solvent in this method [29]. A uniform monolayer of functionalized groups is formed in the surfactant displacement method. The functionalization of MSNs can be categorized depending on different components, such as functional groups, target sites, imaging agents, etc. These components are discussed below.

12.4.1 Functional Groups

Among the functional group, the amine group is the most common group for the modification of MSNs' surface. This group provides great help in the grafting of another group on the surface of MSNs [28]. In a study, aminopropyltriethoxysilane (APTES), an amino silane was introduced on the hollow surface of MSNs by the post-synthetic grafting process. They also studied that increased APTES concentration resulted in increased particle size [30]. The MSNs can be functionalized by thiol or carboxyl group [28], acrylate group [31], aldehyde group, or disulfide group [32]. These functional groups enhance the performance of nanocarriers as drug-delivery agents in cancer treatment.

12.4.2 Targeting Agents

The targeting agent can be used as functional groups at the surface of MSNs to improve the targeted drug delivery of these nanocarriers as it helps them to identify diseased cells [33]. Different ligands, which are recognized by receptors present on tumor cells, can be used to functionalize MSNs, such as sulfated glycosaminoglycan, arginine-glycine-aspartic (RGD) peptide, hyaluronic acid, and lectin ulex europaeus agglutinin-1. Sulfated glycosaminoglycan is functionalized at the surface of MSNs following many steps. At first, the amine group is functionalized, which is then converted to a carboxylic group and it is then used to attach cystamine to the nanocarrier's surface where it reacts to glycosaminoglycan [34]. Similarly, the RGD peptide is also functionalized with an amine group, which is then oxidized to a carboxyl group. This carboxyl group attaches covalently to the amine group of RGD peptide, making it functional [35]. Hyaluronic acid is the ligand recognized by CD44 receptors that are present in cancer cells and help in targeted drug delivery through MSNs.

12.4.3 Imaging Agent

Imaging agents are used to functionalize MSNs to visualize the movement of the particles throughout the system and their uptake by cells. Fluorescein isothiocyanate (FITC) is commonly used as an imaging agent. The co-condensation process was used to attach FITC to the MSNs [36]. In a study, due to its inherent brightness, FITC was commonly used for imaging purposes, and by functionalizing it on MSNs, we can get a brighter contrast for diagnostic purposes [37]. In another study, the natural substance emodin (EO) was employed as a fluorescence agent alongside N-methyl isatoic anhydride and lissamine rhodamine B sulfonyl moieties, two more fluorescence agents. In another study, the natural substance emodin (EO) was employed as a fluorescence compound alongside N-methyl isatoic anhydride and lissamine rhodamine B sulfonyl moieties, two more fluorescence agents. Combining different imaging agents made it possible to examine different wavelengths while avoiding contact with quenching [38]. In addition to fluorescent agents, T1 MRI contrast agents have been gaining prominence as imaging agents. As a T1 MRI contrast agent, Du and coworkers reported hybridizing MSNs with manganese oxide nanoparticles. Because manganese is a physiological regulator of enzymes, they chose manganese oxide nanoparticles as imaging agents because they demonstrated reduced toxicity [39].

12.4.4 POLYMERS

Functionalization of MSNs is typically done with polymer to serve as drug carriers because it is more likely to increase the carrier's overall efficiency and therapeutic effect [40]. For choosing an appropriate type of functionalization, many factors should be considered, e.g., the intended outcome, biocompatibility, precise targeting, stimuli-responsiveness, or prolonged drug release from the MSNs [41]. By utilizing the post-grafting approach, Plohl et al. activated MSNs with branched polyethyleneimine (bPEI). The surface area of these activated MSNs ranged from 706 to 724 m^2/g, with a particle size of 80 to 180 nm [42]. Polyethylene glycol is one of the most utilized polymers for MSN functionalization (PEG). When a carrier is PEG functionalized, non-specific protein adsorption is prevented, and blood circulation duration is increased, which is crucial for an efficient drug delivery agent [43, 44]. In a study, modified MSNs that include both amine and disulfide groups were used to functionalize PEG on the surface of MSNs. The research showed that PEG was connected to the MSNs by a disulfide link in a covalent manner [44]. Biopolymers can also be utilized to functionalize MSNs in addition to synthetic polymers. For example, chitosan was used to functionalize the surface of MSNs by grafting technique to build a pH-responsive system. These chitosan-functionalized MSNs have a particle size ranging from 80 to 130 nm [45].

12.4.5 ZWITTERION

Zwitterions can also be used to functionalize MSNs, making the materials both bioinert and biocompatible. An electrically neutral molecule called zwitterion is one in which the positive and negative charges are balanced. They are hydrophilic in nature and MSNs coated with the zwitterion have a comparable structure to a cell phospholipid membrane. The MSN's contact with the cell membrane is facilitated by the surface's various charges, which may lead to a greater amount of MSN internalization [43, 44].

12.4.6 MISCELLANEOUS MSNs

Inorganic groups like metal and metal oxides have also been used to functionalize MSNs. According to numerous studies, gold and MSNs work well together. To develop a stimuli active release carrier, gold nanoparticles were utilized as a cap to seal the pores of MSNs [46]. Iron oxide is also a commonly used inorganic compound to create magnetic MSNs. Moreover, titanium, titanium dioxide, magnesium, calcium gallium, etc., are also used in hybridization of MSNs [47, 48].

Another class that is organic-inorganic hybrid MSNs was discovered around 1999. There are two types of this substance: periodic mesoporous organosilica and mesoporous organosilica nanoparticles (MONs) (PMO). The main difference between the manufacturing of MONs and PMOs and the sol-gel synthesis of MSNs is the silica supply.

12.5 APPLICATIONS OF MSNS AS DRUG DELIVERY SYSTEM

MSNs are unique due to their high surface area, biocompatibility, ease of functionalization, and other characteristics. Due to these qualities, they are suitable for use as a medication delivery agent. The increased surface area made it possible to combine a high concentration of medications, although the premature release is still the problem. The medicine can, however, be loaded into the pores because of the material's porous nature, and the pore opening can be closed with other molecules. The closed pores can be opened by a particular stimulus in order to increase the MSNs' capacity as carriers. Applications for MSNs make them unique for use.

12.5.1 PASSIVE TARGETING

It is possible to define passive targeting as the buildup of nanoparticles in solid tumors. Generally, and briefly saying tumor growth at specific sites results in solid stress due to an increase in cell numbers and tumor size. There is less nutrient supply, which results in hypoxia, which results in the production of vascular endothelial growth factor (VEGF). VEGF along with vascular permeability enhancers like bradykinin, nitric oxide, and prostaglandin increase these tight junctions between endothelial linings. The matrix metalloproteinases (MMP) along with these factors result in disorientation and histopathological changes in the tumor area. This disturbance in the microtumor environment inhibits lymph drainage. Therefore, the retention of the drug carrier due to impaired lymphatic drainage and spontaneous drug carrier buildup in areas of solid tumors with leaky vasculature are the two characteristics that favor passive targeting. These two findings lead to the conception of the enhanced permeation and retention (EPR) effect.

For MSNs to be used as a drug delivery agents via passive targeting, three aspects must be under control: particle size, shape, and surface characteristics. The particle size needs to be between 50 and 300 nm, which is roughly between the renal clearance level and small enough to diffuse to the tumor cell through the leaky channel for spontaneous accumulation. The second crucial factor for a considerable EPR effect is the surface features of MSNs, which must be regulated as secondary parameters. After the intravenous administration, the MSNs can be recognized by the reticuloendothelial system (RES). Therefore, by surface alteration of MSNs by any macromolecule, these particles can be saved from RES clearance. It is discovered that MSNs when surface functionalized with polyethylene glycol (PEG) can lessen RES absorption and increase MSN's overall stability, which can boost the EPR effect [49, 50]. Although the EPR effect's passive targeting is an effective method of medication delivery, it nevertheless has a number of drawbacks. Small animal xenograft tumor models, which are used in the in vivo investigation, have a more complex method of nanoparticle admission to the tumor, and the EPR effect is more evident in these animals. Although this EPR effect happens in humans, it varies widely depending on the individual and the type of tumor [51]. This heterogeneity lessens the therapeutic effect by preventing an even dispersion of carriers [52]. Therefore, a more effective medication delivery method is required to solve this problem through passive targeting.

12.5.2 ACTIVE TARGETING

The active targeting technique is based on the exploitation of the tumor cell-specific receptors. The receptors are highly expressed on the tumor cell surface, hence it is an easy task to achieve active targeting. The uptake and EPR impact can be improved as more carriers accumulate at the tumor location by functionalizing the MSNs' surface with a targeted ligand that can bind with the receptors. This will increase the effectiveness of the therapy [53, 54]. Additionally, by adding the targeting agent, medication delivery is no longer entirely dependent on the EPR effect, and this active targeting can reach cancers such as hematological malignancies and tiny metastatic tumors that do not exhibit the EPR effect [55]. The ligand density is a key factor in creating a successful targeting approach. Increased clearance potential, bigger particles that reduce the EPR effect, steric hindrances that lower binding potential and decreased cellular uptake are all effects of high-density targeted ligands [56, 57].

12.5.2.1 Antibody Targeting Agent

Immunoglobulin (Ig), another name for antibodies, is one of the key components in the creation of active targeted drug delivery systems. Complement antibodies can direct the carrier to the tumor site by locating an antigen that is selectively overexpressed on cancer cells. Due to their specificity and

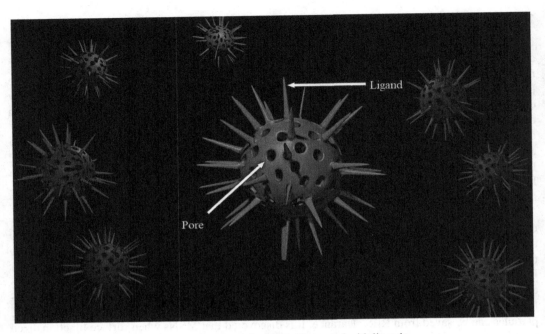

FIGURE 12.1 A typical mesoporous nanoparticle surface decorated with ligands.

selectivity, antibody-targeting agents have a few benefits over other chemicals. A targeted system's effectiveness will depend on a number of variables, including the origin and mechanism of linking the antibodies to the carrier [56].

A number of different pieces of research are present, functionalizing the MSNs with antibodies for active targeting of the tumor (Figure 12.1). Through the esterification reaction between a carboxyl group and an amino group, antibodies can be linked to MSNs [39]. A monoclonal anti-human epidermal growth factor receptor (EGFR) antibody, clone AT6E3, was coupled to MSNs composite to specifically target HeLa cells. The antibody was attached to the graphene oxide surface of the MSNs' composite. The outcome showed that the carrier was internalized and maintained in HeLa cells with antibody conjugation, demonstrating the utility of the antibody in treatment and targeting cancellation [57]. To specifically target breast cancer cells, the HER2 receptor-targeting antibody trastuzumab, which is FDA-approved, was coupled with MSNs [58, 59]. Despite the fact that antibodies are successful at locating the desired cancer cell, their high price and the possibility of an unfavorable immune reaction have prompted research into an alternative targeting agent.

12.5.2.2 Aptamers and Receptor Targeting

Aptamers are single-stranded DNA/RNA oligonucleotide sequences with binding affinity to different molecules and receptors of cell. To treat colorectal adenocarcinoma, MSNs were functionalized with AS1411 DNA aptamer (targeting agent) that was bonded to the PEG covers the MSNs surface [60]. Mucin-1 is highly expressed on the surface of various ovarian cancers, breast and lung cancer. In a study, MSNs were successfully functionalized with DNA aptamer specifically targeting MUC-1, and the capability of this hybrid system was determined against MCF-7 human breast cancer cell [61].

In active targeting, various chemotherapeutic agents can also be attached to the surface of MSNs to functionalize them for targeting different receptors, which may include folate receptors, transferrin receptors, CD44 receptors, and integrin receptors. Hybrid MSNs with various compounds used to functionalize them are discussed in Table 12.1.

TABLE 12.1
Mesoporous Nanoparticle-Based Cancer Drug Delivery Dystems

Functionalized MSN	Ligand/ Encapsulating Material	Drug	Cancer Cells	Reference
Cellulose -conjugated MSNs	Cellulose	DOX	Human liver cancer cells	[74]
GSH-conjugated MSNs	RGD peptide	DOX	U87 MG cell line	[75]
MSNs	Hyaluronic acid	DOX	HCT-116	[76]
PEG-functionalized polydopamine coated MSNs	-	DOX+Quercetin	HCT-8	[77]
Chitosan- capped hollow MSNs	Folic acid	Pheophorbide+DOX	KB-cells & L-02 cells	[4]
MSNs	Hyaluronic acid	DOX	Prostate cancer	[78]
Polydopamine (PDA)- modified mesoporous silica nanoparticles (MSNs)	Folic acid	DOX	Hela cells	[79]
MSNs	-	DOX	MCF-7 cells	[80]
Hollow MSNs	Dopamine-modified hyaluronic acid	DOX+indocyanine green	Mammary carcinoma cells	[80]
MSNs	Anti-B220 anti body	Daunorubicin	Acute myloid leukemia cells	[81]
MSNs	Anti-CD133	HNF4α+Cisplatin	Liver cancer cells Huh7	[82]
FITC-MSNs	-	Cisplatin	Hela, A549 cells	[83]
LPEI-MSNs	-	DOX	A549 cells	[84]
MSNs	Transferrin	DOX	Huh7 cells	[85]
MSNs	Folic acid	CMP	Hela cells	[86]
MSNs	Hyaluronic acid	DOX	Hela cells	[87]
MSNs	Folic acid	CMP	Panc1 cells	[88]
Hollow MSNs	-	DOX+CMP	A549 cells	[89]
MSN-DPH	Hyaluronic acid	DOX	Cos7 and MGC-803	[90]
MSNs	Hyaluronic acid	DOX	Hela cells	[68]

12.5.2.3 Stimulus Responsive MSNs

An extra chemical agent is used to trap the cargo in the general form of a stimulus-responsive system, which concurrently employs passive targeting and active targeting. After it enters the target areas through a particular stimulus, this gate will become open. The many types of stimuli can be categorized as internal (pH, redox, and enzymes) or external (light, temperature), or even on the basis of how many stimuli are present, such as one or many.

12.5.2.4 Single Stimuli

One of the potential methods for delivering anticancer medications to the intended area is pH-responsive MSNs. This technique was created by taking advantage of the fact that most cancers have lower pH levels than normal cells. Due to the Warburg effect, which occurs when cancer cells make energy through glycolysis with or without oxygen, acidic lactate is produced, resulting in the pH being lower (about 6.5) [62]. Polyacrylic acid, a pH-sensitive polymer, was used to seal the MSNs' pores, and folic acid was grafted onto the surface as a targeting agent. Due to decreased electrostatic interaction and the dissolution of the amide link between the MSNs and the polymer, the medication was released under an acidic pH [63].

Another method for creating a stimulus-responsive drug delivery agent uses redox potential. Reactive oxygen species (ROS) are produced at higher levels in malignant cells as a result of genetic mutation, mitochondrial malfunction, and altered metabolism. In order to combat this, ROS scavenger synthesis is also enhanced, with tripeptide glutathione (GSH) being the most notable. Although GSH is present in both normal and malignant cells, it is in cancerous cells that it contributes to the development of radio- and chemo-resistance [56]. One of the most popular linkers used to create redox-responsive MSNs is the thiol-linker. GSH will cause this linker to break, which will cause the medication to release. Gold (Au) nanoparticles served as the gate to the MSNs in the redox-responsive system described by Zhang and colleagues. When the carrier was exposed to an environment with a high concentration of GSH, the thiol-linker that had attached the Au to the MSNs surface disintegrated, releasing the medication doxorubicin [46].

In addition to the previously mentioned internal stimulus, it was discovered that external stimuli like light and temperature were frequently used in the creation of a responsive delivery system using MSNs. Functionalization with a photoactive group is required to produce light-responsive MSNs. Light of various wavelengths, such as ultraviolet (UV), visible (VIS), and near-infrared (NIR), will be the catalyst for medication release [53].

Another stimulus utilized to create MSNs that are responsive to stimuli is temperature. It must be stable during circulation (37°C) and the drug must be delivered at the locally heated tumor (40–45°C) in order to produce thermo-responsive MSNs [64]. It is possible to add a lipid bilayer to the surface of MSNs to create thermos-sensitive MSNs. The lipid bilayer will dissolve when these particles are exposed to high temperatures, releasing the medication at the tumor location [65]. The thermos-sensitive polymer can be used to coat MSNs, acting as a gate until the particles arrive at their destination.

12.5.2.5 Multiple Stimuli

Now the stimulus-responsive-MSNs used as drug delivery agents are not limited to single stimuli only. Most studies have discussed the use of two responsive systems, and some have mentioned as many as three. The pH and redox stimuli are most frequently utilized simultaneously. There have been reports on the creation of pH and redox-responsive MSNs using chitosan and disulfide bonds. A biopolymer that responds to pH is chitosan. Chitosan may break down in an acidic environment, causing the pore to open and the release of the medication. A redox-responsive system was developed by joining the MSNs and chitosan together via a disulfide bond. When the disulfide link was broken by a significant amount of GSH, the chitosan gate opened, and the medication was released [66, 67].

Dual and multi-responsive nanoparticles generally link to the advanced theranostics system comprising therapy and diagnosis [37]. It has been reported that the drug delivery capsule is formulated with a combination of rapid blood circulation time, effective transportation to the tumor, and enzyme-sensitive release of the drug. Hence three-layered MSNs are prepared where degradation of each layer takes place depending upon the sensitivity to the specific stimulus. Doxorubicin (DOX)-loaded MSN was first coated with hyaluronic acid, the second layer consisted of silica and the third layer is made up of a zwitterion 2,3-dimethylmaleic anhydride. This nanocarrier was highly permeable to the tumor cells, then the zwitterion layer was disrupted due to pH sensitivity and led to the internalization of MSNs. Afterward, a high amount of glutathione in the cytoplasm of tumor cells caused the breakdown of the disulfide bond of the silica shell. After this, the hyaluronic acid surface was exposed and attached to its receptor and released the DOX into the cells [68].

12.5.2.6 Multidrug Carrier

Chemotherapy is a systemic medication that treats malignancies that have a tendency to spread into more advanced tumors. To attain optimal efficacy, there are a number of challenges that must be solved, including the following:

- Bad side effects.
- Most chemotherapeutic medicines have low water solubility and poor stability.
- Ineffective distribution.
- Multidrug resistance (MDR).

In a typical chemotherapy regimen, several medicines are administered in a sequence [69], to boost treatment efficacy and delay. While with the help of MSNs, two or more drugs can be administered in one carrier. According to multiple reports, two anticancer medications were delivered using MSNs as a single carrier in order to provide a possible solution to these problems.

In a study, acute promyelocytic leukemia was treated by MSNs coated with folic acid-modified PEGylated lipid bilayer membrane to carry paclitaxel and tanshinone IIA drugs [70]. Specifically, to reduce the MDR of cancer stem cells, MSNs were used to deliver doxorubicin and tariquidar [71]. In another study, Zhu and coworkers developed a MSN-based platform for the co-delivery of DOX and cisplatin. The MSNs showed a synergistic effect on cytotoxicity in ovarian cancer cells, and the co-delivery of the two drugs resulted in a higher tumor inhibition rate compared to the single-drug-loaded MSNs [72].

In addition to conventional chemotherapeutic drugs, MSNs have also been used for the delivery of other types of drugs, such as proteins and nucleic acids. For example, Wang et al. developed a MSN-based system for the co-delivery of siRNA and DOX for the treatment of breast cancer. The MSNs showed a sustained release of both drugs and effectively downregulated the expression of the target gene and induced cell apoptosis in vitro and in vivo [73]. Many other studies have also been reported about the success of MSNs as a multidrug carrier. These are summarized in Table 12.1.

12.6 CHEMOTHERAPEUTIC DRUG DELIVERY

Mesoporous silica nanoparticles (MSNs) are promising nanomaterials for various biomedical applications, including cancer therapy. Due to their unique structural properties, MSNs have been extensively studied as drug delivery systems for various cancer therapies. Here are some examples of how MSNs are used in different cancer therapies:

12.6.1 CHEMOTHERAPY

MSNs can be used to deliver chemotherapeutic drugs to cancer cells (Table 12.1). The porous structure of MSNs allows for high drug loading, while the surface functionalization of MSNs can increase drug specificity to cancer cells. Additionally, MSNs can protect the drug from degradation and improve drug stability [91].

12.6.2 PHOTODYNAMIC THERAPY

MSNs can be loaded with photosensitizers and used for photodynamic therapy. Photosensitizers (PS) are activated by infrared light (650–900 nm), generating reactive oxygen species that can kill cancer cells. MSNs can protect photosensitizers from degradation and increase their accumulation in cancer cells [92]. MSNs can be used to incorporate PS alone as well as in combination with some of the chemotherapeutic agents. A group of researchers developed MSNs using methylene blue as PS and DOX was the drug of choice. They further surface-functionalized the MSNs with PEG for the escape of these particles from RES. These particles not only caused tumor cell death due to photodynamic therapy but also caused matrix degradation and drug release via ROS production [93]. A number of different PS can be used for this purpose like chlorin e6 (excited at 660 nm), zinc phthalocyanine (excited at 680 nm), protoporphyrin IX (excited at 630 nm), hematoporphyrin (excited at 630 nm), etc [94].

12.6.3 RADIATION THERAPY

MSNs can be used to enhance the effect of radiation therapy. By loading radio sensitizers into MSNs, cancer cells can be sensitized to radiation, leading to increased cell death [95, 96]. Bismuth base MSNs have been extensively studied for their effect under the influence of x-rays. In 2015, a research group prepared such particles using bismuth neodecanoate, CTAB, and DOX as a chemotherapeutic agent. They found a 1.55- to 4.40-fold increase in the cytotoxic effect of these particles in the presence of x-rays [97].

12.6.4 IMMUNOTHERAPY

MSNs can be used to deliver immunotherapeutic agents to cancer cells. By delivering immunotherapeutic agents directly to cancer cells, MSNs can enhance the immune response against cancer cells [96, 98]. Antiprogrammed cell death protein 1 (PD-1) resistance may be faced in immunologically cold tumor cells, therefore, the anti-PD-1 antibody was combined with CTAB MSNs. These were evaluated in vitro and in vivo and results revealed that despite immunologically cold state, these particles killed tumor [99].

12.6.5 GENE THERAPY

MSNs can be used to deliver nucleic acids to cancer cells for gene therapy. The porous structure of MSNs allows for high nucleic acid loading, while the surface functionalization of MSNs can increase the specificity of gene delivery to cancer cells [100].

In summary, MSNs have various applications in cancer therapy due to their unique structural properties. MSNs can be used to deliver chemotherapeutic drugs, photosensitizers, radio sensitizers, immunotherapeutic agents, and nucleic acids to cancer cells.

12.7 BENEFITS, LIMITATIONS, AND CHALLENGES

Over the past years, different nanoparticles have been utilized for delivering many anticancer drugs for curing various cancers in vivo and in vitro [83]. One of the most suitable alternatives among various nanoparticles is mesoporous silica nanoparticles. The main properties of MSNs are their strength and stability to deliver the drug at a site of action without prior release. They are not utilized just as delivering agents for chemotherapeutic drugs but are also famous for their diagnostic ability. Many studies revealed that MSNs also play an important role in the treatment of other diseases along with their working potential as diagnostic and curative agents in cancer treatment. It is proved by recent studies in which MSNs served as both controlled released delivery and imaging agent, respectively. In a study pH-responsive carrier was made by luminescent MSNs, which were developed by adding 10-phenylphenothiazine as the aggregation-induced emission (AIE) molecule, and the coating was done by a pH-sensitive polymer [101]. In another study, the role of MSNs was studied for therapeutic and ultrasound imaging purpose by Mira and coworkers. Gas capable of starting cavitation at both low and high sonic intensities was used to stabilize them. According to their findings, ultrasound imaging was created at low acoustic pressure, but at high acoustic pressure, the microbubbles collapsed, creating shockwaves that temporarily produce pores in the membranes of adjacent cells or ablated them [102].

MSNs are biocompatible and gradually break down into the non-toxic chemical silicic acid [103]. Due to MSN's quick bodily clearance following injection, their application as nanocarriers becomes restricted [104]. Better delivery of these particles through the cell membrane is achieved by fusing liposomes to MSN surfaces. This fusion product, known as a protocell, is a more efficient carrier with less toxicity [105].

For the high drug-loading capacity nanoparticles must be stable, repeatable, and scalable in fabrication. As MSNs can be replicated on a local scale but not a big one, this is an important problem that needs to be solved. The overall concentration of MSNs that must be delivered to the tissue site to provide therapeutic effects is strongly impacted by the concentration of the drug of choice. Moreover, studies on the biodistribution and excretion of these NPs have primarily been conducted in mice; nevertheless, human trials are necessary to identify the immune response and any potential negative effects. The surface of MSNPs also contains silanol groups that interact with the phospholipids in red blood cell membranes to cause hemolysis. Therefore, due to these difficulties and restrictions, the FDA has not yet approved any MSNs formulation.

12.8 CONCLUSION

Conventional chemotherapies do not show good biocompatibility, biodegradability, and clearance of the drugs. Additionally, they are unable to transport the drug to the intended site, endangering healthy cells as well. Multidrug resistance is another limitation of most cancer therapies. Therefore, it was the need of time to develop some cost-effective controlled-drug delivery system that may be able to overcome these drawbacks. MSNs have been used as an efficient drug delivery system for multiple purposes including controlled drug delivery, chemotherapy, and diagnostics due to their specificity, stability, and low toxicity. These nanoparticles are intriguing for controlled drug loading and its release with some specialized tunable properties such as chemical stability, drug loading capacity, size, pore volume and diameter, shape, number of accessible hydroxyl groups, and surface modification. Utilizing different strategies including surface engineering, attachment of targeting moieties, combinatorial delivery of numerous therapeutic agents, and stimuli-responsive drug administration, the efficacy of MSNP-based nanomedicines for disease detection, therapy, and theranostics may be further studied.

REFERENCES

1. Dayana, E., H. Ahmad, and M. Rahman, *Optimization of synthesis parameters of mesoporous silica nanoparticles based on ionic liquid by experimental design and its application as a drug delivery agent. Journal of Nanomaterials*, 2019. **2019**: pp. 1–8.
2. Kresge, A.C., et al., *Ordered mesoporous molecular sieves synthesized by a liquid-crystal template mechanism. Nature*, 1992. **359**(6397): pp. 710–712.
3. Zhou, Y., et al., *Mesoporous silica nanoparticles for drug and gene delivery. Acta Pharmaceutica Sinica B*, 2018. **8**(2): pp. 165–177.
4. Yan, T., et al., *Chitosan capped pH-responsive hollow mesoporous silica nanoparticles for targeted chemo-photo combination therapy. Carbohydrate Polymers*, 2020. **231**: pp. 115706.
5. Kao, K.-C. and C.-Y. Mou, *Pore-expanded mesoporous silica nanoparticles with alkanes/ethanol as pore expanding agent. Microporous and Mesoporous Materials*, 2013. **169**: pp. 7–15.
6. Li, H., et al., *A sulfonated mesoporous silica nanoparticle for enzyme protection against denaturants and controlled release under reducing conditions. Journal of Colloid and Interface Science*, 2019. **556**: pp. 292–300.
7. Raza, A., et al., *Solid nanoparticles for oral antimicrobial drug delivery: a review. Drug Discovery Today*, 2019. **24**(3): pp. 858–866.
8. Ali, O.M., et al., *Synthesis of lactoferrin mesoporous silica nanoparticles for pemetrexed/ellagic acid synergistic breast cancer therapy. Colloids and Surfaces B: Biointerfaces*, 2020. **188**(110824): p. 24.
9. Al-Asmar, A., et al., *Effect of mesoporous silica nanoparticles on the physicochemical properties of pectin packaging material for strawberry wrapping. Nanomaterials*, 2019. **10**(1): p. 52.
10. Mehmood, Y., et al., *Amino-decorated mesoporous silica nanoparticles for controlled sofosbuvir delivery. European Journal of Pharmaceutical Science*, 2020. **143**(105184): p. 14.

11. Cao, Y., et al., *Folate functionalized pH-sensitive photothermal therapy traceable hollow mesoporous silica nanoparticles as a targeted drug carrier to improve the antitumor effect of doxorubicin in the hepatoma cell line SMMC-7721. Drug Delivery*, 2020. **27**(1): pp. 258–268.

12. Saini, K., R.S. Prabhuraj, and R. Bandyopadhyaya, *Development of mesoporous silica nanoparticles of tunable pore diameter for superior gemcitabine drug delivery in pancreatic cancer cells. Journal of Nanoscience and Nanotechnology*, 2020. **20**(5): pp. 3084–3096.

13. Xu, C., et al., *Rod-like mesoporous silica nanoparticles with rough surfaces for enhanced cellular delivery. Journal of Material Chemistry B*, 2014. **2**(3): pp. 253–256.

14. Yu, F., et al., *Temperature-sensitive copolymer-coated fluorescent mesoporous silica nanoparticles as a reactive oxygen species activated drug delivery system. International Journal of Pharmaceuticals*, 2018. **536**(1): pp. 11–20.

15. Tawfeek, G.M., et al., *Enhancement of the therapeutic efficacy of praziquantel in murine Schistosomiasis mansoni using silica nanocarrier. Parasitol Research*, 2019. **118**(12): pp. 3519–3533.

16. Valtchev, V. and L. Tosheva, *Porous nanosized particles: preparation, properties, and applications. Chemical Reviews*, 2013. **113**(8): pp. 6734–6760.

17. Singh, L.P., et al., *Sol-gel processing of silica nanoparticles and their applications. Advances in Colloid and Interface Science*, 2014. **214**: pp. 17–37.

18. Grün, M., I. Lauer, and K.K. Unger, *The synthesis of micrometer- and submicrometer-size spheres of ordered mesoporous oxide MCM-41. Advanced Materials*, 1997. **9**(3): pp. 254–257.

19. Lv, X., et al., *Controlled synthesis of monodispersed mesoporous silica nanoparticles: particle size tuning and formation mechanism investigation. Microporous and Mesoporous Materials*, 2016. **225**: pp. 238–244.

20. Lv, C., et al., *Constructing highly dispersed Ni based catalysts supported on fibrous silica nanosphere for low-temperature CO_2 methanation. Fuel*, 2020. **278**: p. 118333.

21. Soares, D.C.F., et al., *Mesoporous SBA-16 silica nanoparticles as a potential vaccine adjuvant against Paracoccidioides brasiliensis. Microporous and Mesoporous Materials*, 2020. **291**: pp. 109676.

22. Abburi, A., M. Ali, and P.V. Moriya, *Synthesis of mesoporous silica nanoparticles from waste hexafluorosilicic acid of fertilizer industry. Journal of Materials Research and Technology*, 2020. **9**(4): pp. 8074–8080.

23. Mohamad, D.F., et al., *Synthesis of mesoporous silica nanoparticle from banana peel ash for removal of phenol and methyl orange in aqueous solution. Materials Today: Proceedings*, 2019. **19**: pp. 1119–1125.

24. Li, H., et al., *Evaluation of biomimetically synthesized mesoporous silica nanoparticles as drug carriers: structure, wettability, degradation, biocompatibility and brain distribution. Materials Science and Engineering: C*, 2019. **94**: pp. 453–464.

25. Möller, K. and T. Bein, *Degradable drug carriers: vanishing mesoporous silica nanoparticles. Chemistry of Materials*, 2019. **31**(12): pp. 4364–4378.

26. Thi, T.T.H., et al., *Functionalized mesoporous silica nanoparticles and biomedical applications. Materials Science and Engineering: C*, 2019. **99**: pp. 631–656.

27. Zhang, R., et al., *How to design nanoporous silica nanoparticles in regulating drug delivery: surface modification and porous control. Materials Science and Engineering: B*, 2021. **263**: p. 114835.

28. Zaharudin, N.S., et al., *Functionalized mesoporous silica nanoparticles templated by pyridinium ionic liquid for hydrophilic and hydrophobic drug release application. Journal of Saudi Chemical Society*, 2020. **24**(3): pp. 289–302.

29. Wu, S.-H., Y. Hung, and C.-Y. Mou, *Mesoporous silica nanoparticles as nanocarriers. Chemical Communications*, 2011. **47**(36): pp. 9972–9985.

30. Nguyen, T.N.T., et al., *Aminated hollow mesoporous silica nanoparticles as an enhanced loading and sustained releasing carrier for doxorubicin delivery. Microporous and Mesoporous Materials*, 2020. **309**: p. 110543.

31. Yismaw, S., et al., *Selective functionalization of the outer surface of MCM-48-type mesoporous silica nanoparticles at room temperature. Journal of Nanoparticle Research*, 2020. **22**: pp. 1–15.

32. Tian, Z., Y. Xu, and Y. Zhu, *Aldehyde-functionalized dendritic mesoporous silica nanoparticles as potential nanocarriers for pH-responsive protein drug delivery. Materials Science and Engineering: C*, 2017. **71**: pp. 452–459.

33. Hu, J.J., D. Xiao, and X.Z. Zhang, *Advances in peptide functionalization on mesoporous silica nanoparticles for controlled drug release. Small*, 2016. **12**(25): pp. 3344–3359.

34. Liu, M., et al., *Paclitaxel and quercetin co-loaded functional mesoporous silica nanoparticles overcoming multidrug resistance in breast cancer. Colloids and Surfaces B: Biointerfaces*, 2020. **196**: p. 111284.

35. Niu, B., et al., *Proper functional modification and optimized adsorption conditions improved the DNA loading capacity of mesoporous silica nanoparticles. Colloids and Surfaces A: Physicochemical and Engineering Aspects*, 2018. **548**: pp. 98–107.

36. Vares, G., et al., *Functionalized mesoporous silica nanoparticles for innovative boron-neutron capture therapy of resistant cancers. Nanomedicine: Nanotechnology, Biology and Medicine*, 2020. **27**: p. 102195.

37. Chen, N.-T., et al., *Lectin-functionalized mesoporous silica nanoparticles for endoscopic detection of premalignant colonic lesions. Nanomedicine: Nanotechnology, Biology and Medicine*, 2017. **13**(6): pp. 1941–1952.

38. Jänicke, P., et al., *Fluorescent spherical mesoporous silica nanoparticles loaded with emodin: synthesis, cellular uptake and anticancer activity. Materials Science and Engineering: C*, 2021. **119**: p. 111619.

39. Du, D., et al., *PSA targeted dual-modality manganese oxide–mesoporous silica nanoparticles for prostate cancer imaging. Biomedicine & Pharmacotherapy*, 2020. **121**: p. 109614.

40. Kankala, R.K., et al., *Nanoarchitectured structure and surface biofunctionality of mesoporous silica nanoparticles. Advanced Materials*, 2020. **32**(23): p. 1907035.

41. Bansal, K.K., et al., *Therapeutic potential of polymer-coated mesoporous silica nanoparticles. Applied Sciences*, 2020. **10**(1): p. 289.

42. Plohl, O., S. Gyergyek, and L.F. Zemljič, *Mesoporous silica nanoparticles modified with N-rich polymer as a potentially environmentally-friendly delivery system for pesticides. Microporous and Mesoporous Materials*, 2021. **310**: p. 110663.

43. Castillo, R.R., et al., *Advances in mesoporous silica nanoparticles for targeted stimuli-responsive drug delivery: An update. Expert Opinion on Drug Delivery*, 2019. **16**(4): pp. 415–439.

44. Garrido-Cano, I., et al., *Biocompatibility and internalization assessment of bare and functionalised mesoporous silica nanoparticles. Microporous and Mesoporous Materials*, 2021. **310**: p. 110593.

45. Nairi, V., et al., *Interactions between bovine serum albumin and mesoporous silica nanoparticles functionalized with biopolymers. Chemical Engineering Journal*, 2018. **340**: pp. 42–50.

46. Zhang, L., et al., *An optimized mesoporous silica nanosphere-based carrier system with chemically removable Au nanoparticle caps for redox-stimulated and targeted drug delivery. Nanotechnology*, 2020. **31**(47): p. 475102.

47. Wang, Y., et al., *Structure-dependent adsorptive or photocatalytic performances of solid and hollow dendritic mesoporous silica & titania nanospheres. Microporous and Mesoporous Materials*, 2020. **305**: p. 110326.

48. Du, X., et al., *Mesoporous silica nanoparticles with organo-bridged silsesquioxane framework as innovative platforms for bioimaging and therapeutic agent delivery. Biomaterials*, 2016. **91**: pp. 90–127.

49. Ku, S., et al., *The blood-brain barrier penetration and distribution of PEGylated fluorescein-doped magnetic silica nanoparticles in rat brain. Biochem Biophys Res Commun*, 2010. **394**(4): pp. 871–6.

50. Watermann, A. and J. Brieger, *Mesoporous silica nanoparticles as drug delivery vehicles in cancer. Nanomaterials*, 2017. **7**(7): p. 189.

51. Shi, Y., et al., *The EPR effect and beyond: strategies to improve tumor targeting and cancer nanomedicine treatment efficacy. Theranostics*, 2020. **10**(17): pp. 7921–7924.

52. Narum, S.M., et al., *Chapter 4 – passive targeting in nanomedicine: fundamental concepts, body interactions, and clinical potential*, in *Nanoparticles for Biomedical Applications*, E.J. Chung, L. Leon, and C. Rinaldi, Editors. 2020, Amsterdam: Elsevier. pp. 37–53.

53. Barui, S. and V. Cauda, *Multimodal decorations of mesoporous silica nanoparticles for improved cancer therapy. Pharmaceutics*, 2020. **12**(6): pp. 527.

54. Behera, A. and S. Padhi, *Passive and active targeting strategies for the delivery of the camptothecin anticancer drug: A review. Environmental Chemistry Letters*, 2020. **18**(5): pp. 1557–1567.

55. Tarudji, A.W. and F.M. Kievit, *Chapter 3 – active targeting and transport*, in *Nanoparticles for Biomedical Applications*, E.J. Chung, L. Leon, and C. Rinaldi, Editors. 2020, Amsterdam: Elsevier. pp. 19–36.

56. Gisbert-Garzarán, M. and M. Vallet-Regí, *Influence of the surface functionalization on the fate and performance of mesoporous silica nanoparticles. Nanomaterials*, 2020. **10**(5): p. 916.

57. Attarwala, H., *Role of antibodies in cancer targeting. Journal of Natural Science, Biology and Medicine*, 2010. **1**(1): pp. 53–6.

58. Yamaguchi, H., et al., *HER2-targeted multifunctional silica nanoparticles specifically enhance the radiosensitivity of HER2-overexpressing breast cancer cells. International Journal of Molecular Science*, 2018. **19**(3): p. 908.

59. Li, L., et al., *Actively targeted deep tissue imaging and photothermal-chemo therapy of breast cancer by antibody-functionalized drug-loaded x-ray-responsive bismuth sulfide@mesoporous silica core-shell nanoparticles. Advances in Functional Materials*, 2018. **28**(5): p. 11.

60. Babaei, M., et al., *Targeted rod-shaped mesoporous silica nanoparticles for the co-delivery of camptothecin and survivin shRNA in to colon adenocarcinoma in vitro and in vivo. European Journal of Pharmaceutics and Biopharmaceutics*, 2020. **156**: pp. 84–96.

61. Si, P., et al., *MUC-1 recognition-based activated drug nanoplatform improves doxorubicin chemotherapy in breast cancer. Cancer Letters*, 2020. **472**: pp. 165–174.

62. Iturrioz-Rodríguez, N., M.A. Correa-Duarte, and M.L. Fanarraga, *Controlled drug delivery systems for cancer based on mesoporous silica nanoparticles. International Journal of Nanomedicine*, 2019. **14**: pp. 3389–3401.

63. Kundu, M., et al., *Tumor targeted delivery of umbelliferone via a smart mesoporous silica nanoparticles controlled-release drug delivery system for increased anticancer efficiency. Materials Science and Engineering: C*, 2020. **116**(111239): p. 24.

64. Ghosh Dastidar, D. and G. Chakrabarti, *Chapter 6 – thermoresponsive Drug Delivery Systems, Characterization and Application*, in *Applications of Targeted Nano Drugs and Delivery Systems*, S.S. Mohapatra, et al., Editors. 2019, Amsterdam: Elsevier. pp. 133–155.

65. Zhang, Q., et al., *Thermo-responsive mesoporous silica/lipid bilayer hybrid nanoparticles for doxorubicin on-demand delivery and reduced premature release. Colloids and Surfaces B: Biointerfaces*, 2017. **160**: pp. 527–534.

66. Xu, Y., et al., *pH and redox dual-responsive MSN-S-S-CS as a drug delivery system in cancer therapy. Materials*, 2020. **13**(6): p. 1279.

67. Zhang, K., et al., *A redox and pH dual-triggered drug delivery platform based on chitosan grafted tubular mesoporous silica. Ceramics International*, 2019. **45**(17, Part B): pp. 22603–22609.

68. Lin, J.-T., et al., *pH and redox dual stimulate-responsive nanocarriers based on hyaluronic acid coated mesoporous silica for targeted drug delivery. Materials Science and Engineering: C*, 2017. **81**: pp. 478–484.

69. Meng, Q.Y., et al., *Rational design and latest advances of codelivery systems for cancer therapy. Materials Today Bio*, 2020. **7**: p. 100056.

70. Li, Z., et al., *Folic acid modified lipid-bilayer coated mesoporous silica nanoparticles co-loading paclitaxel and tanshinone IIA for the treatment of acute promyelocytic leukemia. International Journal of Pharmaceutics*, 2020. **586**: pp. 119576.

71. Pan, Y., et al., *Novel dendritic polyglycerol-conjugated, mesoporous silica-based targeting nanocarriers for co-delivery of doxorubicin and tariquidar to overcome multidrug resistance in breast cancer stem cells. Journal of Controlled Release*, 2021. **330**: pp. 1106–1117.

72. Alyassin, Y., et al., *Application of mesoporous silica nanoparticles as drug delivery carriers for chemotherapeutic agents. Drug Discovery Today*, 2020. **25**(8): pp. 1513–1520.

73. Zhuang, J., et al., *Tumour-targeted and redox-responsive mesoporous silica nanoparticles for controlled release of doxorubicin and an siRNA against metastatic breast cancer. International Journal of Nanomedicine*, 2021. **16**: p. 1961.

74. Hakeem, A., et al., *Cellulose conjugated FITC-labelled mesoporous silica nanoparticles: intracellular accumulation and stimuli responsive doxorubicin release. Nanoscale*, 2016. **8**(9): pp. 5089–5097.

75. Li, Z.-Y., et al., *A redox-responsive drug delivery system based on RGD containing peptide-capped mesoporous silica nanoparticles. Journal of Materials Chemistry B*, 2015. **3**(1): pp. 39–44.

76. Zhao, Q., et al., *Dual-stimuli responsive hyaluronic acid-conjugated mesoporous silica for targeted delivery to CD44-overexpressing cancer cells. Acta Biomaterialia*, 2015. **23**: pp. 147–156.
77. Shao, M., et al., *Polydopamine coated hollow mesoporous silica nanoparticles as pH-sensitive nanocarriers for overcoming multidrug resistance. Colloids and Surfaces B: Biointerfaces*, 2019. **183**: p. 110427.
78. Liu, C.-M., et al., *Cancer cell membrane-cloaked mesoporous silica nanoparticles with a pH-sensitive gatekeeper for cancer treatment. Colloids and Surfaces B: Biointerfaces*, 2019. **175**: pp. 477–486.
79. Cheng, W., et al., *pH-sensitive delivery vehicle based on folic acid-conjugated polydopamine-modified mesoporous silica nanoparticles for targeted cancer therapy. ACS Applied Materials & Interfaces*, 2017. **9**(22): pp. 18462–18473.
80. Wang, M., et al., *Acid and light stimuli-responsive mesoporous silica nanoparticles for controlled release. Journal of Materials Science*, 2019. **54**(8): pp. 6199–6211.
81. Mandal, T., et al., *Targeting murine leukemic stem cells by antibody functionalized mesoporous silica nanoparticles. Scientific Reports*, 2018. **8**(1): p. 989.
82. Tsai, P.-H., et al., *Dual delivery of HNF4α and cisplatin by mesoporous silica nanoparticles inhibits cancer pluripotency and tumorigenicity in hepatoma-derived CD133-expressing stem cells. ACS Applied Materials & Interfaces*, 2019. **11**(22): pp. 19808–19818.
83. Alavi, S.E., et al., *Archaeosome: as new drug carrier for delivery of paclitaxel to breast cancer. Indian Journal of Clinical Biochemistry*, 2014. **29**(2): pp. 150–153.
84. Wang, Y., et al., *In situ biodegradable crosslinking of cationic oligomer coating on mesoporous silica nanoparticles for drug delivery. Colloids and Surfaces B: Biointerfaces*, 2017. **153**: pp. 272–279.
85. Chen, X., et al., *Transferrin gated mesoporous silica nanoparticles for redox-responsive and targeted drug delivery. Colloids and Surfaces B: Biointerfaces*, 2017. **152**: pp. 77–84.
86. Sahu, S., et al., *Luminescent magnetic hollow mesoporous silica nanotheranostics for camptothecin delivery and multimodal imaging. Journal of Materials Chemistry B*, 2014. **2**(24): pp. 3799–3808.
87. Chen, C., et al., *Hyaluronic acid conjugated polydopamine functionalized mesoporous silica nanoparticles for synergistic targeted chemo-photothermal therapy. Nanoscale*, 2019. **11**(22): pp. 11012–11024.
88. Liong, M., et al., *Multifunctional inorganic nanoparticles for imaging, targeting, and drug delivery. ACS Nano*, 2008. **2**(5): pp. 889–896.
89. Wei, Z., et al., *A pH-sensitive prodrug nanocarrier based on diosgenin for doxorubicin delivery to efficiently inhibit tumor metastasis. International Journal of Nanomedicine*, 2020. **15**: pp. 6545–6560.
90. Naz, S., et al., *Enzyme-responsive mesoporous silica nanoparticles for tumor cells and mitochondria multistage-targeted drug delivery. International Journal of Nanomedicine*, 2019. **14**: pp. 2533–2542.
91. Hom, C., et al., *Mesoporous silica nanoparticles facilitate delivery of siRNA to shutdown signaling pathways in mammalian cells. Small*, 2010. **6**(11): pp. 1185–1190.
92. Huang, X., et al., *Cancer cell imaging and photothermal therapy in the near-infrared region by using gold nanorods. Journal of the American Chemical Society*, 2006. **128**(6): pp. 2115–2120.
93. Yang, Y., et al., *Red-light-triggered self-destructive mesoporous silica nanoparticles for cascade-amplifying chemo-photodynamic therapy favoring antitumor immune responses. Biomaterials*, 2022. **281**: p. 121368.
94. Hong, S.H. and Y. Choi, *Mesoporous silica-based nanoplatforms for the delivery of photodynamic therapy agents. Journal of Pharmaceutical Investigations*, 2018. **48**(1): pp. 3–17.
95. Hainfeld, J.F., et al., *Gold nanoparticles: a new x-ray contrast agent. British Journal of Radiology*, 2006. **79**(939): pp. 248–53.
96. Wang, X., et al., *Comprehensive Mechanism Analysis of Mesoporous-Silica-Nanoparticle-Induced Cancer Immunotherapy. Advanced Healthcare Materials*, 2016. **5**(10): pp. 1169–1176.
97. Ma, M., et al., *Bi2S3-embedded mesoporous silica nanoparticles for efficient drug delivery and interstitial radiotherapy sensitization. Biomaterials*, 2015. **37**: pp. 447–455.
98. Song, Y., et al., *Mesoporous silica nanoparticles for stimuli-responsive controlled drug delivery: advances, challenges, and outlook. International Journal of Nanomedicine*, 2017. **12**: p. 87.
99. Sun, M., et al., *Mesoporous silica nanoparticles inflame tumors to overcome anti-PD-1 resistance through TLR4-NFκB axis. Journal for ImmunoTherapy of Cancer*, 2021. **9**(6). p. e002508.
100. Lu, J., et al., *Light-activated nanoimpeller-controlled drug release in cancer cells. Small*, 2008. **4**(4): pp. 421–426.

101. Huang, L., et al., *The utilization of multifunctional organic dye with aggregation-induced emission feature to fabricate luminescent mesoporous silica nanoparticles based polymeric composites for controlled drug delivery. Microporous and Mesoporous Materials*, 2020. **308**: p. 110520.

102. Montoya Mira, J., et al., *Gas-stabilizing sub-100 nm mesoporous silica nanoparticles for ultrasound theranostics. ACS Omega*, 2020. **5**(38): pp. 24762–24772.

103. He, Q., et al., *In vivo biodistribution and urinary excretion of mesoporous silica nanoparticles: effects of particle size and PEGylation. Small*, 2011. **7**(2): pp. 271–80.

104. Wang, L.S., et al., *Biofunctionalized phospholipid-capped mesoporous silica nanoshuttles for targeted drug delivery: improved water suspensibility and decreased nonspecific protein binding. ACS Nano*, 2010. **4**(8): pp. 4371–4379.

105. Al Harthi, S., et al., *Nasal delivery of donepezil HCl-loaded hydrogels for the treatment of Alzheimer's disease. Scientific Reports*, 2019. **9**(1): p. 9563.

13 Antibody-Based Cancer Therapies

Malik Saadullah, Hafsa Tariq, Mavra Rubab,
Muhammad Yasir Ali, Saeed Ahmad,
and Nisar ur Rahman

13.1 INTRODUCTION

Antibodies are safeguard proteins produced by the immune system. These have a pivotal role in the treatment of cancer. Antibodies were discovered in the late nineteenth century, and soon afterward, there was speculation that they would be "magic bullets" for cancer diagnosis and treatment. In the following decades, a significant effort was made to immunize numerous animal species with human cancer in the hopes of producing antisera with some level of disease specificity [1]. This strategy produced little of lasting significance despite repeated claims of success and much disagreement, with the notable exception of the discovery of carcinoembryonic antigen (CEA), a marker for colon cancer and other cancers, and -fetoprotein, a marker for hepatocellular cancer [2].

Polyclonal anti-lymphocyte and anti-thymocyte sera, as well as anti-IgG, assisted in the prevention of graft vs. host disease in the fields of stem cell and organ transplantation, as well as in the treatment of anaplastic anemia. With the 1975 development of a monoclonal antibody (mAb) production technique, antibodies were investigated as highly selective targeting and effector agents for cancer therapy [3]. Murine mAbs were used in the early attempts at mAb-based cancer therapy, however, clinical trials frequently revealed poor results. This result was frequently brought about by the production of neutralizing antibodies that were directed against the therapeutic antibody made by the host. Yet with the development of antibody engineering, numerous mAb changes were made possible and important advancements were realized [4].

The creation of chimeric antibodies, which combine murine antigen recognition domains with a human Ig Fc domain, was the first significant step [5]. Because of the presence of the human Fc domain, chimeric antibodies are more similar to human antibodies and work better with effector cells to activate their anticancer action. Moreover, chimeric mAbs have a serum half-life that is typically between 2 and 4 weeks and is less immunogenic, less likely to be neutralized by host antibodies, and less immunogenic than fully human antibodies. As evidenced by the FDA's 1997 approval of the CD20 antibody rituximab for the treatment of B cell lymphomas, which pioneered the field of antibody-based cancer therapy, chimeric mAbs were the first clinically successful antibodies in oncology [6]. Rituximab is a chimeric human IgG1-containing monoclonal antibody (mAb) that binds to tetraspanin CD20, an essential transmembrane protein produced on the surface of both healthy and cancerous B-lineage cells. Soon after that, the chimeric EGFR antibody cetuximab was authorized for the treatment of colorectal cancer [7, 8]. Epithelial cells express the growth factor receptor EGFR, which is frequently overexpressed in epithelial malignancies. The cancer cell is deprived of vital growth factor signals by the antibody's blocking of this receptor, which is

DOI: 10.1201/9781003363958-16

necessary for its survival. Currently (July 2016), the United States and Europe have approved the use of more than 47 mAbs for therapeutic purposes [9].

Bispecific antibodies (bsAbs), bispecific fusion proteins of antibody fragments, antibody fragments carrying toxins or cytokines, and tri- or tetra-specific antibody derivatives are just a few of the additional antibody modifications and therapeutic agents derived from antibodies that have been created. Lastly, antibody fragments are employed to drive T cells towards cancerous target cells in chimeric antigen receptors (CAR)-transfected T cells.

13.2 ADVANTAGES AND DISADVANTAGES OF ANTIBODIES

13.2.1 ADVANTAGES

13.2.1.1 Targeted Therapy
Antibody-based cancer therapies are designed to specifically target cancer cells while sparing healthy cells, minimizing side effects, and reducing damage to healthy tissues.

13.2.1.2 Specificity
Antibodies can be engineered to target specific cancer cell surface proteins or receptors, which allows for a highly specific approach to cancer treatment.

13.2.1.3 Diversity
Antibodies can be designed to target different types of cancer, making them a potentially useful treatment option for a wide range of cancers.

13.2.1.4 Immune System Support
Some antibody-based therapies can also stimulate the immune system to recognize and attack cancer cells, leading to a more robust and effective response to cancer.

13.2.1.5 Efficacy
Antibody-based therapies have shown promising results in clinical trials, with some demonstrating high response rates and prolonged survival for patients with certain types of cancer.

13.2.1.6 Convenience
Antibody-based therapies can be administered via injection or infusion, making them a more convenient treatment option for patients compared to some other cancer therapies that require hospitalization or complex administration protocols. Overall, antibody-based cancer therapies offer a targeted, effective, and potentially a less toxic approach to cancer treatment, making them an important tool in the fight against cancer.

13.2.2 DISADVANTAGES

Antibody-based cancer therapies, also known as immunotherapies, have been a breakthrough in cancer treatment in recent years. However, like any medical treatment, there are also potential disadvantages to consider. Here are some of the disadvantages of antibody-based cancer therapies:

13.2.2.1 Limited Efficacy
Although antibody-based therapies have shown remarkable results in some patients, they may not work for everyone. Response rates vary depending on the cancer type and stage, and some patients may not respond at all.

13.2.2.2 Side Effects

Antibody-based therapies can cause side effects, which can range from mild to severe. These may include fatigue, nausea, fever, rash, and diarrhea. In some cases, the immune system can overreact and cause autoimmune side effects, such as inflammation of organs and tissues.

13.2.2.3 Cost

Antibody-based therapies are expensive, and the cost may be a barrier for some patients, as insurance may not always cover the full cost.

13.2.2.4 Resistance

Some cancers can become resistant to antibody-based therapies over time, making them less effective.

13.2.2.5 Long-Term Safety

The long-term safety of antibody-based therapies is not yet fully understood, as these treatments are relatively new. There is a need for more research to understand the long-term safety and potential risks associated with these therapies.

13.3 ANTIBODY STRUCTURE

There are five classes of immunoglobin family (IgA, IgD, IgE, IgM, and IgG), and IgG is the most effective antibody for cancer treatment [10]. IgG is comprised of two identical heavy chains (HC, 50000) and two identical light chains (LC, 25000) that are held together by four interchain disulfide bonds and arranged in a Y shape (Figure 13.1) [11]. The HC consists of one variable domain (VH), a discrete folded region containing 110 amino acids, three constant domains (CH1, CH2, and CH3), and a hinge linker. The LC consists of one variable domain (VL) and a constant domain (CL) with two subtypes, lambda, and kappa. The domains of VH, VL, CL, and CH1 form the fragment antigen binding (Fab) region, which recognizes and binds a specific antigen. The CH2 and CH3 form the fragment crystallizable (Fc) region that mediates the recruitment of immune cells through interaction with Fc gamma receptors (FcγR) [12]. The four subclasses of IgG (IgG1-4) are highly conserved and differ in their hinge region length, the number and location of interchain disulfide bonds, and the upper CH2 domains [13]. The Fc region of IgG subclasses leads to their functional difference in ADCC and CDC [12].

13.4 MONOCLONAL ANTIBODY-BASED CANCER THERAPIES

The rate of cancer is becoming increasingly popular among developing and developed countries [14]. Monoclonal antibodies are artificial proteins that have similar functions to actual antibodies. A potent tool for creating novel therapeutic mAbs for clinical use is antibody engineering. For instance, murine mAbs can be further modified to produce chimeric, humanized, complete human or bispecific antibodies following sequencing and cloning [15–18]. By combining the mouse antibody's complementary-determining region (CDR) with the human mAb framework sequence, the first humanized mAb (anti-IL2 daclizumab) was created and given US FDA approval in 1997 [19]. A chimeric mAb-drug conjugate (brentuximab) have the ability to target CD30 hodgkin lymphoma [20, 21], Trastuzumab (humanized mAb) is able to target HER2-positive breast cancer, and stomach cancer [22], inotuzumab ozogamicin (humanized, drug conjugate mAb) target CD22 acute lymphoblastic leukemia [23], humanized mAb (atezolizumab) target PD-L1 urothelial carcinoma, non-small cell lung cancer [24, 25], ado-trastuzumab Emtansine target HER2-positive breast cancer [26], necitumumab (Human mAb) target EGFR squamous non-small cell lung cancer [27]. mAbs have

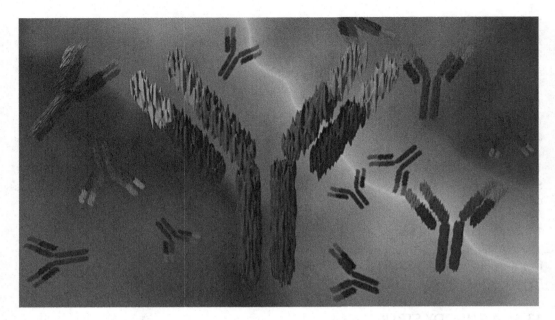

FIGURE 13.1 Structure of a typical antibody.

developed into a key biopharmaceutical for the delivery of targeted anti-cancer treatments in either monotherapy or conjugated therapy [28].

There have been established a number of platforms or technologies for the production of therapeutic antibodies, such as transgenic mice, phage display, and hybridoma technology. To get over murine antibodies' drawbacks, a variety of modified antibodies, including chimeric, humanized, and fully human antibodies, have been created and are frequently utilized in medical settings [28]. The development of further antibody-facilitated targeted therapeutics, including antibody-drug conjugates and antibody-tagged polymeric nanoparticles for drug delivery, has also been rapid [28].

13.4.1 mAbs For Fc-Mediated Effecter

Initially, the creation of mAbs as anticancer medications is mostly centered on Fab binding to antigens, but Fc can be utilized to activate numerous immunological pathways through interactions with Fc receptors [29]. In this manner, the Fc receptor on immune cells binds to Fc, stimulates and activates phagocytes, complement, and effecter cells, leading to the mechanisms of ADCC, ADCP, and CDC to destroy tumor cells. After the antibody attaches to the target antigen, Fc recruits immune cells with Fc receptors, such as T cells, NK cells, and macrophages. It subsequently causes the release of perforin and granzyme, or phagocytosis, to eliminate tumor cells. Also, after Fc and the C1q component engage, the complement system is activated to create the membrane assault complex and damage the membrane of the tumor cell [30].

13.4.2 Tumor Antigen-Targeting mAbs

The bulk of mAbs still utilized in cancer treatment are from the first generation of mAbs to be granted clinical use approval. These mAbs target tumor antigens only. Certain tumor antigens, to a greater or lesser extent, are essential for the development, survival, and invasiveness of the tumor. By interfering with tumor cell signaling pathways, anti-human epidermal growth factor receptor 2

(HER2) and anti-epidermal growth factor receptor (EGFR) antibodies are used to inhibit cell proliferation and induce tumor cell death [31, 32]. Tumor cell-bound antibodies can activate the FcRs on effecter cells such as natural killer (NK) cells, macrophages, or neutrophils, and these effecter cells can then cause tumor cell lysis [33].

Antibody-antigen binding may neutralize circulating targets or cell surface receptors depending on the epitope an antibody is directed towards. When an antibody binds to a receptor, it may block or even encourage receptor activation by ligands. An antibody that identifies a normal or unmodified antigen may no longer bind to the antigen after it has been modified, making the epitope for antibody binding extremely important. This is because some cancers may alter surface proteins by post-translational modification. A humanized IgG1 mAb called bevacizumab targets and prevents VEGF from attaching to its particular receptor on the vascular endothelium. Several tumors release VEGF to promote the growth of new blood vessels [34]. In comparison to chemotherapy alone, bevacizumab and chemotherapy were observed to improve objective responses, the median time to progression, and survival in patients with metastatic cancer. Edrecolomab (17-A mAb) is a murine immunoglobulin G2A (IgG2a) mAb that binds to the extracellular epitope of epithelial cell adhesion molecule (Ep-CAM), a glycoprotein typically present on the basolateral surface of non-squamous epithelium of the lung, gastrointestinal tract, pancreas, prostate, etc [35].

13.5 ANTIBODIES TARGETING TUMOR RECEPTORS

The term "checkpoint inhibitors" refers to a recently discovered class of mAbs used in cancer therapy. These antibodies target immunological checkpoint proteins including programmed cell death 1 (PD-1) or cytotoxic T lymphocyte antigen 4 (CTLA-4) or their ligands, such as programmed cell death ligand 1, to increase anti-tumor immune responses (PD-L1). Checkpoint proteins that regulate excessive T cell responses are expressed on activated T cells. The ligands of PD-1 are frequently produced by tumor cells as well as by myeloid cells invading the tumor microenvironment (TME) as a mechanism of immune resistance. Since checkpoint inhibition increases T cell activation, the clinical launch of checkpoint inhibitors resulted in significant advancement in the treatment of numerous cancer types [36–38].

13.5.1 CD33

A member of the sialic acid-binding Ig-like lectin family, CD33 is a glycoprotein receptor with two tyrosine-based motifs in its cytoplasmic tail. Through interacting with the tyrosine phosphatases SHP-1 and SHP-2, CD33 promotes the release of inflammatory cytokines [39, 40]. A cytotoxic calicheamicin antibiotic derivative and recombinant humanized IgG4 mAb called gemtuzumab ozogamicin targets CD33+ acute myeloid leukemia by binding to the minor groove of the tumor cells' DNA and causing site-specific double-strand breaks [41].

13.5.2 CD30

When activated by IL-4 during the lineage commitment of human naive T cells, CD45RO+ T cells produce CD30, a cytokine receptor that belongs to the tumor necrosis factor superfamily; the expression of CD30 is increased by CD28 co-stimulatory signals [42, 43]. The ability of CD30 to act as a signal transduction molecule quickly activates nuclear factor-B in T cells, raising intracellular $Ca2+$ levels, encouraging the growth of T helper 2 cells, and balancing the response of T helper 1 and 2 cells are its key functional properties [44]. For the treatment of non-Hodgkin and Hodgkin lymphomas, brentuximab vedotin, an antibody-drug conjugate that targets CD30, consists of a chimeric IgG1 mAb conjugated to the microtubule-disrupting substance MMAE [45].

13.5.3 IL-6

The Kaposi sarcoma herpes virus (HHV8)-associated and idiopathic subtypes of multicentric castleman disease (MCD) are lymph proliferative disorders. Germinal center atrophy and hypervascularization to germinal center hyperplasia and polytypic plasmacytosis are all examples of histology [46]. Both subtypes of MCD are associated with high levels of the cytokine IL-6, which contributes to the predominated inflammatory symptoms and causes anemia by inducing the expression of the antimicrobial peptide hepcidin, even if the exact cause of MCD is still unknown [47]. By control of regulatory T/T helper 17 cells, L-6 plays a critical role in regulating autoimmunity by activating the Janus kinase/signal transducer and activator of transcription and mitogen-activated protein kinase pathways. For the treatment of MCD, the chimeric mAb siltuximab inhibits the extracellular signal-regulated kinase 1/2, the phosphorylation of the signal transducer and activator of transcription 1 and 3, and the overexpression of heat shock protein 70 [48, 49]. Maculopapular cAEs, pigmentary change, psoriasis, and eczema are examples of dermatological toxicities brought on by the usage of siltuximab [50–53].

13.5.4 CD79B

As a crucial checkpoint during the transition of pro-B- and pre-B cells to B cells, CD79B, a B cell lineage-restricted subunit of the heterodimeric protein CD79, mediates communication between the B cell receptor complex and downstream signaling pathways. It also controls the expression of genes and cytoskeleton reordering [54, 55]. An anti-CD79B mAb conjugated to the antimitotic, cytotoxic drug MMAE was created for the treatment of non-Hodgkin lymphoma, and is known as polatuzumab vedotin [56]. Rare reports of Maculopapular cAEs and alopecia associated with the administration of polatuzumab vedotin comprise dermatologic effects [57].

13.5.5 CCR4

The non-Hodgkin lymphoma known as cutaneous T cell lymphoma (CTCL) is characterized by the unchecked growth of neoplastic T cells in the skin. Skin-homing molecules, such as CCR4 and cutaneous lymphocyte antigen, which are typically present on T helper 2 and regulatory T cells, are highly expressed in these cells. As a result, the CCR4-directed mAb mogamulizumab was created to treat advanced CTCL [58, 59]. Clinical features alone make it difficult to differentiate mogamulizumab-associated cAEs from CTCL/mycosis fungoides (MF), and they manifest histopathologically as psoriasiform, spongiotic, interface, or granulomatous dermatitis. These response patterns could also heavily overlap. Histopathologically, the CD4:CD8 ratio is typically reversed or leveled with dermatologic toxicities related to mogamulizumab, contrary to the predicted preponderance of CD4+ over CD8+ T cells in the majority of cases with CTCL/MF [60].

In the superficial dermis, psoriasiform reactions show parakeratosis, acanthosis, spongiosis, and lymphocytic infiltrates. Lichenoid reactions include phototoxic eruptions and display Civatte bodies, moderate/lymphohistiocytic infiltrates at the dermal-epidermal junction and hyperplastic orthokeratotic epidermis. A vacuolar variant of interface dermatitis with exocytosis of CD8+ (rather than CD4+) T cells and granzyme+ B cells occurred in one patient who received mogamulizumab treatment [61–63]. The presence of superficial and/or deep granulomatous infiltration with eosinophils and multinucleated giant cells, which can clinically resemble CTCL progression, distinguishes granulomatous reactions from CTCL progression [64]. However, there was a normal CD4:CD8 T cell ratio in the dermis and TCR polyclonality, which distinguished this dermatologic toxicity from CTCL [65, 66]. Another study found a cAE with MF-like features in patients treated with mogamulizumab, including exocytosis of lymphocytes into the epidermis and follicular epithelium as well as lamellar fibroplasia. However, results from the MAVORIC trial revealed that there may not be a single form of mogamulizumab-associated cA that is the most common [66].

13.5.6 Nectin-4

Nectin-4 is a transmembrane Ig-like cellular adhesion molecule that aids in the formation and maintenance of adheren junctions in skin tissues. In healthy skin, nectin-4 is expressed, and keratinocyte differentiation is associated with its expression [67]. On the surface of many different cancer cell types, including lung, breast, gastric, and urothelial cancer cells, it is a tumor-associated antigen that is abundantly expressed. Enfortumab vedotin is a nectin-4-targeting mAb that has been successfully used to treat metastatic Urothelial cancer [68]. It is conjugated to the cytotoxic microtubule-disrupting compound monomethyl auristatin E (MMAE). A number of dermatologic toxicities, such as alopecia and Maculopapular, interface, urticarial, and erythematous cAE, have been linked to the use of this mAb [69]. In other studies, patients who received enfortumab had keratinocyte dysmaturation, perivascular lymphocytic infiltrates with neutrophils and eosinophils, and vacuolar interface dermatitis or epidermal spongiosis [70, 71]. Enfortumab vedotin-related severe dermatologic toxicities vary from bullous dermatitis and erythema multiform-like cAE to deadly SJS/TEN [72, 73]. Immunofluorescence investigations indicate that the majority of vesiculobullous lesions associated with enfortumab therapy do not appear to be autoimmune reactions; nonetheless, a patient's adverse reaction that resembled pemphigoid was described during treatment [74, 75].

13.5.7 TROP2

As intracellular calcium concentrations rise and signaling pathways for cell migration, proliferation, apoptosis prevention, and epithelial-mesenchymal transition are modulated, TROP2—a transmembrane calcium signal transducer—increases intracellular calcium levels—is implicated. A mAb against TROP2 conjugated to SN-38, the active metabolite of the topoisomerase inhibitor irinotecan, is called sacituzumab govitecan. When SN-38 is internalized, it is released within the tumor cell and uses the "bystander effect" to help destroy nearby cancer cells [76]. Sacituzumab govitecan's clinical studies for metastatic Urothelial, lung, and triple-negative breast malignancies have demonstrated a comparatively low safety profile as a result of this selectivity. The most frequent dermatologic toxicity is alopecia, which is followed by a poorly understood Maculopapular cAE. These toxicities are most likely caused by a high expression of TROP2 in keratinocytes, inner root sheaths, and the infundibulum/isthmus of hair follicles [77, 78].

13.5.8 EGFR

Around 3% of all malignancies have EGFR mutations, making it a key target for cancer treatments. Together with Nibs, a number of mAbs (such as cetuximab, Necitumumab, and panitumumab) also target the EGFR. A novel bispecific antibody called amivantamab [EGFR + MET (mesenchymal-epithelial transition)] targets the tyrosine protein kinase MET and EGFR signaling pathways [79, 80]. Up to 80% of patients treated with mAbs targeting EGFR experience dermatological toxicities, including acneiform/papulopustular dermatitis. These toxicities result from altered EGFR signaling, which causes irregularities in growth and migration as well as the release of inflammatory cytokines and sensitization to UV rays. EGFR is extensively expressed in keratinocytes within the epidermis and at the hair follicle roots [81–84]. These lesions show as superficial or suppurative perifolliculitis with neutrophilic infiltrates, rupture of the epithelial lining, and follicular hyperkeratosis and are histopathologically similar to those seen with usage of mitogen-activated protein kinase kinase (MAPKK or MEK) inhibitors [85].

13.5.9 VEGF Receptors

VEGFR1, VEGFR2, and VEGFR3 are the three receptor tyrosine kinases that control the angiogenic activities of VEGF family members. Although they enhance a variety of downstream processes, these receptors are physically extremely similar. Each VEGF receptor has a split intra-cellular protein tyrosine kinase domain, a carboxyterminal tail, a single transmembrane domain segment, a juxtamembrane segment, and a seven-member immunoglobulin-like domain extracel-lular region [86].

13.5.9.1 VEGFR1

Fms-like tyrosyl kinase-1, commonly known as VEGFR1, binds VEGF, VEGF-B, and PlGF [87, 88]. The first six of the seven immunoglobulin domains are present in the soluble version of the receptor (sVEGFR1) that is created by alternative splicing of VEGFR1. This form of the receptor binds to and suppresses the activity of VEGF [89]. As a decoy receptor, VEGFR1 can sequester the ligand and stop it from signaling through other receptors by using its great affinity for VEGF (about 10 times stronger than that of VEGFR2 for VEGF) [90]. Making it challenging to assess the degree of VEGFR1 auto-phosphorylation in cells, that are not designed to produce the receptor at high levels. The VEGFR1 protein is crucial for development. Animals without VEGFR1 are embryonically fatal, and they lack a structured, organized vascular network [91]. It is interesting to note that VEGFR1-TK-/- mice, which retain the transmembrane segment and ligand-binding extra-cellular domains but lack the tyrosine kinase domain of VEGFR1, are alive, highlighting the sig-nificance of ligand sequestration in VEGFR1 function [92]. VEGFR2 small molecule inhibitors can reverse the mutant phenotype brought on by VEGFR1 loss in blood vessels produced from embry-onic stem cells. Although the exact mechanism of VEGFR1 signaling is still unknown, evidence suggests that the receptor is involved in hematopoiesis, monocyte migration, and the attraction of bone marrow-derived progenitor cells [93, 94]. Furthermore, matrix metalloproteinase-9, uPA, and plasminogen activator inhibitor-1, molecules crucial for ECM breakdown that might enhance VEGF release and cell motility, have been linked to VEGFR1 through VEGF-B-mediated EC expression. Moreover, it has been demonstrated that VEGF binding to VEGFR1 causes SHP-1 phosphatase activity, which in turn lowers VEGFR2 phosphorylation levels. These findings suggest that VEGFR1 controls VEGFR2 activity adversely, which may have significant implications for inhibiting the VEGF pathway in malignancies [95].

13.5.9.2 VEGFR2

VEGFR2 [kinase domain-containing receptor (KDR)/fetal liver kinase-1 (Flk-1)] is primarily responsible for VEGF-induced angiogenic signaling [96]. EC survival, migration, proliferation, and vascular permeability are among the tasks performed by VEGFR2 [97]. Both VEGF-C and VEGF-D are bound by VEGFR2. VEGR2 has a greater kinase activity than VEGFR1, although having a lower affinity for VEGF. VEGF causes receptor dimerization and trans-auto-phosphorylation when it binds to VEGFR2. Recent research has shown that macrophage infiltration in tumor-bearing animals is mediated by the expression of VEGFR2 by macrophages [98]. VEGFR2 Between days E8.5 and E9.5, null mice are embryonic fatal. These animals lack structured blood vessels at any phase in the developing embryo or yolk sac, and they show severe abnormalities in the development of endothelial and hematopoietic cells.

13.5.9.3 VEGFR-3

With sustained functions in adult angiogenesis and lymphangiogenesis, VEGFR-3 (Flt-4) binds both VEGF-C and VEGF-D and contributes to the remodeling of the primary capillary plexus throughout embryonic development [99]. VEGFR3 null mice exhibit cardiovascular failure and are embryonic lethal at day E9.5 as a result of abnormal large vessel structure and organization that causes defective vessel lumens and an accumulation of fluid in the pericardial cavity [100]. As a result of inactivating mutations in the catalytic loop of the VEGFR3 kinase domain, Milroy disease—a hereditary form of lymphedema—occurs in humans. It is characterized by chronic swelling of the extremities due to malfunctioning lymphatic veins [101]. The phenotype of VEGFR3 null mice and the lymphatic abnormalities of Milroy disease suggest that VEGFR3 functions initially in the development of the cardiovascular system and subsequently in the adult lymphatic vasculature.

13.5.9.3.1 Antibodies Targeting the VEGF Receptors

MF1/IMC-18F1: In an autoimmune arthritis paradigm, the rat anti-mouse VEGFR1 IgG1 mAb, MF1, was initially demonstrated to inhibit tumor and ischemia retinal angiogenesis as well as inflammation. When Kaplan et al. suppressed VEGFR1 with MF1, they were able to show that VEGFR1 participates in the premetastatic niche in animal models more efficiently than when they inhibited VEGFR2 [102]. A fully human mAb against human VEGFR1 was created as a result of these studies (mAb 6.12, IMC-18F1, ImClone Systems), which inhibited tumor growth in vivo and blocked VEGFR1 signaling in breast cancer cell lines that expressed VEGFR1.

DC101/IMC-1C11: DC101 is a monoclonal antibody that targets the vascular endothelial growth factor receptor 2 (VEGFR2), a protein that is expressed on the surface of cells that line blood vessels. VEGF is a signaling protein that promotes the growth of blood vessels, a process known as angiogenesis. In cancer, angiogenesis is essential for tumor growth and spread, and targeting VEGF signaling has emerged as an effective strategy for cancer treatment.

DC101 works by binding to VEGFR2 on the surface of cells, thereby preventing the binding of VEGF and inhibiting angiogenesis. By blocking the growth of blood vessels, DC101 can prevent the delivery of nutrients and oxygen to the tumor, ultimately leading to tumor cell death.

DC101 has been studied extensively in preclinical models and has shown promising results in several clinical trials. In a phase II trial in patients with metastatic renal cell carcinoma, DC101 in combination with interferon-alpha resulted in a significant improvement in progression-free survival compared to interferon-alpha alone. Similarly, in a phase II trial in patients with metastatic colorectal cancer, DC101 in combination with chemotherapy improved progression-free survival compared to chemotherapy alone.

Overall, DC101 is an exciting new treatment option for cancer that targets the VEGF signaling pathway, an important driver of angiogenesis and tumor growth. Ongoing clinical trials are exploring the use of DC101 in combination with other therapies, and it will be interesting to see how this drug is integrated into the treatment landscape for various types of cancer.

IMC-1121B: IMC-1121B is a monoclonal antibody that targets the VEGF (vascular endothelial growth factor) receptor. VEGF is a protein that plays a key role in the formation of new blood vessels (angiogenesis). It is involved in the growth and spread of tumors, as well as in the development of certain ocular conditions, such as macular degeneration.

IMC-1121B works by binding to the VEGF receptor, which prevents the receptor from interacting with VEGF and thus inhibits the downstream signaling that leads to angiogenesis. This can potentially slow or halt the growth and spread of tumors, as well as reduce the risk of vision loss in patients with certain ocular conditions.

Clinical studies have shown that IMC-1121B has promising results in the treatment of various cancers, including lung, breast, and colorectal cancers. It has also shown potential in the treatment of ocular conditions, such as neovascular age-related macular degeneration.

However, like any medication, IMC-1121B can have side effects. Some of the most common side effects include hypertension, fatigue, and gastrointestinal disturbances. Rarely, more serious side effects, such as bleeding or blood clotting disorders may occur.

13.5.10 FcΓRs IN ANTIBODY-BASED CANCER THERAPY

Early preclinical studies confirmed the significance of Fc: FcγR interactions in direct tumor targeting. Rituximab and trastuzumab's full in vivo activity was shown by Clynes et al. to need activating Fc: FcγR engagement [103]. Compared to wild-type mice, mice lacking the c signaling chain were unable to stop tumor growth in vivo. Additionally, these antibodies' tumor-killing effectiveness was decreased in modified Fc versions that could not activate FcγRs. These findings suggested that, given the different anticancer activity attributed to these mAbs. As a result of this observation, it was hypothesized that the ideal anti-cancer mAb would preferentially bind activating FcγR rather than inhibitory FcγR. The potential of TAA-specific mAbs to prevent tumor development and metastasis in vivo was later demonstrated to be substantially more powerful. These mAbs have murine FCS that selectively binds activating FcγRs as opposed to inhibitory FcγRs. This suggested that the variation in activity was caused by isotypes that activate FccR with a high activating to inhibitory ratio (A/I) [104, 105].

13.5.10.1 FcγR Genetic Polymorphism

In addition to inhibiting growth factor/receptor interactions and/or down-regulating oncogenic proteins (such as growth factor receptors) on the surface of tumor cells, mAbs also have the ability to activate immune system effecters mechanisms like antibody-dependent cellular cytotoxicity (ADCC) and complement-mediated cytotoxicity (CMC). IgG antibodies operate as a mediator of such immune responses by activating the cellular immune system and interacting with the Fc domain of immune cells' Fc gamma receptors (FcγRs). The most important receptors for controlling antibody-directed cytotoxicity are activating receptors FcγRIIa and FcγRIIIa and inactivating receptor FcγRIIb [106]. There are several methods that have been established to change the affinity of human antibodies to different FcγRs. They can be divided into two categories: methods that alter the Fc amino acid sequence and methods that alter the state of glycosylation. It has been successful to produce antibodies with altered binding to particular FcγRs by modifying the amino acid sequence of the Fc section of antibodies using information obtained from screening libraries of Fc variants and/or through computational design based on structural understanding. A number of these antibodies have been tested in vivo, and it has been shown that they have the anticipated effects on ADCC [107, 108]. It has been shown that glycosylation, including fucosylation, sialylation, and mannose structures, affects Fc binding to FcRs and ADCC. Fucose content seems to be a significant contributor to ADCC in vitro. Fucose removal has been shown to significantly boost FcγRIIIa affinity and enhance ADCC. More than 90% of the recombinant immunoglobulin G's (rIgGs) produced in normal chinese hamster ovary (CHO) cells are fucosylated; consequently, a number of methods have been developed to lessen fucosylation of rIgGs, including the development of CHO cell lines that lack or express 1, 6-fucosyltransferase less than normal or in which the enzyme can be overexpressed inducibly. Clinical trials are now being conducted on a number of rIgGs that have been designed to contain little or no fucose [109, 110].

13.5.11 HGF–cMET

Hepatocyte growth factor (HGF), the only known ligand of the receptor tyrosine kinase cMET, is essential for cellular proliferation, survival, invasion, tissue development, and organ regeneration [111]. A single-chain precursor of cMET is created, and through post-translational modification, it is changed into a structure connected by disulfide bonds. A 140-kDa transmembrane chain and a 50-kDa extracellular chain make up mature cMET [112]. Pro-HGF, an inactive precursor of HGF that is secreted, is cleaved by serine proteases to become active HGF. Hence, the N-terminal domain, cringle domains (K1–K4) in the -chain, and a serine protease-like domain in the -chain make up the active ligand structure of HGF [113]. High-affinity binding to cMET is mediated by the N-terminal domain and the K1, which also appears to cause the creation of a secondary binding site within the HGF -chain. HGF then binds to cMET to create a potent complex that can activate signal transduction. Active HGF binds to cMET, causing the receptor to multimerize and internalize, phosphorylate tyrosine residues in the intracellular kinase domain repeatedly, and activate a variety of signaling pathways involved in the invasion, growth, and metastasis of cancer [114].

Although HGF-induced cMET activation is tightly controlled, dysregulated HGF-cMET signaling is seen in a variety of malignant neoplasm's [115]. By HGF-independent mechanisms such MET mutations, gene amplification, and transcriptional upregulation, abnormal cMET activation can take place [116].

13.5.11.1 HGF/c-Met Signaling Pathway

To regulate many biological processes such as embryonic development, epithelial branching morphogenesis, postnatal organ regeneration, and wound healing, the HGF/c-Met signaling pathway has an impact on a range of cellular activities [117, 118]. HGF is a paracrine signaling substance that mesenchymal cells make and secrete to influence nearby epithelial cells that express c-Met. HGF has been shown to play protective functions in endothelial damage, tissue fibrosis, liver cirrhosis, and lung fibrosis [119, 120]. Inactive single-chain precursors of HGF are synthesized, and after processing, they are converted into active heterodimers of one alpha and one beta chain connected by a disulfide bond [121]. A mature receptor made of a transmembrane beta subunit that is disulfide-bonded to a glycosylated, extracellular alpha subunit is formed from c-Met as well as a single-chain precursor [122]. A Sema domain (homologous to semaphorins), a cysteine-rich Met-related-sequence domain, and four immunoglobulin (Ig)-like modules (IgG domains), that bind HGF make up the extracellular component of c-Met. A juxtamembrane domain, a tyrosine kinase domain, and a C-terminal regulatory tail that is in charge of signal transduction make up the intracellular component of c-Met [123].

13.5.11.2 Antibody-Based Therapeutics Targeting HGF and c-Met

There are two categories of HGF/c-Met signaling pathway inhibitors: Although biologics, such as c-Met, disrupt the signaling pathway by reducing c-Met autophosphorylation and tyrosine kinase activity in small-molecule drugs. By preventing interactions between HGF and c-Met, shortened HGF, the N-terminal Sema domain of HGF, the soluble extracellular domain of c-Met (decoy Met), and antibodies against both HGF and c-Met disrupt the signaling pathway. Biologics more precisely inhibit the HGF/c-Met signaling pathway than do small-molecule drugs, which frequently target numerous RTKs. Many anti-tumor therapeutic antibodies that target the HGF/c-Met signaling pathway are presently being developed in preclinical and clinical settings [124].

13.6 ANTIBODY-DRUG CONJUGATES FOR CANCER THERAPY

ADCs are the most popular format for antibody-based cancer immunotherapeutic medicines, aside from monoclonal antibodies [125]. Ten ADCs have received FDA approval to date. Moreover, more than 80 ADCs are being developed in clinical settings as single-agent or multiple-agent therapies for the treatment of various cancer types [126]. ADCs are intricate molecules that use a chemical linker to attach a strong cytotoxic drug to particular locations on an antibody. The cytotoxic substance is also known as the "payload," which consists of toll-like receptor agonists, DNA alkylating agents, RNA polymerase II, and anti-mitotic tubulin disruptors [127]. ADCs rely on antibodie's ability to target tumor cells specifically in order to internalize the ADC, release the payload, and then cause cytotoxicity. Despite the fact that the majority of FDA-approved ADCs are used to treat hematological malignancies, more ADCs are being developed to treat solid tumors. For instance, well-defined ADCs for breast cancer such as trastuzumab emtansine (T-DM1) and sacituzumab govitecan can dramatically increase progression-free and overall survival in patients with metastatic triple-negative breast cancer [128]. As ADCs might cause greater cytotoxicity than mAbs, this side effect continues to be the main obstacle for ADCs. Target selection, linker chemistry, innovative payload development, conjugation process improvement, and improving internalization are some of the engineering prospects for ADCs in the future. Proteolysis-targeting chimaera (PROTAC), also known as degrader-antibody conjugates, has recently been used as a payload for ADC (DAC) [129].

13.7 BSABS AND CAR-BASED THERAPIES

BsAbs directly detect two separate antigens on tumor or immune cells. In contrast to monospecific antibodies, BsAbs are artificially created to function as a synergistic mechanism or to increase the therapy index. BsAbs have been widely researched for usage in cancer, hemophilia, and auto-immune illnesses, among others. They are typically made with one antigen-binding site against the CD3 receptor on cytotoxic T lymphocytes and the other against the receptor on the surface of tumour cells for the purpose of treating tumours. BsAbs attract T lymphocytes to tumors, where they are eventually induced to release granzymes and perforin to kill cancer cells. Although more and more BsAbs and multi-specific antibodies are being developed and entered into clinical trials, only blinatumomab is commercially accessible. The first BsAb approved for cancer treatment was catumaxomab, which activates endogenous T cells by connecting CD3 with epithelial cell adhesion molecule (EpCAM) on cancer cells, indicating for malignant ascites therapy. Catumaxomab was only used for intraperitoneal injection because intravenous administration may cause severe toxicity at low doses, related to Fc-mediated off-target T cell activation in the liver [8]. However, catumaxomab was withdrawn from the market in 2017 for commercial reasons. A CD19- and CD3-targeting antibody fragment without an Fc region, blincyto® (blinatumomab) differs from catumaxomab and is currently indicated primarily for the treatment of adults and children with B cell ALL. As a result, blinatumomab has a brief half-life and requires long-term intravenous administration to maintain stable plasma concentrations. Long-term follow-up survival data showed that the overall survival (OS) of 8–10 years after treatment was more than 50%, but the neurological adverse events and CRS are common adverse reactions.

13.8 DEVELOPMENT OF ANTIBODY-BASED C-MET INHIBITORS

Cellular activities such as development, differentiation, migration, and death depend heavily on communication between individual cells and between cells and their environments in living things. Receptor tyrosine kinase (RTK) interactions with their ligands initiate signaling pathways that in turn regulate these physiological functions [130]. These cellular functions are mostly controlled by signaling pathways that are activated by interactions between receptor tyrosine kinases (RTKs) and their ligands.

RTKs on the cell surface trigger downstream signaling cascades and control target gene expression in a paracrine or autocrine manner upon ligand interaction. The growth and spread of malignancies as well as the regulation of several cellular functions depend on these signaling pathways, which are mediated by RTKs and their ligands. RTK-mediated signaling pathways are closely controlled in accordance with the physiological state of normal cells. In contrast, gain-of-function mutations, gene rearrangements, gene amplifications, excessive expression, or aberrant stimulation of receptors/ligands cause RTK signaling pathways to be dysregulated or hyper activated in a variety of malignancies [131, 132]. To create anti-cancer therapeutic drugs that inhibit the signaling pathways by preventing interactions between RTKs and their ligands, dimerizing and phosphorylating RTKs, and activating downstream components, specific RTK-mediated signaling cascades can be targeted at various levels. RTK-mediated signaling pathways are primarily suppressed for monoclonal antibody-based therapies by preventing interactions between RTKs and their ligands. Antibody inhibitors have higher target selectivity for certain RTKs and/or ligands in comparison to small-molecule drugs that block the kinase activity and autophosphorylation of a variety of RTKs.

13.9 CONCLUSION

All the various strategies discussed in this chapter have produced lead candidates that exhibit promising clinical activity, mostly in trials with patients who have been heavily pretreated and are refractory, demonstrating the clear maturation of antibody-based therapy. The continued progress in design, engineering and insights in the tumor-immune interaction will aid further optimization of antibody-based approaches. One of the important challenges in the upcoming years is to incorporate the advances in antibody engineering into optimal combinations with standard-of-care treatment such as chemo- and/or radiotherapy, to achieve curative treatment.

REFERENCES

1. Rettig, W.J. and L.J. Old, *Immunogenetics of human cell surface differentiation. Annual Review of Immunology*, 1989. **7**(1): pp. 481–511.
2. Van den Eynde, B. and A. Scott, *Encyclopedia of Immunology (eds Roitt, DPJ & Roitt, IM) 2424–2431*. 1998, Academic Press, London.
3. Finke, J., et al., *Standard graft-versus-host disease prophylaxis with or without anti-T-cell globulin in haematopoietic cell transplantation from matched unrelated donors: a randomised, open-label, multicentre phase 3 trial. The Lancet Oncology*, 2009. **10**(9): pp. 855–864.
4. Vaickus, L. and K.A. Foon, *Biotechnology update: overview of monoclonal antibodies in the diagnosis and therapy of cancer. Cancer Investigation*, 1991. **9**(2): pp. 195–209.
5. LoBuglio, A.F., et al., *Mouse/human chimeric monoclonal antibody in man: kinetics and immune response. Proceedings of the National Academy of Sciences*, 1989. **86**(11): pp. 4220–4224.
6. Maloney, D.G., et al., *IDEC-C2B8 (Rituximab) anti-CD20 monoclonal antibody therapy in patients with relapsed low-grade non-Hodgkin's lymphoma. Blood, The Journal of the American Society of Hematology*, 1997. **90**(6): pp. 2188–2195.
7. Cunningham, D., et al., *Cetuximab monotherapy and cetuximab plus irinotecan in irinotecan-refractory metastatic colorectal cancer. New England Journal of Medicine*, 2004. **351**(4): pp. 337–345.
8. Reff, M.E., et al., *Depletion of B cells in vivo by a chimeric mouse human monoclonal antibody to CD20. Blood*, 1994. **83**(2): pp. 435–445.
9. Reichert, J.M. *Antibodies to watch in 2015. MAbs*. 2015. **7**(1): pp. 1–8.
10. Wang, W., et al., *Antibody structure, instability, and formulation. Journal of Pharmaceutical Sciences*, 2007. **96**(1): pp. 1–26.
11. Liu, H. and K. May. *Disulfide bond structures of IgG molecules: structural variations, chemical modifications and possible impacts to stability and biological function. MAbs*, 2012. **4**(1): pp. 17–23.
12. Indik, Z.K., et al., *The molecular dissection of Fc gamma receptor mediated phagocytosis. Blood*, 1995. **86**(12): pp. 4389–4399.
13. Vidarsson, G., G. Dekkers, and T. Rispens, *IgG subclasses and allotypes: from structure to effector functions. Frontiers in Immunology*, 2014. **5**: p. 520.
14. Jemal, A., et al., *Global cancer statistics. CA: A Cancer Journal for Clinicians*, 2011. **61**(2): pp. 69–90.
15. Gilliland, G.L., *Engineering antibody therapeutics Mark L Chiu and Gary L Gilliland. Current Opinion in Structural Biology*, 2016. **38**: pp. 163–173.
16. Chiu, M.L. and G.L. Gilliland, *Engineering antibody therapeutics. Current Opinion in Structural Biology*, 2016. **38**: pp. 163–173.
17. Sievers, S.A., et al., *Antibody engineering for increased potency, breadth and half-life. Current Opinion in HIV and AIDS*, 2015. **10**(3): pp. 151.
18. Liu, Z., et al., *A novel antibody engineering strategy for making monovalent bispecific heterodimeric IgG antibodies by electrostatic steering mechanism. Journal of Biological Chemistry*, 2015. **290**(12): pp. 7535–7562.
19. Tsurushita, N., P.R. Hinton, and S. Kumar, *Design of humanized antibodies: from anti-Tac to Zenapax. Methods*, 2005. **36**(1): pp. 69–83.
20. Hoberg, E., et al., *Monoclonal antibodies specific for human cardiac myosin: selection, characterization and experimental myocardial infarct imaging. European Heart Journal*, 1988. **9**(3): pp. 328–336.
21. Zaroff, S. and G. Tan, *Hybridoma technology: the preferred method for monoclonal antibody generation for in vivo applications. Biotechniques*, 2019. **67**(3): pp. 90–92.
22. Stergiou, N., et al., *Evaluation of a novel monoclonal antibody against tumor-associated MUC1 for diagnosis and prognosis of breast cancer. International Journal of Medical Sciences*, 2019. **16**(9): p. 1188.

23. Waldmann, H., *Human monoclonal antibodies: the benefits of humanization. Human Monoclonal Antibodies: Methods and Protocols*, 2019: pp. 1–10.

24. Rogers, L.M., S. Veeramani, and G.J. Weiner, *Complement in monoclonal antibody therapy of cancer. Immunologic Research*, 2014. **59**: pp. 203–210.

25. Winkler, M.T., et al., *Enhanced CDC of B cell chronic lymphocytic leukemia cells mediated by rituximab combined with a novel anti-complement factor H antibody. Plos One*, 2017. **12**(6): p. e0179841.

26. Thakur, A., M. Huang, and L.G. Lum, *Bispecific antibody based therapeutics: strengths and challenges. Blood Reviews*, 2018. **32**(4): pp. 339–347.

27. Alfaleh, M.A., et al., *Phage display derived monoclonal antibodies: from bench to bedside. Frontiers in Immunology*, 2020. **11**: p. 1986.

28. Si, Y., et al., *Monoclonal antibody-based cancer therapies. Chinese Journal of Chemical Engineering*, 2021. **30**: pp. 301–307.

29. Li, W., et al., *Antibody and cellular-based therapies for pediatric acute lymphoblastic leukemia: mechanisms and prospects. Pharmacology*, 2022. **107**(7–8): pp. 368–375.

30. Chen, W., Y. Yuan, and X. Jiang, *Antibody and antibody fragments for cancer immunotherapy. Journal of Controlled Release*, 2020. **328**: pp. 395–406.

31. Hudis, C.A., *Trastuzumab—mechanism of action and use in clinical practice. New England Journal of Medicine*, 2007. **357**(1): pp. 39–51.

32. Weiner, G.J., *Monoclonal antibody mechanisms of action in cancer. Immunologic Research*, 2007. **39**: pp. 271–278.

33. Chenoweth, A.M., et al., *Harnessing the immune system via FcγR function in immune therapy: a pathway to next-gen mAbs. Immunology and Cell Biology*, 2020. **98**(4): pp. 287–304.

34. Kanai, T., et al., *Anti-tumor and anti-metastatic effects of human-vascular-endothelial-growth-factor-neutralizing antibody on human colon and gastric carcinoma xenotransplanted orthotopically into nude mice. International Journal of Cancer*, 1998. **77**(6): pp. 933–936.

35. Riethmüller, G., et al., *Monoclonal antibody therapy for resected Dukes' C colorectal cancer: seven-year outcome of a multicenter randomized trial. Journal of Clinical Oncology*, 1998. **16**(5): pp. 1788–1794.

36. Pohl, R., et al., *Muonic hydrogen and the proton radius puzzle. Annual Review of Nuclear and Particle Science*, 2013. **63**: pp. 175–204.

37. Sow, H.S., et al., *FcγR interaction is not required for effective anti-PD-L1 immunotherapy but can add additional benefit depending on the tumor model. International Journal of Cancer*, 2019. **144**(2): pp. 345–354.

38. Walunas, T.L., et al., *CTLA-4 can function as a negative regulator of T cell activation. Immunity*, 1994. **1**(5): pp. 405–413.

39. Paul, S.P., et al., *Myeloid specific human CD33 is an inhibitory receptor with differential ITIM function in recruiting the phosphatases SHP-1 and SHP-2. Blood, The Journal of the American Society of Hematology*, 2000. **96**(2): pp. 483–490.

40. Gonzalez, Y., et al., *High glucose concentrations induce TNF-α production through the down-regulation of CD33 in primary human monocytes. BMC Immunology*, 2012. **13**: pp. 1–14.

41. Fenton, C. and C.M. Perry, *Gemtuzumab ozogamicin: a review of its use in acute myeloid leukaemia. Drugs*, 2005. **65**: pp. 2405–2427.

42. Dürkop, H., et al., *Expression of the CD30 antigen in non-lymphoid tissues and cells. The Journal of Pathology: A Journal of the Pathological Society of Great Britain and Ireland*, 2000. **190**(5): pp. 613–618.

43. Kadin, M.E., *Regulation of CD30 antigen expression and its potential significance for human disease. The American Journal of Pathology*, 2000. **156**(5): pp. 1479–1484.

44. Pellegrini, P., et al., *CD30 antigen: not a physiological marker for TH2 cells but an important costimulator molecule in the regulation of the balance between TH1/TH2 response. Transplant Immunology*, 2003. **12**(1): pp. 49–61.

45. Younes, A., U. Yasothan, and P. Kirkpatrick, *Brentuximab vedotin. Nature Reviews. Drug Discovery*, 2012. **11**(1): p. 19.

46. Fajgenbaum, D.C., F. van Rhee, and C.S. Nabel, *HHV-8-negative, idiopathic multicentric Castleman disease: novel insights into biology, pathogenesis, and therapy. Blood, The Journal of the American Society of Hematology*, 2014. **123**(19): pp. 2924–2933.

47. Song, S.-N.J., et al., *Down-regulation of hepcidin resulting from long-term treatment with an anti–IL-6 receptor antibody (tocilizumab) improves anemia of inflammation in multicentric Castleman disease.* Blood, The Journal of the American Society of Hematology, 2010. **116**(18): pp. 3627–3634.

48. Chen, R. and B. Chen, *Siltuximab (CNTO 328): A promising option for human malignancies.* Drug Design, Development and Therapy, 2015. **9**: p. 3455.

49. Rose-John, S., *IL-6 trans-signaling via the soluble IL-6 receptor: importance for the pro-inflammatory activities of IL-6.* International Journal of Biological Sciences, 2012. **8**(9): pp. 1237–1247.

50. Davis, C.C., K.S. Shah, and M.J. Lechowicz, *Clinical development of siltuximab.* Current Oncology Reports, 2015. **17**: pp. 1–9.

51. Van Rhee, F., et al., *A phase 2, open-label, multicenter study of the long-term safety of siltuximab (an anti-interleukin-6 monoclonal antibody) in patients with multicentric Castleman disease.* Oncotarget, 2015. **6**(30): p. 30408.

52. Van Rhee, F., et al., *Siltuximab for multicentric Castleman's disease: a randomised, double-blind, placebo-controlled trial.* The Lancet Oncology, 2014. **15**(9): pp. 966–974.

53. Keating, M., et al., *Management guidelines for use of alemtuzumab in B-cell chronic lymphocytic leukemia.* Clinical Lymphoma, 2004. **4**(4): pp. 220–227.

54. Visco, C., et al., *Oncogenic mutations of MYD88 and CD79B in diffuse large B-cell lymphoma and implications for clinical practice.* Cancers, 2020. **12**(10): p. 2913.

55. Kouro, T., et al., *Bruton's tyrosine kinase is required for signaling the CD79b-mediated pro-B to pre-B cell transition.* International Immunology, 2001. **13**(4): pp. 485–493.

56. Choi, Y. and C.S. Diefenbach, *Polatuzumab Vedotin: a new target for B cell malignancies.* Current Hematologic Malignancy Reports, 2020. **15**: pp. 125–129.

57. Palanca-Wessels, M.C.A., et al., *Safety and activity of the anti-CD79B antibody–drug conjugate polatuzumab vedotin in relapsed or refractory B-cell non-Hodgkin lymphoma and chronic lymphocytic leukaemia: a phase 1 study.* The Lancet Oncology, 2015. **16**(6): pp. 704–715.

58. Duvic, M. and F.M. Foss. *Mycosis fungoides: pathophysiology and emerging therapies.* In Seminars in Oncology. 2007. Amsterdam: Elsevier.

59. Watson, S. and J.B. Marx, *Mogamulizumab-kpkc: a novel therapy for the treatment of cutaneous T-cell lymphoma.* Journal of the Advanced Practitioner in Oncology, 2019. **10**(8): p. 883.

60. Wang, J.Y., et al., *Histopathologic characterization of mogamulizumab-associated rash.* The American Journal of Surgical Pathology, 2020. **44**(12): pp. 1666–1676.

61. Ito, A., et al., *CD8+ T-cell-mediated interface dermatitis after CCR4+ T-cell depletion by mogamulizumab treatment of adult T-cell leukaemia/lymphoma.* Acta Dermato-Venereologica, 2017. **97**(3): pp. 377–378.

62. Trum, N.A., et al., *Dupilumab as a therapy option for treatment refractory mogamulizumab-associated rash.* JAAD Case Reports, 2021. **14**: pp. 37–42.

63. Lehner, G.M., et al., *Psoriasis vulgaris triggered by treatment with mogamulizumab in a patient with cutaneous T-cell lymphoma.* JDDG: Journal der Deutschen Dermatologischen Gesellschaft, 2021. **19**(9): pp. 1355–1358.

64. Chen, L., et al., *Mogamulizumab-associated cutaneous granulomatous drug eruption mimicking mycosis fungoides but possibly indicating durable clinical response.* JAMA Dermatology, 2019. **155**(8): pp. 968–971.

65. Hirotsu, K.E., et al., *Clinical characterization of mogamulizumab-associated rash during treatment of mycosis fungoides or Sézary syndrome.* JAMA Dermatology, 2021. **157**(6): pp. 700–707.

66. Musiek, A.C., et al., *Characterization and outcomes in patients with mogamulizumab-associated skin reactions in the MAVORIC trial.* Blood, 2020. **136**: pp. 23–24.

67. Heath, E.I. and J.E. Rosenberg, *The biology and rationale of targeting nectin-4 in urothelial carcinoma.* Nature Reviews Urology, 2021. **18**(2): pp. 93–103.

68. Mollo, M.R., et al., *p63-dependent and independent mechanisms of nectin-1 and nectin-4 regulation in the epidermis.* Experimental Dermatology, 2015. **24**(2): pp. 114–119.

69. Takahashi, S., et al., *A phase I study of enfortumab vedotin in Japanese patients with locally advanced or metastatic urothelial carcinoma.* Investigational New Drugs, 2020. **38**: pp. 1056–1066.

70. Ungaro, A., et al., *Antibody-drug conjugates in urothelial carcinoma: a new therapeutic opportunity moves from bench to bedside.* Cells, 2022. **11**(5): p. 803.

71. Dobry, A.S., et al., *Cutaneous reactions with enfortumab vedotin: A case series and review of the literature. JAAD Case Reports*, 2021. **14**: pp. 7–9.

72. Nguyen, M.N., M. Reyes, and S.C. Jones, *Postmarketing Cases of Enfortumab Vedotin-Associated Skin Reactions Reported as Stevens-Johnson Syndrome or Toxic Epidermal Necrolysis. JAMA Dermatology*, 2021. **157**(10): pp. 1237–1239.

73. Yu, A.L., et al., *Anti-GD2 antibody with GM-CSF, interleukin-2, and isotretinoin for neuroblastoma. New England Journal of Medicine*, 2010. **363**(14): pp. 1324–1334.

74. Powles, T., et al., *Enfortumab vedotin in previously treated advanced urothelial carcinoma. New England Journal of Medicine*, 2021. **384**(12): pp. 1125–1135.

75. Rosenberg, J., et al., *EV-101: a phase i study of single-agent enfortumab vedotin in patients with nectin-4-positive solid tumors, including metastatic urothelial carcinoma. Journal of Clinical Oncology*, 2020. **38**(10): pp. 1041–1049.

76. Goldenberg, D.M., R. Stein, and R.M. Sharkey, *The emergence of trophoblast cell-surface antigen 2 (TROP-2) as a novel cancer target. Oncotarget*, 2018. **9**(48): pp. 28989–29006.

77. Bardia, A., et al., *Sacituzumab govitecan, a Trop-2-directed antibody-drug conjugate, for patients with epithelial cancer: final safety and efficacy results from the phase I/II IMMU-132-01 basket trial. Annuals of Oncology*, 2021. **32**(6): pp. 746–756.

78. Ito, T., K. Tanegashima, and Y. Tanaka, *Trop2 expression in extramammary Paget's disease and normal skin. International Journal of Molecular Sciences* 2021. **22**(14). p. 7706.

79. Salamone, J.M., et al., *Promoting scientist–advocate collaborations in cancer research: why and how. Cancer research*, 2018. **78**(20): pp. 5723–5728.

80. Friedlaender, A. and V. Subbiah, *EGFR and HER2 exon 20 insertions in solid tumours: From biology to treatment. Nature Reviews Clinical Oncology*, 2022. **19**(1): pp. 51–69.

81. Curry, J.L., et al., *Dermatologic toxicities to targeted cancer therapy: shared clinical and histologic adverse skin reactions. International Journal of Dermatology*, 2014. **53**(3): pp. 376–384.

82. Li, J. and H. Yan, *Skin toxicity with anti-EGFR monoclonal antibody in cancer patients: a meta-analysis of 65 randomized controlled trials. Cancer Chemotherapy Pharmacology*, 2018. **82**(4): pp. 571–583.

83. Seervai, R.N., et al., *The diverse landscape of dermatologic toxicities of non-immune checkpoint inhibitor monoclonal antibody-based cancer therapy. Journal of Cutaneous Pathology*, 2023. **50**(1): pp. 72–95.

84. Paz-Ares, L., et al., *Necitumumab plus pemetrexed and cisplatin as first-line therapy in patients with stage IV non-squamous non-small-cell lung cancer (INSPIRE): an open-label, randomised, controlled phase 3 study. The Lancet Oncology*, 2015. **16**(3): pp. 328–337.

85. Brodell, L.A., et al., *Histopathology of acneiform eruptions in patients treated with epidermal growth factor receptor inhibitors. Journal of Cutaneous Pathology*, 2013. **40**(10): pp. 865–870.

86. Roskoski Jr, R., *Vascular endothelial growth factor (VEGF) signaling in tumor progression. Critical Reviews in Oncology/Hematology*, 2007. **62**(3): pp. 179–213.

87. De Vries, C., et al., *The fms-like tyrosine kinase, a receptor for vascular endothelial growth factor. Science*, 1992. **255**(5047): pp. 989–991.

88. Park, J.E., et al., *Placenta growth factor. Potentiation of vascular endothelial growth factor bioactivity, in vitro and in vivo, and high affinity binding to Flt-1 but not to Flk-1/KDR. Journal of Biological Chemistry*, 1994. **269**(41): pp. 25646–25654.

89. Kendall, R.L. and K.A. Thomas, *Inhibition of vascular endothelial cell growth factor activity by an endogenously encoded soluble receptor. Proceedings of the National Academy of Sciences*, 1993. **90**(22): pp. 10705–10709.

90. Waltenberger, J., et al., *Different signal transduction properties of KDR and Flt1, two receptors for vascular endothelial growth factor. Journal of Biological Chemistry*, 1994. **269**(43): pp. 26988–26995.

91. Fong, G.-H., et al., *Role of the Flt-1 receptor tyrosine kinase in regulating the assembly of vascular endothelium. Nature*, 1995. **376**(6535): pp. 66–70.

92. Hiratsuka, S., et al., *Flt-1 lacking the tyrosine kinase domain is sufficient for normal development and angiogenesis in mice. Proceedings of the National Academy of Sciences*, 1998. **95**(16): pp. 9349–9354.

93. Gerber, H.-P., et al., *VEGF regulates haematopoietic stem cell survival by an internal autocrine loop mechanism. Nature*, 2002. **417**(6892): pp. 954–958.

94. Luttun, A., et al., *Revascularization of ischemic tissues by PlGF treatment, and inhibition of tumor angiogenesis, arthritis and atherosclerosis by anti-Flt1. Nature Medicine*, 2002. **8**(8): pp. 831–840.

95. LeCouter, J., et al., *Angiogenesis-independent endothelial protection of liver: role of VEGFR-1. Science*, 2003. **299**(5608): pp. 890–893.

96. Quinn, T.P., et al., *Fetal liver kinase 1 is a receptor for vascular endothelial growth factor and is selectively expressed in vascular endothelium. Proceedings of the National Academy of Sciences*, 1993. **90**(16): pp. 7533–7537.

97. Takahashi, T., et al., *A single autophosphorylation site on KDR/Flk-1 is essential for VEGF-A-dependent activation of PLC-γ and DNA synthesis in vascular endothelial cells. The EMBO Journal*, 2001. **20**(11): pp. 2768–2778.

98. Dineen, S.P., et al., *Vascular endothelial growth factor receptor 2 mediates macrophage infiltration into orthotopic pancreatic tumors in mice. Cancer Research*, 2008. **68**(11): pp. 4340–4346.

99. Galland, F., et al., *The FLT4 gene encodes a transmembrane tyrosine kinase related to the vascular endothelial growth factor receptor. Oncogene*, 1993. **8**(5): pp. 1233–1240.

100. Dumont, D.J., et al., *Cardiovascular failure in mouse embryos deficient in VEGF receptor-3. Science*, 1998. **282**(5390): pp. 946–949.

101. Olsson, A.-K., et al., *VEGF receptor signalling? In control of vascular function. Nature Reviews Molecular Cell Biology*, 2006. **7**(5): pp. 359–371.

102. Kaplan, R.N., et al., *VEGFR1-positive haematopoietic bone marrow progenitors initiate the pre-metastatic niche. Nature*, 2005. **438**(7069): pp. 820–827.

103. Clynes, R.A., et al., *Inhibitory Fc receptors modulate in vivo cytotoxicity against tumor targets. Nature Medicine*, 2000. **6**(4): pp. 443–446.

104. Ravetch, J.V. and L.L. Lanier, *Immune inhibitory receptors. Science*, 2000. **290**(5489): p. 84–89.

105. Nimmerjahn, F. and J.V. Ravetch, *Divergent immunoglobulin g subclass activity through selective Fc receptor binding. Science*, 2005. **310**(5753): pp. 1510–1512.

106. Presta, L.G., *Molecular engineering and design of therapeutic antibodies. Current Opinion in Immunology*, 2008. **20**(4): pp. 460–470.

107. Yan, L., et al. *How can we improve antibody-based cancer therapy? MAbs.* 2009. **1**(1): pp. 67–70.

108. Stavenhagen, J.B., et al., *Fc optimization of therapeutic antibodies enhances their ability to kill tumor cells in vitro and controls tumor expansion in vivo via low-affinity activating Fcγ receptors. Cancer Research*, 2007. **67**(18): pp. 8882–8890.

109. Satoh, M., S. Iida, and K. Shitara, *Non-fucosylated therapeutic antibodies as next-generation therapeutic antibodies. Expert Opinion on Biological Therapy*, 2006. **6**(11): pp. 1161–1173.

110. Shields, R.L., et al., *Lack of fucose on human IgG1 N-linked oligosaccharide improves binding to human FcγRIII and antibody-dependent cellular toxicity. Journal of Biological Chemistry*, 2002. **277**(30): pp. 26733–26740.

111. Tempest, P., M. Stratton, and C. Cooper, *Structure of the met protein and variation of met protein kinase activity among human tumour cell lines. British Journal of Cancer*, 1988. **58**(1): pp. 3–7.

112. Donate, L.E., et al., *Molecular evolution and domain structure of plasminogen-related growth factors (HGF/SF and HGF1/MSP). Protein Science*, 1994. **3**(12): pp. 2378–2394.

113. Kirchhofer, D., et al., *Structural and functional basis of the serine protease-like hepatocyte growth factor β-chain in Met binding and signaling. Journal of Biological Chemistry*, 2004. **279**(38): pp. 39915–39924.

114. Birchmeier, C., et al., *Met, metastasis, motility and more. Nature Reviews Molecular Cell Biology*, 2003. **4**(12): pp. 915–925.

115. Blumenschein Jr, G.R., G.B. Mills, and A.M. Gonzalez-Angulo, *Targeting the hepatocyte growth factor–cMET axis in cancer therapy. Journal of Clinical Oncology*, 2012. **30**(26): p. 3287.

116. Sattler, M., et al., *The role of the c-Met pathway in lung cancer and the potential for targeted therapy. Therapeutic Advances in Medical Oncology*, 2011. **3**(4): pp. 171–184.

117. You, W.-K. and D.M. McDonald, *The hepatocyte growth factor/c-Met signaling pathway as a therapeutic target to inhibit angiogenesis. BMB Reports*, 2008. **41**(12): p. 833.

118. Cecchi, F., D.C. Rabe, and D.P. Bottaro, *Targeting the HGF/Met signaling pathway in cancer therapy. Expert Opinion on Therapeutic Targets*, 2012. **16**(6): pp. 553–572.

119. Ueki, T., et al., *Hepatocyte growth factor gene therapy of liver cirrhosis in rats. Nature Medicine*, 1999. **5**(2): pp. 226–230.

120. Kusumoto, K., et al., *Repeated intravenous injection of recombinant human hepatocyte growth factor ameliorates liver cirrhosis but causes albuminuria in rats. International Journal of Molecular Medicine*, 2006. **17**(3): pp. 503–509.

121. Nakamura, T., et al., *Molecular cloning and expression of human hepatocyte growth factor. Nature*, 1989. **342**(6248): pp. 440–443.

122. Rodrigues, G.A., M.A. Naujokas, and M. Park, *Alternative splicing generates isoforms of the met receptor tyrosine kinase which undergo differential processing. Molecular and Cellular Biology*, 1991. **11**(6): pp. 2962–2970.

123. Bardelli, A., C. Ponzetto, and P. Comoglio, *Identification of functional domains in the hepatocyte growth factor and its receptor by molecular engineering. Journal of Biotechnology*, 1994. **37**(2): pp. 109–122.

124. Lee, D., et al., *Development of antibody-based c-Met inhibitors for targeted cancer therapy. Immunotargets and Therapy*, 2015: pp. 35–44.

125. Khongorzul, P., et al., *Antibody–Drug Conjugates: A Comprehensive Review Antibody–Drug Conjugates in Cancer Immunotherapy. Molecular Cancer Research*, 2020. **18**(1): pp. 3–19.

126. Dean, A.Q., et al. *Targeting cancer with antibody-drug conjugates: Promises and challenges. MAbs.* 2021. **13**(1): p. 1951427.

127. Su, D. and D. Zhang, *Linker design impacts antibody-drug conjugate pharmacokinetics and efficacy via modulating the stability and payload release efficiency. Frontiers in Pharmacology*, 2021. **12**: p. 687926.

128. Cortés, J., et al. *Post-Progression Therapy Outcomes in Patients From the Phase 3 ASCENT Study of Sacituzumab Govitecan in Metastatic Triple-Negative Breast Cancer.* In *Poster Presented at the San Antonio Breast Cancer Symposium 2021 Annual Meeting*. 2021.

129. Ocaña, A. and A. Pandiella, *Proteolysis targeting chimeras (PROTACs) in cancer therapy. Journal of Experimental & Clinical Cancer Research*, 2020. **39**(1): p. 189.

130. Lemmon, M.A. and J. Schlessinger, *Cell signaling by receptor tyrosine kinases. Cell*, 2010. **141**(7): pp. 1117–1134.

131. Xu, A.M. and P.H. Huang, *Receptor tyrosine kinase coactivation networks in cancerRTK coactivation networks. Cancer Research*, 2010. **70**(10): pp. 3857–3860.

132. Fauvel, B. and A. Yasri. *Antibodies directed against receptor tyrosine kinases: current and future strategies to fight cancer. MAbs.* 2014. **6**(4): pp. 838–851.

14 Aptamer-Based Anticancer Therapies

Muhammad Yasir Ali, Ummaima Shahzad,
Maryam Shabir, Nisar ur Rahman, Saeed Ahmad,
Udo Bakowsky, Muhammad Umair Amin, Imran Tariq,
and Ghazala Ambreen

14.1 INTRODUCTION

Among the deadliest diseases that majorly affect the world, cancer remains at the top of the list. In 2008, there were 7.6 million cancer-related deaths and an estimated 12.7 million new cases [1]. About 56% of the cases and 64% of the deaths happened in poor countries. According to the CDC (http://www.cdc.gov), cancer is the second largest cause of death in the US. A total of 1,529,560 new cancer cases and 569,490 cancer-related deaths were anticipated to occur in 2010 [2]. The "war on cancer," which has become one of the top goals in the pharmaceutical industry and the National Institutes of Health (NIH), has received enormous investment and effort over the previous four decades. Early detection and effective treatment were the key points over the last decades in the research field. For a more detailed understanding of the disease, the researchers focus on advances in molecular biology and the steps involved in the cellular basis of cancer progression and development [3, 4].

Most of the treatment options available currently in clinical practice for cancer, such as radiotherapy, immunotherapy, and conventional chemotherapy are unfortunately unable to selectively target the specific site. To date, all these treatment options against cancer have serious limitations such as poor selectivity of cancerous tissues, very rapid clearance from the systemic circulation, low intratumoral accumulation, and drug resistance [5, 6]. The non-specificity ultimately leads to uneven bio-distribution of agents in the body, which results in unexpected side effects and harm to normal tissues and cells, which is challenging and problematic. Therefore, targeted therapy to minimize the unwanted side effects is highly desirable. The targeted strategies are extensively based on specific ligand-directed recognition steps in which the target ligand recognizes and binds to receptors that are expressed on the diseased cells or tissues. Various techniques have been developed for targeting specific tumor cells by conjugating drug delivery material to different biomolecules and ligands that are specific to cancer cells. Surface modification is another technique for nano-sized carriers such as liposomes, micelles, and polymeric nanoparticles with cancer cell-specific antibodies that can target cancer cells via receptor-mediated endocytosis [7].

Chemotherapy is the basic and powerful treatment for targeting highly proliferative cancerous cells and is associated with so many significant limitations in the treatment. The dose-limiting toxicity, poor specificity concerning the target site, and frequently emerging drug resistance are the major limitations of cancerous cell therapy. To overcome all these drawbacks associated with conventional cancer therapy there is a need to be more specific in terms of improving diagnostic techniques for better detection of cancer cells and avoiding drug-induced toxicity in non-neoplastic tissues. For this reason, researchers are more focused on the development of novel and more specific strategies to target malignant cells [8].

DOI: 10.1201/9781003363958-17

The ray of hope arrived with the technology of using monoclonal antibodies (mAbs) for the targeted treatment of cancerous cells was the breakthrough in cancer treatment in the 1970s. The target-specific property of mAbs is capable of binding specific targets such as tumor antigens and carrying anti-cancer agents to the cancerous cells and less damage to the normal healthy cells. For the few following years, mAbs' usefulness for clinical diagnoses and treatment of a few types of cancers remains exceptional among biomedical researchers. Although mAbs fail to achieve the expected wonders due to many limitations associated with the therapy and the unsuccessfulness of the treatment for many cancer types [9].

With the advance of research in the following years, the 1990s of the last century comes up with another technology of making bimolecular targeting specific sites. The technique was named systematic evolution of ligands by exponential enrichment (SELEX) and the molecules produced by this technology were named "aptamers" [10].

14.2 ADVANTAGES AND LIMITATIONS OF APTAMERS OVER ANTIBODIES

Aptamers are single-stranded (either DNA or RNA) oligonucleotides usually 25–90 nucleotide bases with unique three-dimensional configurations. Aptamers are capable of recognizing targets through three-dimensional complementarily instead of base pairs and specifically bind with high affinity to a broad range of targets such as proteins, viruses, cells, and small organic molecules [11]. They are described as nucleic acid antibodies. Thus nucleic acid aptamers developed as alternatives to antibodies for targeted therapy. Aptamers act similarly as antibodies do, but with some advantages over mAbs or protein antibodies in terms of in vivo applications and several other advantages, one of which is no or very little immunogenicity. No immunogenicity makes it favorable for repeated use with fewer side effects as it does not undergo immunological rejection. The production of aptamers does not rely on their biological system so it is much easier to increase its production with minimum batch-to-batch variability. The smaller size of aptamers (150 kDa) can lead to better penetration into the solid tumor. During chemical synthesis, the various functional groups can easily bind to aptamers due to orthogonal conjugation chemistry to orthogonal nucleic acid chemistry. Aptamers can be synthesized in large quantities through a chemical process and are much more resistant to heat and pH changes than protein antibodies so they can be denatured and renatured without loss of activity. The surface modification of functional groups through the chemical process makes them more favorable in terms of target-specific treatment [12]. On the other side, there are several disadvantages associated with aptamers that need the attention of researchers in the future. Few of them are faster excretion from system circulation than the antibodies, and unmodified aptamers undergo serum degradation, unpredictable toxicity, and intellectual property-related issues [13].

Many aptamers already have been approved by the US Food and Drug Administration (FDA), e.g. The aptamer mucagen (pegaptanib sodium injection), which is used to treat age-related macular degeneration. Mucagen antagonizes the binding of vascular endothelial growth factor (VEGF) to its receptor [14, 15]. Various cancer-targeting aptamers are under clinical investigation. A nucleolin aptamer named AS1411, NucA is in a phase II trial for the treatment of metastatic renal cell carcinoma with remarkable tumor-targeting properties and is nontoxic [16].

14.3 APTAMER PRODUCTION PROCESSES

The systematic evolution of ligands by exponential enrichment (SELEX) technique is used for the generation and isolation of aptamers. The whole process consists of repeated binding, partitioning, and amplification [17]. The procedure of specific oligonucleotide selection by the SELEX process is a combinatorial biochemical technique and will go through many rounds of selection. The initial random library contains 1014–1015 oligonucleotides, which are incubated with target molecules. After a specified time the unbound sequences are separated by multiple washing. The bound aptamers are then amplified by polymerase chain reaction (PCR). The resultant pool is then used for subsequent selection cycles (Figure 14.1). Sometimes, one step of negative selection is also added to remove the unwanted aptamers present due to their attachment to the solid support used to fix target molecules. Finally, sequencing and characterization are done (Table 14.1) and different modifying groups are attached, i.e., functional groups like carboxylic or amine groups or fluorescent probes. These modifications are meant for the attachment of aptamers on nano-scale formulations and fluorescent detection in experimental samples. Furthermore, this modification prevents the major limitation associated with exonuclease digestion of aptamers, which results in the instability of nucleic acid aptamers. As cancer-targeted therapy, aptamers can guide drugs to specific cancer sites by acting as a molecular probe to recognize and bind specific targets [18, 19].

14.4 DIAGNOSTIC APTAMERS

In-time diagnosis will only be possible if precise and sensitive methodologies having appropriate detecting agents are used. Aptamers have become a traditional tool in the field of diagnosis. The functional groups present on the aptamers are structurally quite similar to those of antibodies,

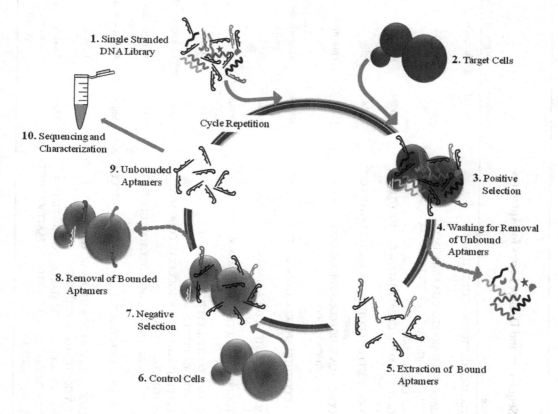

FIGURE 14.1 Selection of DNA aptamer using SELEX.

Note: For the selection of RNA aptamer, the DNA oligonucleotide pool must be in vitro transcribed into RNA oligonucleotide pool before selection, and the collected oligonucleotides must be reverse transcribe-amplified with TR-PCR into DNA and then be in-vitro transcribed into RNA for the next round of selection [9].

TABLE 14.1

Examples of Sequences and Dosage Forms for Aptamers

Sr. No.	Sequence	Names	Targeting Moiety	Disease	Dosage Forms	Reference
1.	5'-GGTGGTGGTGGTTGTGGTGGTGGTGG-3'	AS1411	Nucleolin	Cancer	Aptamer functionalized exosomes	[20, 21]
2.	5'-GGGAGGACGAUGCGGACCGAAAAAGACCU GACUUCUAUACUAAAGUCUACGUUCCCAGA CGACUCGCCCGA-3'	A10	PSMA	Cancer	Docetaxel-encapsulated nanoparticle-aptamer bio-conjugate	[22, 23]
3.	5'-ACGGGCCACATCAACTCATTGATAGACAATGCGTCCAC TGCCCGT-3'	aptPD-L1	PD-L1	Immune diseases, cancer	Aptamer-based spherical nucleic acids	[24]
4.	5'-GGGGCACGTTTATCCGTCCCTCCTAGTGGCGTGCCCC-3'	D17.4	IgE	Allergy	Aptamer/ protein complex	[25, 26]
5.	5'-UGCCGCUAUAAUGCACGGAUUUAAUCGCCGUAG AAAGCAUGUCAAAGCCG-3'	E07	Epidermal growth factor receptor (EGFR) cells	Cancer	Aptamer-drug conjugates	[27, 28]
6.	5'-CATGCCCCTGTAATCGCCCATGGGTAGC-3'	HM69	Mesenchymal stem cells (MSCs)	Bone repair	HM69-functionalized nanoparticles	[29, 30]
7.	5'-GTACAGTTCCCGTCCCTGCACTACA-3'	MP7	PD-1	Immune diseases, cancer	Aptamer–polymer conjugates	[31, 32]
8.	5'-TGTGGGGGTGGACGGGCCGGGTAGA-3'-	Pegaptanib, VEap121	VEGF	AMD, Cancer	Sterile solution	[33, 34]
9.	5'-TCTCTAGTTATTGAGTTTTCTTTTATGGGT GGGTGGGGGTTTTT-3'	R13	Ovarian cancer cells	Ovarian cancer	Aptamer targeted photodynamic therapy	[35, 36]
10.	5'-TTTTTTTTTTATCTAACTGCTGCGCCGCGGGAAA ATACTGTACGGTTAGA-3'	Sgc8	Leukaemia cells	Blood cancer	Aptamer hybridized DNA dendrimers	[37, 38]
11.	5'-GCACCGGGCAGGACGTCCGGGGTCCTCGGGGGGC-3'	S15	Dengue virus 2 (DENV)	Dengue	Aptamer functionalized quantum dots	[39, 40]
12.	5'-CCTCGGCACGTTCTCAGTAGCGCTCGCTGGTCATCCCAC-A-3'	Seq-3	Gastric cancer cells	Cancer	Activatable aptamer probes	[30, 41]
13.	5'-ACAGCATCCCCATGTGAACAATCGCATTGTGATTGTTACGG TTTCCGCCTCATGGACGTGCTG-3'	TLS11a	HepG2	Liver Cancer	Aptamer conjugated nanoparticles	[42, 43]
14.	5'-AAGGAGCAGCGTGGAGGATACCCATCAATGTTACGA CCCGCTAGGGCTGCTGTGCCATCGGGTAATTAGGGTGT GTCGTCGTGGT-3'	XL-33	Metastatic colon cancer cells (SW620)	Cancer	Aptamer-fluorescein amidite (FAM) conjugate	[44, 45]

mimicking many properties of the antibodies. Hence, these artificially synthesized oligonucleotides are also termed as "chemical antibodies", but they have many advantages over antibodies. Aptamers are more specific, less immunogenic, and have greater target affinity as compared to antibodies. They can fold into different tertiary structures that give them the ability to detect any given target, whether it is a tiny chemical compound or a multi-domain polysaccharide or protein, amino acid, any organic dye, antibody, live cells or tissues, and whatnot. While antibodies can only bind to large molecules or immunogenic proteins. Aptamers are very easily labeled and conjugated, which allows them to be easily paired with many of the advanced technologies such as microfluidic cell separation, endogenous analysis of nucleic acids, flow cytometry, and many more. These properties make them a potentially useful tool for diagnostic purposes [46, 47]. Aptamers can be used for the diagnosis of bacteria, viruses, parasites, etc.

Sometimes the level of infection in a disease is so very less that it will initiate a disease, but the number of toxins is yet to be increased and this will not allow detection of the disease. Traditional diagnostic methods are not as adept and take more time to detect these levels, which can lead to the worsening of the symptoms. But aptamers are highly efficient and can even detect low levels making them a promising tool [47].

As, in case of infection caused by *Staphylococcus aureus*, the detection is mostly done via culturing, which can take days to yield results while the other available methods are not cost-effective. A current low-cost non-PCR methodology is developed, that detects the resonance light scattering indicator of aptamer conjugated with gold nanoparticles and identifies a unit cell of *S. aureus* in 1.5 hours [48].

14.4.1 TUBERCULOSIS (TB)

TB is a fatal disease and pulmonary tuberculosis is its prevalent manifestation. Sputum smear microscopy is its frequently used diagnostic test, despite the suboptimal activity. Lavania, Surabhi et al. reported the successful development of two tests based on DNA aptamers, named electrochemical sensor (ECS) and aptamer-linked immobilized sorbent assay (ALISA). These can directly detect HspX, a TB biomarker in the sputum. ALISA showed a very good sensitivity of approximately 94.1% in the sputum specimens as compared to the anti-HspX polyclonal antibody-based enzyme-linked immunosorbent assay (Antibody ELISA), which only had 68.2% sensitivity. This shows the superiority of the aptamer-based diagnosis of TB over traditional diagnostic tools [49].

Similarly, the regular methods for the detection of viral agents are time-consuming, less sensitive, and sometimes non-specific causing more harm than good. Aptamers are highly specific substances that can effectively detect viruses with increased sensitivity.

14.4.2 HUMAN PAPILLOMAVIRUS (HPV)

HPV belongs to the Papilomavaridie family and is a non-enveloped DNA virus that mostly has no symptoms. Toscano-Garibay et al. formulated an RNA aptamer that specifically binds to HPV-16 E7 oncoprotein and makes its detection easier. Some other aptamers including the slow off-rate modified DNA aptamer (SOMAmer) and reduced graphene oxide-based field-effect transistor (rGO-FET) against HPV-16 VLPs and HPV E7 protein respectively, were also developed [50].

14.4.3 HEPATITIS C VIRUS (HCV)

HCV causes hepatitis C, cirrhosis, liver cancer, and liver fibrosis and is highly variable, which makes its detection troublesome. A chip-based system using RNA aptamers specifically bound with

HCV core antigen was developed by Lee et al. for the detection of HCV. 2'F RNA aptamers were immobilized in the 96-well plate. HCV core antigen was then detected in the patient's blood serum by Cy3-labeled secondary antibodies [51].

14.5　THERAPEUTIC APTAMERS

The targeting specificity and conformational diversity of RNA aptamers show an enhanced potential for their applications in therapy. Aptamers can inhibit protein–protein interactions and for this purpose, several specific features should be present in them. Firstly, the therapeutic aptamers must be highly stable in the body. As natural DNA and RNA molecules are highly susceptible to endogenous nucleases, the chemical modifications of sugar or phosphodiester backbone should necessarily be included. Secondly, the nucleotide length of the aptamers should be adequately shortened. Abridging of aptamers can reduce manufacturing costs, prevent unexpected toxicities, and can help in the assurance of the quality of materials. Thirdly, the aptamers used in therapy must have good pharmacokinetic properties. One example of aptamers being used in therapy is NOX-A12. It is the spiegelmer aptamer, which is 45-nucleotide long and is linked with the 40 kDa PEG. Spieglemers are DNA or RNA-based aptamers, which bind to and inhibit the pharmacologically related molecules of choice. These have a mirror-image backbone of DNA or RNA oligonucleotides-l-stereoisomers. They give the combined advantage of biopharmaceuticals and small molecular drugs and are bio-stable. NOX-A12 possess therapeutic actions for various myelomas and non-Hodgkin's lymphomas and is developed to be used alongside transplants of autologous hematopoietic stem cells [52].

14.6　APTAMERS IN MOLECULAR IMAGING

Aptamers have sparked significant interest in preclinical molecular testing with almost all the imaging modalities and their combinations as in multimodal imaging applications. Molecular imaging probes typically comprise three elements:

1. A targeting moiety that specifically and selectively binds with the molecule of interest.
2. A spacer connecting the targeting ligand and the reporter.
3. A reporter molecule that produces a signal, which can be detected by an appropriate detector.

Moreover, the spacer may be given a functionality itself (such as pH-sensitive cleavage or redox-, quenching/activation potential, modification of the probe's pharmacokinetic characteristics, etc.) [53]. Aptamers are a practical means for gaining insight of molecular processes in a non-invasive way.

The extensive research in RNA field has led to the development of some innovative imaging aptamers including fluorogenic aptamers, which bind to the target fluorophores to get activated, e.g., spinach, broccoli, mango, and corn.

14.6.1　Spinach and Broccoli

These are green fluorogenic aptamers. Spinach binds to a small fluorophore molecule, i.e., 3,5-difluoro-4-hydroxybenzylidene imidazolinone (DFHBI) or its variants. Upon research it was revealed that the original structure of this aptamer is thermally unstable, requires high concentrations of magnesium for working, and has a tendency for misfolding, hence reduced brightness. To overcome these limitations some other variants such as Spinach2, iSpinach, and Baby Spinach have also been designed [54]. Broccoli was also isolated from the same group as that of spinach, but in a different way to avoid the instabilities. It also binds to DHFBI but shows less dependency on magnesium, better thermal stability, and brighter green fluorescence [55].

14.6.2 MANGO

It is the orange fluorogenic aptamer that is nearly two times better at detection than the spinach system. It binds to a series of derivatives of the thiazole orange (TO1) and increases fluorescence up to 1100 folds [56].

14.6.3 CORN

Corn binds to 3,5-difluoro-4-hydroxynenzylidene imidazolinone-2-oxime (DFHO) and activates the yellow fluorescence. It shows better photostability as compared to spinach and mango, allowing quantitative measurement of the RNA levels in living cells. An imaging period of 320 ms was required to measure its fluorescence as compared to the 160 ms period for broccoli [57].

Another aptamer named SRB-2, which was initially discovered to target the fluorophore sulforhodamine B, binds to several dyes with xanthene-like cores, including pyrosin-B, pyrosin-Y, acridine orange, SR-DN, and TMR-DN, and produces a **"rainbow"** of strong fluorescence with a variety of diverse colors [58]. Hence, all of these aptamers can be used for any kind of intracellular live imaging.

Optical imaging (fluorescence and bioluminescence), positron emission tomography (PET), magnetic resonance imaging (MRI), single-photon emission computed tomography (SPECT), computed tomography (CT), and ultrasound (US) are among some of the imaging techniques currently available for the detection and characterization of cancers, as well as for the assessment of therapeutic interventions and all of these can be modified by relevant aptamers to increase their specificity and efficiency [59].

14.7 APTAMERS IN BIO-SENSING

Aptasensors are biosensors that use aptamers as biorecognition components. Typically, a biosensor consists of two basic parts, i.e., a signal transducer (electrochemical, fluorescent, colorimetric, chemiluminescent, etc.) and a recognition element (antigen, antibody, biological tissue, nucleic acid, enzyme, etc.). Aptamers are used in the field of biosensors because of their high affinity and tunable characteristics, while the transducer has a significant impact on their sensitivity. There is an increasing interest in the study and production of aptasensors. These aptasensors were created using a variety of methodologies, including electrochemical aptasensors, surface-enhanced Raman scattering (SERS) aptasensors, chemiluminescent aptasensors, and optical aptasensors (fluorescence-based optical aptasensors and colorimetric-based optical aptasensors). The majority of the fundamental components of these aptasensors are adaptable or analogous. Some sensors were modified as aptamer beacons for the analysis of numerous targets. The aptamer beacon (aptabeacon) has a hairpin-shaped structure, with the loop acting as a target recognition element and the 5′ and 3′ ends being labeled with a fluorophore and quencher that forms the stem of the aptamer-predicted structure. Due to the presence of fluorescence resonance energy transfer (FRET) between the fluorophore and quencher, the fluorescence is low in the absence of the target. Because the fluorophore and quencher are far away after the target is introduced, the rigid structure of the beacon is destroyed, which causes the fluorescence to return [60]. These biosensors can be used for the detection of numerous conditions, including cancer.

14.8   APTAMERS AS CANCER CELL TARGETING AGENT

Cancer biomarkers are molecules that identify malignancies in their aberrant stages and are crucial for a variety of biological functions, such as signal transduction, cell migration, cell proliferation, and cell–cell interactions. Biomarkers that work well include molecules like membrane proteins, transcription factors, and growth factors [61, 62]. Potential targets for cancer therapies include well-characterized membrane proteins that are endogenously over-expressed on the surfaces of cancer cells (Figure 14.2). Because of their strong affinity for target molecules, aptamers have become novel targeting materials that are sensitive to the detection of these cancer biomarkers. To enhance therapeutic benefits and lessen unneeded toxicity to non-cancerous cells, they recognize and bind to appropriate targets by forming spontaneous three-dimensional structures [63].

Finding aptamer sequences that bind to particular biomarkers of cancer cells is the main problem. For the treatment of various malignancies including breast cancer, colorectal adenocarcinoma, lung cancer, and prostate cancer as well as cancer stem cells, numerous aptamers specific to tumor-related biomarkers have been discovered and thoroughly explored in recent years. Numerous aptamers that specifically target cancer-specific hallmark markers have been developed, including immune-inhibitory programmed death-1, immune-stimulating CD137, CD134, tumorigenic platelet-derived growth factor, and vascular endothelial growth factor [64].

AS1411, a 26-nucleotide guanosine-rich DNA sequence that preferentially binds to overexpressed or translocated nucleolin (NCL) in a variety of cancer cells, is a well-known clinical aptamer in anti-cancer research [65]. In addition to being effective against cancer, AS1411 also prevents NCL from attaching to the Bcl-2 oncogene, which prevents cells from escaping apoptosis. At very low

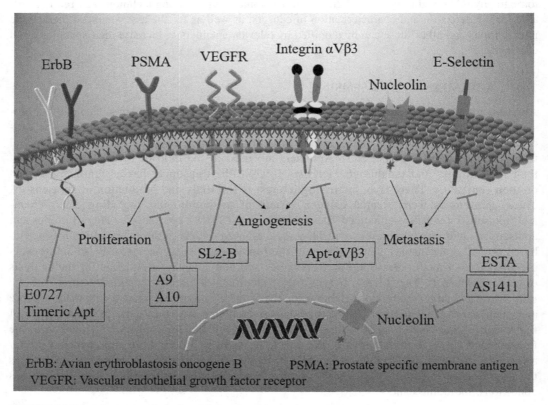

FIGURE 14.2   A few examples of membrane-bound proteins and respective aptamers.

concentrations, AS1411-conjugated nano-vehicles have demonstrated strong inhibitory effects on a number of tumor cell lines with negligible adverse effects [66]. The commercial version of AS1411, developed by Aptamera Inc., Louisville, KY, was motivated by the preclinical success of AS1411 and is currently undergoing phase II clinical studies for its anti-acute myeloid leukemia (AML) and renal cell carcinoma (RC) properties [67].

A10 is a well-known aptamer that binds exclusively to a prostate cancer biomarker and has potential clinical uses. Numerous studies have shown important outcomes, such as specific in vivo therapeutic activity against prostate cancer in a mouse model using LNCaP cells that express PSMA [68].

14.9 DELIVERY OF CHEMOTHERAPEUTIC DRUGS VIA APTAMERS

Targeted therapies using aptamers typically use one of three methods:

(1) Aptamers can be covalently or non-covalently coupled with drugs to generate aptamer-drug conjugates.

(2) Aptamers can serve as antagonists or agonists to inhibit or stimulate, respectively, the interactions of tumor-associated targets (ApDCs). For instance, intercalation at particular paired GC sites in the aptamer sequence successfully load the drug doxorubicin (Dox) onto aptamers. Additionally, aptamers can transport therapeutic compounds to cancer cells.

(3) Aptamers can be included in new nanoparticles to improve therapeutic response. Tumoricidal therapeutic effects are produced by aptamer-conjugated nano-vehicles delivering anti-cancer medicines, in which the aptamers direct the therapeutic agents to the extracellular region of a tumor-specific surface biomarker [64].

Aside from therapies that solely employ aptamers, aptamers can also be utilized to precisely deliver other therapeutic agents, such as chemotherapeutics, small interfering RNAs (siRNAs), micro RNAs (miRNAs), short hairpin RNAs (shRNA), and tiny interfering RNAs (miRNAs). It has proven possible to administer therapeutic drugs with higher local concentrations and treatment efficacy by using a range of aptamers tailored to cancer biomarkers. To create aptamer-drug conjugates (ApDCs) and aptamer-therapeutic oligonucleotide conjugates (ApOCs), respectively, aptamers can be covalently or non-covalently conjugated with medicines and therapeutic oligonucleotides. Covalent conjugation provides the most straightforward connection for aptamer-therapeutic oligonucleotide conjugates. To inhibit the expression of pro-survival genes such as polo-like kinase 1 (PLK1) and B-cell lymphoma 2 (BCL2), a PSMA aptamer-siRNA combination was created that targets prostate cancer [69].

Aptamers can be created chemically and easily altered. In this sense, it is simple to conjugate medicinal compounds to aptamers, including proteins, toxins, and chemotherapeutic molecules (such as Dox). These conjugates have been demonstrated to lessen adverse effects and improve the effectiveness of medication delivery to liver cancer cells in tumor-bearing mice models [70].

Aptamers can also be conjugated non-covalently using "sticky bridges," which are extra-extended strands. To decrease BAFF-R-mediated cancer, for instance, the B-cell-activating factor receptor (BAFF-R) aptamer that can bind to BAFF-R was chosen [70]. Through the use of two complementary stick sequences, the STAT3 siRNA, which is crucial for the development of B-cell lymphoma, was complexed with the BAFF-R aptamer. The GL21.T aptamer that targets the receptor tyrosine kinase Axl was conjugated with anti-miRNA-222 using the same method [71]. The anti-miRNA-222, extended at the 3′ end, and the 17-mer at the 5′ end of the aptamer are completely complimentary to one another.

The resultant aptamer-anti-miRNA combination decreased the levels of miRNA-222 in cells that expressed Axl. Anti-miRNA-10b and anti-miRNA-222 were both combined with aptamer GL21 to boost the therapeutic impact by opposing corresponding onco-miRNAs independently. Bi-modular anti-miRNA-10b and anti-miRNA-222 were non-covalently coupled to the GL21.T aptamer, which antagonized the miRNAs in vitro and in vivo. Additionally, dual-functional CD40 aptamers with two components, such as shRNA with various functionalities, have been developed [72]. To lessen bone marrow aplasia, the agonistic bivalent CD44 RNA aptamer attaches to and activates B cells. Additionally, nonsense-mediated mRNA degradation was prevented by using shRNA against SMG1. It has been noted that the bivalent CD40 aptamer-SMG1 shRNA chimera enhances immunological responses and, as a result, overall survival in vivo. ApOC has been applied as a treatment as well as an imaging technique. Epidermal growth factor receptor (EGFR) aptamers have been produced as targeting molecules, anti-miRNA-21 as therapeutic agents, and Alexa 647 dye as imaging agents into an RNA scaffold in a three-way junction [73]. In a breast cancer-bearing mouse model, it was found that this tri-functional aptamer reduced miRNA-21 levels and inhibited tumor growth while enabling imaging to monitor cancer cells.

Doxorubicin (DOX) is an anthracycline antibiotic that is used in the treatment of many kinds of malignancies including hematological malignancies, soft tissue sarcomas, and carcinomas. Doxorubicin can intercalate within double-stranded GC sequences of DNA and RNA [74]. The use of DOX is also associated with dose-dependent cardiotoxicity, such as dilated congestive heart failure, which urges the need for efficient tumor-targeted delivery strategies for DOX. An aptamer-Dox (Apt-DOX) physical conjugate via intercalation was prepared to fulfill the need for targeted delivery. Aptamer-DIX A10, a 2'-fluoropyrimidine RNA aptamer that binds to the extracellular domain of the prostate-specific membrane antigen (PSMA) with a Kd of 2.1 nM [75], was used in this study. A10 is composed of 57 base pairs and the molecular weight is 18.5 kDa. This Apt-Dox conjugate had the ability of good stability in cell culture medium and was shown to target PSMA-expressing cells with high efficiency [76].

In another research report of aptamer conjugation with DOX, a DNA aptamer termed sgc8c was linked via hydrazones linker for target killing of specific tumor cells. The sgc8c DNA aptamer showed the ability to recognize protein tyrosine kinase 7 (PTK7) with nM binding affinity [77]. The sgc8c was selected by using human T-cell acute lymphoblastic leukemia cells. The highly specific sequence of DNA structure of sgc8c makes it capable of differentiating between target leukemia cells from normal human bone marrow as well as identifying cancer cells closely linked with target cell lines in a clinical specimen. Sometimes, despite higher target cell killing, chemical modifications in the binding sites of aptamers compromise the safety and efficacy of the drug [78]. Therefore, daunorubicin (Dau), which is another drug of the anthracycline family can overcome this issue. The Dau commonly used in the treatment of leukemia can physically bind to sgc8c aptamer via intercalation instead of chemical linkages. It was proved that the sgc8c can deliver Dau into PTK7-positive cells with high potency.

14.10   APTAMERS AS CANCER CELL AGONISTS AND ANTAGONISTS

Very remarkable affinity and specificity of the aptamers towards the targeted ligand make them favorable to inhibit and stimulate the target of interest, such as receptors and growth factors for cancer progression. For example, different forms of RNA aptamers have been developed that can be used against murine CD28. The monomeric aptamer CD28Apt2 can be used to reduce immunogenic signals by acting as an antagonist that inhibits interactions between CD28 and B7.2 ligands. On the other hand, 21-base paired double-stranded bivalent aptamers act as agonists. For the survival of cancerous mice, the agonistic aptamers stimulate CD28 cells and CD4 lymphocytes and promote cellular immune responses. The agonistic properties of OX40 that target CD134 and 4-1BB that target CD137 were proved to enhance the anti-tumor responses through T-cell activation. A bivalent aptamer can also be formed by combining two OX40 aptamers on a scaffold DNA (tandom oligo), which were shown to stimulate primed T-cells both in vitro and in vivo. A bivalent OX40 RNA aptamer was recently created and found to encourage T-cell proliferation and interferon production [79].

The bivalent 4-1BB aptamer and PSMA aptamer make up the bi-specific PSMA-4-1BB aptamer conjugate [80]. It has been demonstrated that using a bivalent 4-1-BB aptamer along with the tumor-targeting PSMA aptamer reduces adverse effects and enhances therapeutic results.

PD-1 is a new target for cancer treatments because it inhibits T cells' inflammatory activity by attaching to PD-L1 [81]. In order to counteract PD-1-mediated immune-suppression, the MP7 aptamer preferentially binds to the extracellular area of the PD-1 receptor on T cells [35]. Additionally, the MP7 aptamer coupled with polyethylene glycol, which increases the aptamer's half-life to up to 24-48 h, inhibits the growth of tumors without inducing signals from the innate immune system that are mediated by TLR9.

The antagonistic aptamers anti-PDGF RNA aptamer (ARC126) and anti-VEGF aptamer (pegaptanib) prevent angiogenesis in a variety of malignancies. The latter has been put on the market, whereas the former has undergone phase II clinical studies. Two anti-VEGF aptamers were attached to a hexaethylene glycol spacer to improve their biocompatibility. An "oligobody" (oligomer + antibody), which has recently been designed for increased in vivo anti-cancer activity [82], is an aptamer-antibody combination.

14.11 DELIVERY OF CHEMOTHERAPEUTIC DRUGS VIA APTAMER-NANOPARTICLE CONJUGATE

Nanotechnology can have a revolutionary impact due to its remarkable property of being smaller than a few hundred nanometers and several orders smaller in magnitude than human cells [83]. Distinct from both molecules and solids nanomaterial can interact with bi-molecules both on the surface of and inside the cells, which may result in improved detection and treatment of cancerous cells. The large surface area, loading capacity, and structural chemistry make them excellent carriers for targeted anti-cancer drug delivery. A variety of nanoparticle-aptamers (NP-Apt) conjugates have been constructed over the last decade, which can have broad applications ranging from diagnostic to targeted delivery of chemotherapeutic drugs [84].

Dox intercalation into DNA duplexes may produce significant DNA structural changes, potentially lowering the selectivity of aptamers, even while Dox-intercalated aptamers decreased off-target cytotoxicity, reducing side effects in comparison to those of the free drug. DNA structural alterations induced by Dox intercalation were investigated by Agudelo et al. [85]. The NH2 group on Dox played a crucial role in the structural change from a partial B to an A-DNA form, which was essential for intercalation. The effectiveness of Dox delivery by Dox-intercalated aptamers and Dox-encapsulating aptamer-conjugated liposomes was also contrasted by Park et al. [86].

For drug delivery and targeted cytotoxicity, Dox-intercalated aptamers performed less well than Dox-encapsulating aptamer-conjugated liposomes. These findings suggested that for aptamers to be used as targeting molecules, their structural integrity must be preserved.

Aptamers can be coupled with nano-vehicles such as liposomes, micelles, polymeric nanoparticles, and quantum dots (QDs), which preserves the aptamer structure, to get over this troublesome distortion in the aptamer structure. For instance, liposomes have been coupled with an anti-VEGF aptamer (NX213) [87]. A chicken chorioallantoic membrane model's in vivo angiogenesis was decreased by the aptamer-conjugated liposomes. Polyethylene glycol (PEG) can be used to easily modify the surfaces of liposomes to reduce non-specific lipid fusion with membranes. Liposomes can transport highly hazardous medicines.

An "aptamosome," as described by Beak et al., is a liposome that has been conjugated with a PSMA RNA aptamer and can contain Dox [88]. This PSMA aptamosome attaches to prostate cancer cells only when they express PSMA, but not when they do not, and it demonstrates selective toxicity for PSMA-positive cells. The bio-distribution and tumor growth reduction by an aptamosome with a therapeutic potential were shown in vivo in an LNCaP cell xenograft mouse model. A simple TDO5 DNA aptamer that targets the immunoglobulin heavy chain receptor was coupled to lipid tails via PEG to create an aptamer-micelle complex [89] for improved penetration and higher binding affinity. When aptamer and aptamer-micelle ability to bind to target cells were evaluated, aptamer-micelle demonstrated faster and more sensitive targeting.

In a research study, the anti-cancer efficacy of a NP-Apt conjugate showed promising both in vitro and in vivo properties. A10 RNA aptamer was used as the targeted ligand. Docetaxel (Dtxl) is an antimitotic chemotherapy drug. The nanoparticle used in NP-Apt conjugation was made up of bio-degradable and biocompatible copolymer, poly (D, L-lactic-co-glycolic acid)-block-poly (ethylene glycol) (i.e., PLGA-b-PEG). It was proved that the NP-Apt-Dtxl conjugate bound to PSMA on the cancer cell's surface. The subsequent endocytosis into cells led to increased cellular toxicity than the non-targeted nanoparticles (i.e., NP-Dtxl). The intratumoral injection of NP-Apt-Dtxl led to a significant anti-tumor effect with excellent therapeutic efficacy and reduced toxicity. The enhanced efficacy of NP-Apt-Dtxl over NP-Dxtl was attributed to targeted delivery and intracellular Dtxl release upon PSMA-mediated endocytosis of the earlier while NP-Dxtl may release the drug in extracellular space causing reduced efficacy and increased toxicity. A similar technique of delivery was used in another study for the delivery of cisplatin, which is another chemotherapeutic drug that can bind to and cause cross-linking of DNA into cancer cells [90, 91].

Another research report described the fabrication of a smart Bi-FRET QD-Apt-Dox conjugate delivery as well as an imaging agent. FRET and QD are fluorescence resonance energy transfer and quantum dot, respectively. Inorganic fluorescent semiconductor nanoparticles known as QDs have numerous desirable characteristics for imaging applications, including high quantum yields, high molar extinction coefficients, strong fluorescent features, narrow emission spectra, substantial size, and resistance to chemical and photochemical deterioration. Dox was intercalated in the double-stranded stem region of the A10 RNA aptamer, which was bonded covalently to the QD surface [92]. This QD-Apt-Dox combination is initially in the fluorescence "OFF" state because the absorbance of Dox quenched the fluorescence of QD and the A10 aptamer quenched the fluorescence of Dox. Dox was progressively released from the conjugate after being taken up by PSMA-positive cancer cells, which caused the fluorescence signal from QD and Dox to recover (i.e., the "ON" state). As a result, this versatile QD-Apt-Dox combination can be utilized to simultaneously image the target cells while also monitoring the transport and release of the medication to the targeted cells.

Comparing PSMA-positive and PSMA-negative cells, it was discovered that PSMA-positive cells had much greater levels of QD-Apt-Dox cytotoxicity. The A10 aptamer was then attached to various nanoparticles, such as thermally cross-linked superparamagnetic iron oxide nanoparticles (TCL-SPION, which could act as both a magnetic resonance contrast agent and a carrier for Dox), and gold nanoparticles (which served as both a contrast agent for computed tomography and a carrier for Dox). Subsequently, similar strategies have also been used for cancer imaging and therapy applications by several other groups [93, 94].

When more than one type of aptamer is bonded to the nanoparticle surface, dual-targeting can be used for drug administration because of the relatively large size and surface area of nanoparticles. One such dual-aptamer combination was recently developed to target prostate cancer cells that are PSMA-positive and PSMA-negative A dual-aptamer complex was created by coupling the A10 RNA aptamer and the DUP-1 peptide aptamer, which are both selective against PSMA-negative cells and can transport medicines to both PSMA-positive and PSMA-negative cells [95] Similar to what was discussed before, Dox was loaded on the A10 aptamer's stem region. A10 RNA aptamer and DUP-1 peptide aptamer loaded with Dox were also immobilized on the TCL-SPION surface to administer Dox to specific cells. This proof-of-research study showed that this dual-aptamer combination may deliver tumor-specific drugs to numerous sites and has potential applications for image-guided drug delivery and therapeutic response monitoring [96, 97].

14.12 APTAMER-BASED BIOSENSING AND BIOIMAGING IN CANCER

Aptamer-based biosensing is a novel technique for cancer diagnosis in its early stages and it involves the use of molecular probes. The tumor cell diagnosis may include the use of electrochemical aptasensors, optical aptasensors, or any other aptamer-based biosensor. The optical sensors use aptamers as their prime recognition agents for the early detection of tumor cells [98]. One example is the detection of breast cancer cells in humans by Li's group. They developed a gold nanorod (GNR) ligated with an aptamer to detect the MCF-7 cells of human breast cancer. Surface localized plasma resonance spectra were utilized to detect the affinities in target tumor cell and mucin-1(MUC-1)-specific aptamer-GNR [99].

Aptamers can not only be used as an exemplary fluorescent probe but can also be applied as novel tools in bioimaging. Silver and gold nanoclusters along with other photoluminescent nanomaterials are widely used in cancer bioimaging. But they are quite pricy and show poor photostability. Quantum dots (QDs) appear to be an attractive alternative to these nanomaterials but they have their limitations. On the other hand, silicon quantum dots (Si QDs) can be an intriguing replacement for QDs containing heavy toxic metals in bioimaging, but in addition to being slightly toxic, they are subject to oxidative biodegradation in biological systems. For cell imaging, biocompatible probes with low toxicity are required, which can be provided by carbon dots (CDs). The excellent photoluminescence properties, low toxicity, high photostability, and biocompatibility of CDs make them an ideal choice for cancer bioimaging. An example is the use of nitrogen and phosphor co-doped carbon dots (N-P doped CDs) for targeting HeLa cells in cancer cell bioimaging with a quantum yield of 9.8% [100].

14.13 CONCLUSION

Aptamer studies are still in their infancy, and to better prepare for clinical application or commercialization, a deeper comprehension of aptamer-target interactions and pharmacokinetics is still required. Even though numerous aptamers have been created and some of them have begun clinical trials, the FDA has only yet to approve one of them for usage in actual clinical settings. The best outcomes are still to come as effective medicines continue to advance, although slowly. In terms of cancer treatment, aptamers have the benefit of having little to no immunogenicity, are relatively simple to penetrate solid tumor tissue due to their lower molecular weight, and are more affordable than mAbs because they are made in vitro. Therefore, additional efforts should be made to find new anti-cancer aptamers, characterize the existing aptamers in-depth, and accelerate the process of advancing anti-cancer aptamers already in use through clinical trials. Despite the abundance of resources in aptamers, there are still several areas where their application may be enhanced. To increase the production of aptamers, oligonucleotide synthesis technology needs to be improved. To make it easier to quickly identify target aptamers, the technology for screening aptamers needs to be improved. Expanding aptamer modification techniques is also necessary to make them available for molecular coupling. The biological stability of aptamers in vivo, which is a requirement for the application of aptamers, should also be seriously considered. We think that improvements in aptamer technology will allow for an effective solution to these issues.

REFERENCES

1. Jemal, A., et al., *Global cancer statistics. CA: A Cancer Journal for Clinicians*, 2011. **61**(2): pp. 69–90.
2. Jemal, A., et al., *Cancer statistics, 2010. CA: A Cancer Journal for Clinicians*, 2010. **60**(5): pp. 277–300.
3. Rajendran, L., H.-J. Knölker, and K. Simons, *Subcellular targeting strategies for drug design and delivery. Nature Reviews Drug Discovery*, 2010. **9**(1): pp. 29–42.

4. Rosen, H. and T. Abribat, *The rise and rise of drug delivery. Nature Reviews Drug Discovery*, 2005. **4**(5): pp. 381–385.

5. Eichler, H.-G., et al., *Assessing the relative efficacy of new drugs: an emerging opportunity. Nature Reviews Drug Discovery*, 2015. **14**(7): pp. 443–444.

6. Liu, Y.P., et al., *Molecular mechanisms of chemo-and radiotherapy resistance and the potential implications for cancer treatment. MedComm*, 2021. **2**(3): pp. 315–340.

7. Zugazagoitia, J., et al., *Current challenges in cancer treatment. Clinical Therapeutics*, 2016. **38**(7): pp. 1551–1566.

8. Diniz, F., et al., *Glycans as targets for drug delivery in cancer. Cancers*, 2022. **14**(4): p. 911.

9. Fu, Z. and J. Xiang, *Aptamers, the nucleic acid antibodies, in cancer therapy. International Journal of Molecular Sciences*, 2020. **21**(8): p. 2793.

10. Fu, Z. and J. Xiang, *Aptamers, the Nucleic Acid Antibodies, in Cancer Therapy*, in *Advances in Medical Biochemistry, Genomics, Physiology, and Pathology*. 2021, New Delhi: Jenny Stanford. pp. 143–175.

11. Nimjee, S.M., C.P. Rusconi, and B.A. Sullenger, *Aptamers: An emerging class of. Annual Review of Medicine*, 2005. **56**: pp. 555–83.

12. Liss, M., et al., *An aptamer-based quartz crystal protein biosensor. Analytical Chemistry*, 2002. **74**(17): pp. 4488–4495.

13. Keefe, A., S. Pal and, A. Ellington, *Aptamers as therapeutics. Nature Reviews Drug Discovery*, 2010. **9**: p. 537.

14. Kourlas, H. and D.S. Schiller, *Pegaptanib sodium for the treatment of neovascular age-related macular degeneration: a review. Clinical Therapeutics*, 2006. **28**(1): pp. 36–44.

15. Ng, E.W., et al., *Pegaptanib, a targeted anti-VEGF aptamer for ocular vascular disease. Nature Reviews Drug Discovery*, 2006. **5**(2): pp. 123–132.

16. Rosenberg, J.E., et al., *A phase II trial of AS1411 (a novel nucleolin-targeted DNA aptamer) in metastatic renal cell carcinoma. Investigational New Drugs*, 2014. **32**(1): pp. 178–187.

17. Sun, H. and Y. Zu, *A highlight of recent advances in aptamer technology and its application. Molecules*, 2015. **20**(7): pp. 11959–11980.

18. Gopinath, S.C.B., *Methods developed for SELEX. Analytical and Bioanalytical Chemistry*, 2007. **387**(1): pp. 171–182.

19. Wu, Y.X. and Y.J. Kwon, *Aptamers: the "evolution" of SELEX. Methods*, 2016. **106**: pp. 21–28.

20. Mosafer, J. and A. Mokhtarzadeh, *Cell surface nucleolin as a promising receptor for effective AS1411 aptamer-mediated targeted drug delivery into cancer cells. Current Drug Delivery*, 2018. **15**(9): pp. 1323–1329.

21. Hosseini, N.F., et al., *AS1411 aptamer-functionalized exosomes in the targeted delivery of doxorubicin in fighting colorectal cancer. Biomedicine & Pharmacotherapy*, 2022. **155**: p. 113690.

22. Choksi, A.U., et al., *Functionalized nanoparticles targeting biomarkers for prostate cancer imaging and therapy. American Journal of Clinical and Experimental Urology*, 2022. **10**(3): p. 142.

23. Farokhzad, O.C., et al., *Targeted nanoparticle-aptamer bioconjugates for cancer chemotherapy in vivo. Proceedings of the National Academy of Sciences*, 2006. **103**(16): pp. 6315–6320.

24. Lai, W.-Y., et al., *A novel PD-L1-targeting antagonistic DNA aptamer with antitumor effects. Molecular Therapy-Nucleic Acids*, 2016. **5**: p. e397.

25. Liang, C., et al., *Aptamer-functionalized lipid nanoparticles targeting osteoblasts as a novel RNA interference–based bone anabolic strategy. Nature Medicine*, 2015. **21**(3): pp. 288–294.

26. Poongavanam, M.-V., et al., *Ensemble and single-molecule biophysical characterization of D17. 4 DNA aptamer–IgE interactions. Biochimica et Biophysica Acta (BBA)-Proteins and Proteomics*, 2016. **1864**(1): pp. 154–164.

27. Li, W., et al., *Aptamers for thrombotic diseases. Aptamers for Medical Applications*, 2021, Singapore: Springer, pp. 279–318.

28. Wang, S.C., et al., *The landscape of nucleic-acid-based aptamers for treatment of hematologic malignancies: challenges and future directions. Bioengineering*, 2022. **9**(11): pp. 635.

29. Wang, M., et al., *Novel aptamer-functionalized nanoparticles enhances bone defect repair by improving stem cell recruitment. International Journal of Nanomedicine*, 2019. **14**: p. 8707.

30. Attia, N., et al., *Mesenchymal stem cells as a gene delivery tool: promise, problems, and prospects. Pharmaceutics*, 2021, 13: p. 843.

31. Heiat, M., et al., *Characterization of pharmacological properties of isolated single-stranded DNA aptamers against angiotensin II. Molecular and Cellular Probes*, 2016. **30**(4): pp. 238–245.
32. Nerantzaki, M., C. Loth, and J.-F. Lutz, *Chemical conjugation of nucleic acid aptamers and synthetic polymers. Polymer Chemistry*, 2021. **12**(24): pp. 3498–3509.
33. Zhu, G., et al., *Combinatorial screening of DNA aptamers for molecular imaging of HER2 in cancer. Bioconjugate Chemistry*, 2017. **28**(4): pp. 1068–1075.
34. Lee, J. and Y.-S. Rhee, *Ophthalmic dosage forms for drug delivery to posterior segment. Journal of Pharmaceutical Investigation*, 2022. **52**(2): pp. 161–173.
35. Prodeus, A., et al., *Targeting the PD-1/PD-L1 immune evasion axis with DNA aptamers as a novel therapeutic strategy for the treatment of disseminated cancers. Molecular Therapy-Nucleic Acids*, 2015. **4**: p. e237.
36. Yan, J., et al., *Aptamer-targeted photodynamic platforms for tumor therapy. ACS Applied Materials & Interfaces*, 2021. **13**(24): pp. 27749–27773.
37. Wong, T.Y., G. Liew, and P. Mitchell, *Clinical update: New treatments for age-related macular degeneration. The Lancet*, 2007. **370**(9583): pp. 204–206.
38. Le, J., et al., *One nanometer self-assembled aptamer-DNA dendrimers carry 350 doxorubicin: Super-stability and intra-nuclear DNA comet tail. Chemical Engineering Journal*, 2020. **388**: p. 124170.
39. Li, F., et al., *Characterization of a DNA aptamer for ovarian cancer clinical tissue recognition and in vivo imaging. Cellular Physiology and Biochemistry*, 2018. **51**(6): pp. 2564–2574.
40. Ulusoy, M., et al., *One-pot aqueous synthesis of highly strained CdTe/CdS/ZnS nanocrystals and their interactions with cells. RSC Advances*, 2015. **5**(10): pp. 7485–7494.
41. Tan, J., et al., *Aptamer-functionalized fluorescent silica nanoparticles for highly sensitive detection of leukemia cells. Nanoscale Research Letters*, 2016. **11**(1): pp. 1–8.
42. Chen, H.-L., et al., *Selection and characterization of DNA aptamers targeting all four serotypes of dengue viruses. PLoS one*, 2015. **10**(6): p. e0131240.
43. Chakraborty, S., et al., *A comparative investigation of the ability of various aptamer-functionalized drug nanocarriers to induce selective apoptosis in neoplastic hepatocytes: in vitro and in vivo outcome. AAPS Pharmscitech*, 2020. **21**(3): pp. 1–13.
44. Zheng, Y., et al., *DNA aptamers from whole-serum SELEX as new diagnostic agents against gastric cancer. RSC Advances*, 2019. **9**(2): pp. 950–957.
45. Zhuo, Z., et al., *Recent advances in SELEX technology and aptamer applications in biomedicine. International Journal of Molecular Sciences*, 2017. **18**(10): pp. 2142.
46. Hu, Z., et al., *Aptamer combined with fluorescent silica nanoparticles for detection of hepatoma cells. Nanoscale Research Letters*, 2017. **12**(1): pp. 1–8.
47. Li, X., et al., *Evolution of DNA aptamers through in vitro metastatic-cell-based systematic evolution of ligands by exponential enrichment for metastatic cancer recognition and imaging. Analytical Chemistry*, 2015. **87**(9): pp. 4941–4948.
48. Khoee, S. and S. Khezrian, *Applications of aptamers for the diagnosis and therapy of different diseases*, in *Nanostructures for Novel Therapy*. 2017, Amsterdam: Elsevier. pp. 591–619.
49. Chandola, C., et al., *Application of aptamers in diagnostics, drug-delivery and imaging. Journal of Biosciences*, 2016. **41**(3): pp. 535–561.
50. Chang, Y.-C., et al., *Rapid single cell detection of Staphylococcus aureus by aptamer-conjugated gold nanoparticles. Scientific Reports*, 2013. **3**(1): pp. 1–7.
51. Lavania, S., et al., *Aptamer-based TB antigen tests for the rapid diagnosis of pulmonary tuberculosis: potential utility in screening for tuberculosis. ACS Infectious Diseases*, 2018. **4**(12): pp. 1718–1726.
52. Hong, E.J., et al., *Cancer-targeted photothermal therapy using aptamer-conjugated gold nanoparticles. Journal of Industrial and Engineering Chemistry*, 2018. **67**: pp. 429–436.
53. Bohrmann, L., et al., *Aptamers used for molecular imaging and theranostics-recent developments. Theranostics*, 2022. **12**(9): p. 4010.
54. Okuda, M., D. Fourmy, and S. Yoshizawa, *Use of Baby Spinach and Broccoli for imaging of structured cellular RNAs. Nucleic Acids Research*, 2017. **45**(3): pp. 1404–1415.

55. Filonov, G.S., et al., *Broccoli: rapid selection of an RNA mimic of green fluorescent protein by fluorescence-based selection and directed evolution. Journal of the American Chemical Society*, 2014. **136**(46): pp. 16299–16308.

56. Dolgosheina, E.V., et al., *RNA mango aptamer-fluorophore: a bright, high-affinity complex for RNA labeling and tracking. ACS Chemical Biology*, 2014. **9**(10): pp. 2412–2420.

57. Song, W., et al., *Imaging RNA polymerase III transcription using a photostable RNA–fluorophore complex. Nature Chemical Biology*, 2017. **13**(11): pp. 1187–1194.

58. Sunbul, M. and A. Jäschke, *SRB-2: a promiscuous rainbow aptamer for live-cell RNA imaging. Nucleic Acids Research*, 2018. **46**(18): p. e110.

59. Yoon, S. and J.J. Rossi, *Targeted molecular imaging using aptamers in cancer. Pharmaceuticals*, 2018. **11**(3): p. 71.

60. Ning, Y., J. Hu, and F. Lu, *Aptamers used for biosensors and targeted therapy. Biomedicine & Pharmacotherapy*, 2020. **132**: p. 110902.

61. Goossens, N., et al., *Cancer biomarker discovery and validation. Translational Cancer Research*, 2015. **4**(3): p. 256.

62. Sawyers, C.L., *The cancer biomarker problem. Nature*, 2008. **452**(7187): pp. 548–552.

63. Tesmer, V.M., et al., *Molecular mechanism for inhibition of g protein-coupled receptor kinase 2 by a selective RNA aptamer. Structure*, 2012. **20**(8): pp. 1300–1309.

64. Kim, M., et al., *Applications of cancer cell-specific aptamers in targeted delivery of anticancer therapeutic agents. Molecules*, 2018. **23**(4): p. 830.

65. Hovanessian, A.G., et al., *Surface expressed nucleolin is constantly induced in tumor cells to mediate calcium-dependent ligand internalization. PloS one*, 2010. **5**(12): p. e15787.

66. Xing, H., et al., *Selective delivery of an anticancer drug with aptamer-functionalized liposomes to breast cancer cells in vitro and in vivo. Journal of Materials Chemistry B*, 2013. **1**(39): pp. 5288–5297.

67. Mongelard, F. and P. Bouvet, *AS-1411, a guanosine-rich oligonucleotide aptamer targeting nucleolin for the potential treatment of cancer, including acute myeloid leukemia. Current Opinion in Molecular Therapeutics*, 2010. **12**(1): pp. 107–114.

68. Ristau, B.T., D.S. O'Keefe, and D.J. Bacich. *The prostate-specific membrane antigen: lessons and current clinical implications from 20 years of research.* In *Urologic Oncology: Seminars and Original Investigations.* 2014. Amsterdam: Elsevier.

69. Dassie, J.P., et al., *Systemic administration of optimized aptamer-siRNA chimeras promotes regression of PSMA-expressing tumors. Nature Biotechnology*, 2009. **27**(9): pp. 839–846.

70. Zhou, J., et al., *Dual functional BAFF receptor aptamers inhibit ligand-induced proliferation and deliver siRNAs to NHL cells. Nucleic Acids Research*, 2013. **41**(7): pp. 4266–4283.

71. Catuogno, S., et al., *Selective delivery of therapeutic single strand antimiRs by aptamer-based conjugates. Journal of Controlled Release*, 2015. **210**: pp. 147–159.

72. Soldevilla, M.M., et al., *2-fluoro-RNA oligonucleotide CD40 targeted aptamers for the control of B lymphoma and bone-marrow aplasia. Biomaterials*, 2015. **67**: pp. 274–285.

73. Shu, D., et al., *Systemic delivery of anti-miRNA for suppression of triple negative breast cancer utilizing RNA nanotechnology. ACS Nano*, 2015. **9**(10): pp. 9731–9740.

74. Toma, S., et al., *Doxorubicin (or epidoxorubicin) combined with ifosfamide in the treatment of adult advanced soft tissue sarcomas. Annals of Oncology*, 1992. **3**: pp. S119–S123.

75. Lupold, S.E., et al., *Identification and characterization of nuclease-stabilized RNA molecules that bind human prostate cancer cells via the prostate-specific membrane antigen. Cancer Research*, 2002. **62**(14): pp. 4029–4033.

76. Bagalkot, V., et al., *An aptamer–doxorubicin physical conjugate as a novel targeted drug-delivery platform. Angewandte Chemie International Edition*, 2006. **45**(48): pp. 8149–8152.

77. Huang, Y.F., et al., *Molecular assembly of an aptamer–drug conjugate for targeted drug delivery to tumor cells. Chembiochem*, 2009. **10**(5): pp. 862–868.

78. Shangguan, D., et al., *Aptamers evolved from live cells as effective molecular probes for cancer study. Proceedings of the National Academy of Sciences*, 2006. **103**(32): pp. 11838–11843.

79. Pratico, E.D., B.A. Sullenger, and S.K. Nair, *Identification and characterization of an agonistic aptamer against the T cell costimulatory receptor, OX40. Nucleic Acid Therapeutics*, 2013. **23**(1): pp. 35–43.

80. Pastor, F., et al., *Targeting 4-1BB costimulation to disseminated tumor lesions with bi-specific oligonucleotide aptamers. Molecular Therapy*, 2011. **19**(10): pp. 1878–1886.

81. Chen, L. and X. Han, *Anti–PD-1/PD-L1 therapy of human cancer: past, present, and future*. The *Journal of Clinical Investigation*, 2015. **125**(9): pp. 3384–3391.

82. Heo, K., et al., *An aptamer-antibody complex (oligobody) as a novel delivery platform for targeted cancer therapies*. *Journal of Controlled Release*, 2016. **229**: pp. 1–9.

83. Davis, M.E., Z.G. Chen, and D.M. Shin, *Nanoparticle therapeutics: an emerging treatment modality for cancer*. *Nature Reviews Drug Discovery*, 2008. **7**(9): pp. 771–782.

84. Farokhzad, O.C., J.M. Karp, and R. Langer, *Nanoparticle–aptamer bioconjugates for cancer targeting*. *Expert Opinion on Drug Delivery*, 2006. **3**(3): pp. 311–324.

85. Agudelo, D., et al., *Intercalation of antitumor drug doxorubicin and its analogue by DNA duplex: structural features and biological implications*. *International Journal of Biological Macromolecules*, 2014. **66**: pp. 144–150.

86. Park, H., et al., *Comparison of Drug Delivery Efficiency between Doxorubicin Intercalated in RNA Aptamer and One Encapsulated in RNA Aptamer-Conjugated Liposome*. *Bulletin of the Korean Chemical Society*, 2015. **36**(10): pp. 2494–2500.

87. Willis, M.C., et al., *Liposome-anchored vascular endothelial growth factor aptamers*. *Bioconjugate Chemistry*, 1998. **9**(5): pp. 573–582.

88. Baek, S.E., et al., *RNA aptamer-conjugated liposome as an efficient anticancer drug delivery vehicle targeting cancer cells in vivo*. *Journal of Controlled Release*, 2014. **196**: pp. 234–242.

89. Wu, Y., et al., *DNA aptamer–micelle as an efficient detection/delivery vehicle toward cancer cells*. *Proceedings of the National Academy of Sciences*, 2010. **107**(1): pp. 5–10.

90. Sedletska, Y., M.-J. Giraud-Panis, and J.-M. Malinge, *Cisplatin is a DNA-damaging antitumour compound triggering multifactorial biochemical responses in cancer cells: importance of apoptotic pathways*. *Current Medicinal Chemistry-Anti-Cancer Agents*, 2005. **5**(3): pp. 251–265.

91. Dhar, S., et al., *Targeted delivery of cisplatin to prostate cancer cells by aptamer functionalized Pt (IV) prodrug-PLGA–PEG nanoparticles*. *Proceedings of the National Academy of Sciences*, 2008. **105**(45): pp. 17356–17361.

92. Bagalkot, V., et al., *Quantum dot– aptamer conjugates for synchronous cancer imaging, therapy, and sensing of drug delivery based on bi-fluorescence resonance energy transfer*. *Nano Letters*, 2007. **7**(10): pp. 3065–3070.

93. Wang, A.Z., et al., *Superparamagnetic iron oxide nanoparticle–aptamer bioconjugates for combined prostate cancer imaging and therapy*. *Chemmedchem: Chemistry Enabling Drug Discovery*, 2008. **3**(9): pp. 1311–1315.

94. Kim, D., Y.Y. Jeong, and S. Jon, *A drug-loaded aptamer– gold nanoparticle bioconjugate for combined CT imaging and therapy of prostate cancer*. *ACS Nano*, 2010. **4**(7): pp. 3689–3696.

95. Min, K., et al., *Dual-aptamer-based delivery vehicle of doxorubicin to both PSMA (+) and PSMA (−) prostate cancers*. *Biomaterials*, 2011. **32**(8): pp. 2124–2132.

96. Zitzmann, S., et al., *A new prostate carcinoma binding peptide (DUP-1) for tumor imaging and therapy*. *Clinical Cancer Research*, 2005. **11**(1): pp. 139–146.

97. Zhang, L., et al., *Quantum dot-aptamer conjugates for synchronous cancer imaging and therapy based on bi-fluorescence resonance energy transfer*. *Clinical Cancer Research*, 2007. **13**(19_ Supplement): pp. A19–A19.

98. Zhou, Z., M. Liu, and J. Jiang, *The potential of aptamers for cancer research*. *Analytical Biochemistry*, 2018. **549**: pp. 91–95.

99. Li, Y., et al., *A simple aptamer-functionalized gold nanorods based biosensor for the sensitive detection of MCF-7 breast cancer cells*. *Chemical Communications*, 2016. **52**(20): pp. 3959–3961.

100. Pirsaheb, M., S. Mohammadi, and A. Salimi, *Current advances of carbon dots based biosensors for tumor marker detection, cancer cells analysis and bioimaging*. *TrAC Trends in Analytical Chemistry*, 2019. **115**: pp. 83–99.

15 Polyamidoamine-Based Anticancer Therapies

Maria Manan, Rida Siddique, Maryam Shabir,
Azhar Rasul, Nosheen Aslam, Uzma Saleem,
Muhammad Yasir Ali, Shazia Anwer Bukhari,
and Mulazim Hussain Asim

15.1 INTRODUCTION

The terminology "dendrimer," which derives from the Greek terms "dendron" and "mer," which mean "tree" and "part," respectively, was used by chemists to characterize molecules having dendritic features resembling trees [1]. PAMAM has continued to be one of the most often utilized systems among the several varieties of dendrimers [2]. The polyamidoamine (PAMAM) dendrimer is a polymeric molecule that branches out into several monomers from a central core that has a large number of active amine groups and a large number of reactive groups on the surface [3]. For precise targeting, PAMAM dendrimers can be engineered with a variety of functional groups [3–6]. PAMAM dendrimers were not without limitations too, which hindered their commercial acceptability [4]. For instance, PAMAM is cytotoxic and is quickly excreted from the body's circulation after being supplied intravenously because it has positive amine groups on its surface. Drugs can be distributed throughout the dendritic structure, trapped on the surface, or enclosed within the PAMAM's enormous interior cavity to prevent physiological degradation. It is also suitable for passive drug targeting because it increases tumor cell permeation and retention, enhanced permeation and retention (EPR), which reduces the negative effects of loaded drugs. The PAMAM dendrimers' acceptable biodegradation, regulated drug release, and limited non-specific blood-protein binding capabilities are further benefits [7]. PAMAM dendrimers are useful in many investigations and applications because of their dendritic characteristics, peptide/protein mimic qualities, and reliable production, with certain PAMAM dendrimers being commercially accessible at reasonable prices [1, 8, 9]. In this study, we will focus on the most aggressive and commonly diagnosed types of cancer are of brain, breast, ovarian, and gastric, where PAMAM dendrimer has recently made success. We emphasize PAMAM dendrimers' potential to deliver gene therapies and anticancer medications [3].

15.2 STRUCTURE OF PAMAM DENDRIMERS

The first family of absolute PAMAM dendrimers was created, described, published, and marketed in 1984 by Tomalia and colleagues [5]. PAMAM dendrimers are distinguished by their three distinct structural elements: (1) a core, (2) branches made up of amide groups that branch out from a tertiary amine and create cavities, and (3) terminal groups. The ethylenediamine core was the first to be reported, which is abbreviated as EDA. Later, PAMAM dendrimers were created using several other cores, including cystamine, diaminobutane (DAB), diaminohexane, and diaminododecane [6]. Amido linkages seen in PAMAM dendrimer branches resemble the peptide backbones of

 DOI: 10.1201/9781003363958-18

proteins [6]. Several functional groups, such as NH2, OH, CHO, COOMe, Boc, COONa, or CH3 groups, might end PAMAM's superficial branches. PAMAM dendrimers are a class of artificial macromolecules that are highly branching and monodisperse [10], meaning that they have a consistent size and shape throughout their whole surface [8] and well-defined structures and makeup [10]. To create homo-structural layers (branching units), "wedges" or "dendrons" extend outward from the central core [11, 12]. PAMAMs are cationic dendrimers of the polyamidoamine type that may produce up to ten generations [9]. These are three-dimensional, 1–10 nm-sized molecules with distinct physiochemical characteristics [13].

Dendrimers grow in size when new generations are produced. The density of the molecules packed onto the surface of the dendrimer will determine the size of the dendrimer. With PAMAM dendrimers, Tomalia et al. reported an exponential rise in the number of surface groups and a linear rise in the diameter [9]. The fact that the flexibility of peripheral groups increases with generation and the distance between functional groups on the dendrimer's perimeter reduces as a result is a significant result [7]. After PAMAM G7, this steric crowding of branches intensifies, which results in the creation of a faulty structure (De Gennes dense packing effect). Following the eleventh generation, the synthetic yield has decreased [14]. Dendrimers cannot develop at this point due to a lack of available space. The "starburst effect" is the name given to this phenomenon [12]. The number of generations has an impact on the morphology of the polymer.

15.3 POLY (AMIDOAMINE) DENDRIMER

One of the most often utilized compounds in research, created on an industrial scale, is polyamidoamine (PAMAM) dendrimers (Figure 15.1). The PAMAM family of dendrimers was among the first to be completely characterized, synthesized, and marketed [15–18]. Methyl acrylate and ethylenediamine are the two substances that are most frequently used to create internal branches, whereas substances with a lot of amide or carboxylic groups are typically used to build surface groups [11].

The linear chain molecules accumulate to form the PAMAM core to start the most important structural variation process called stepwise polymerization with each generation G0 to G6 the molecular weight and number of active surfaces increased exponentially and their diameter increased linearly [19].

15.4 PHYSICOCHEMICAL PROPERTIES

15.4.1 Size

Dendrimers and biological polymers are extremely similar in their topologies, roles, and physical characteristics. They have several characteristics similar to proteins. Due to their nanometric dimensions and other protein-like characteristics, dendrimers can be identified as synthetic proteins with biomimetic characteristics [20].

15.4.2 Higher Solubilization Potential

PAMAM dendrimers may be changed to bind different targeted or guest molecules and are biocompatible, non-immunogenic, water-soluble, and have amine functional groups at the end. Several factors, including generation type, temperature, pH, core, dendrimer concentration, and terminal functionality, can affect dendrimer-mediated solubility [21].

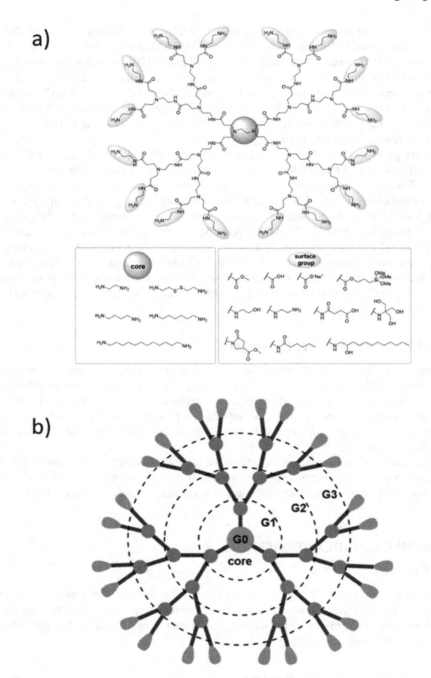

FIGURE 15.1 (a) Chemical structure of poly(amidoamine) dendrimer with a core and surface functional group; (b) cartoon illustration of dendrimer structure shows the generations. The central core is generation 0 (G0); generation 1 (G1), generation 2 (G2), and generation 3 (G3) of dendrimer refer to the first, second, and third levels of branching, respectively [1].

15.4.3 HIGH CAPACITY FOR LOADING

The structure of dendrimers may be used to load and store a variety of inorganic and organic chemicals through covalent bonding with the surface and electrostatic interactions on the surface [22].

15.5 SYNTHESIS OF POLYAMIDOAMINE DENDRIMERS

Throughout the years, different techniques have been created to create PAMAM dendrimers [23]. There are four well-known methods for making PAMAM dendrimers [24]. They are described as follows:

15.5.1 SYNTHESIS OF PAMAM BY CONVERGENT METHOD

To overcome some of the drawbacks of the divergent technique, Hawker and Frechet created the convergent method in 1990. In contrast to the divergent technique, the top-down approach creates dendritic segments, or dendrons, of increasing size as the synthesis proceeds by "one-to-one" coupling of monomers from the surface to the center of a dendrimer [17]. While there are minor flaws in branch development during synthesis brought on by retro-Micheal reactions and intramolecular lactam production, the quality of the dendrimer is around 98% [18]. This results in fewer reactive sites throughout the proliferation process, which speeds up response rates and yields [17]. Several non-symmetrically internally branched PAMAM-type dendrimers were synthesized via convergence, according to Pittelkow and Christensen. In this synthesis, a very effective peptide coupling reagent is combined with extremely effective protection group chemistry. This process may be thought of as a unique convergent strategy for creating a number of internally branched PAMAM dendrimers in the solution phase [25].

15.5.2 SYNTHESIS OF PAMAM BY THE DIVERGENT METHOD

The "divergent technique" was the first approach Tomalia proposed. In divergent synthesis, the monomer molecules with one reactive and two dormant groups react with the core to create the PAMAM dendrimer, which grows from a multifunctional core. First-generation PAMAM dendrimer is created as a result of this reaction. The molecule's newly activated perimeter then reacts with more monomers, and this cycle is continued until the necessary number of generations is reached [26, 27]. Unfortunately, this synthesis approach can be stopped by side reactions that result in imperfect or incomplete dendrimers. The inability to completely purify the end products and the lengthy multistep reactions are further limitations of this approach [28]. By combining a protection/ deprotection technique with a divergent/divergent approach, Martin and Twyman were able to synthesize unsymmetrical dendrimers. Excellent yields were achieved for all dendrimers, necessitating little to no purification [29].

15.5.3 SYNTHESIS OF PAMAM BY COMBINED CONVERGENT-DIVERGENT METHOD

In this method, the building monomers are first synthesized by a divergent approach followed by dendrimers' assembly by the convergent process. Higher-generation dendrimers can be prepared more quickly than divergent or convergent synthesis because of the possibility of reducing the number of reactions necessary for dendrimer synthesis and purification. This method also has the benefit of allowing for the structural variety of the dendrimers to be added by altering the building blocks during dendrimer synthesis [1]. It is a sophisticated technique of dendrimer synthesis that creates a triangle known as a "dendrimer" using both divergent and convergent approaches. Repetition of the growing process might be done using the triangle, resulting in the exponential growth of the dendrimers and therefore is called as double exponential growth [30].

15.5.4 Synthesis of PAMAM by the Click Chemistry Method

The copper-catalyzed azide-alkyne cycloaddition (CuAAC) reaction is used in the click chemistry process, which is one of the most widely used approaches for the synthesis of PAMAM dendrimers. This process produces a dendrimer by reacting an azide-functionalized dendron with an alkyne-functionalized core molecule in the presence of a copper catalyst. This method was quoted to be the most efficient one [31]. A connection between dendritic structures and nanomaterials is made possible by the click dendrimers [32].

15.6 POLYAMIDOAMINE-BASED CANCER THERAPIES

Cancer is a very traumatic disorder and every year millions of cases are being documented [33]. Tumor treatment utilizing traditional anticancer drugs has been impeded by many problems like acute side effects, less permeability, quick elimination, and short therapeutic index. Drugs are available that show excellent efficacy in cancer but the effectiveness of current chemotherapeutics is restricted by their inability to go to the targeted site in adequate quantity to be effective [33].

Most patients are given an increased dose of medicines, which are distributed throughout the body, and also distributes in healthy cells and tissues, causing immune system depression. These drugs also possess a short therapeutic index and huge side effects [34]. A major problem happens when these drugs affect healthy cells of the body like red and white blood cells and cause nausea and diarrhea [35]. To decrease these side effects drug administration to the cancerous area is maximized by designing vectors containing a drug capable of precisely targeting tumor cells [36–38].

On this subject, a huge range of nanosystems like micelles, dendrimers, liposomes, nanoparticles, and carbon nanotubes can be used to increase drug loading and allow drug deposition in target tumor cells while decreasing absorption in healthy cells [39, 40]. The design of smart cancer therapies involves planning such nanosystems' loading medicine and gene, which can target tumor tissues both actively and passively [41]. Gene and novel antitumor strategies constitute the use of strong and unstable agents like aptamers, miRNA, antibodies, and siRNA that rapidly break down and have less stability [42]. The big drawback of traditional antitumor agents is inadequate therapeutic response and side effects involving normal tissues. To overwhelm these problems investigation for new efficacious vectors is very crucial [43].

They may save the unstable agents from breaking down, increasing targeting efficacy, maximizing drug release, and decreasing the side effects like healthy tissue deposition of antitumor drugs [44–46]. The most extensively analyzed dendrimers used as vectors for medical uses are polyamidoamine (PAMAM) and poly (propylene imine) (PPI) [47, 48]. Dendrimers on account of their right, advanced, and consistent drug design variables, overwhelming the physicochemical drawbacks of conventional drugs (specificity, solubility, stability, biodistribution, and clinical effectiveness) are promising. They can also bypass the biological issues to go to the targeted site like immune system excretion, cell penetration, first-pass metabolism, and binding with untargeted sites [49].

Polyamidoamine dendrimers can be effectively utilized in tumor treatment on account of physical encapsulation and covalent conjugation [9, 50]. Additionally, dendrimers are progressively utilized in cancer treatment. They accumulate in cancerous areas that confirm the release of specified drugs in specified doses. In traditional medicines, the issue comes out to be less efficient in the delivery of drugs to the cancerous site [51].

These days many polyamidoamine-based drug vectors have been prepared to investigate their potential for cancer treatment. In previous research work, various types of entities like targeting and therapeutic agents have been complexed with polyamidoamine for preparing more soluble and non-toxic nanovectors. Polyamidoamine dendrimers exhibit selective administration of drugs to the cancerous site in comparison with free drugs [52, 53].

15.6.1 POLYAMIDOAMINE-BASED DRUG ADMINISTRATION

15.6.1.1 Passive Targeting

A cardinal passive targeting strategy was established by Maeda and Matsumura, called the enhanced permeability and retention (EPR) effect [10, 54]. This ERP has been extensively utilized for treating tumors.

A few unique characteristics of tumors like flaws in blood vessel construction, leaky vasculature due to hyperproliferative blood vessels, and malfunctioning lymphatic drainage are accountable for the EPR effect. Tumor management by intravenous delivery of a polymer-based transport system can generate upto 100 fold increased concentration of drug on account of this EPR effect [55]. That is why scientists frequently utilized these polymer-based delivery systems.

15.6.1.2 Active Targeting

In active targeting, a specific ligand is covalently attached to a drug carrier, which can be identified by the receptor, that is over-expressed in the target sites as compared to healthy tissues [10] (Table 15.1). Identification of ligands by receptor causes slow aggregation of polymer-based nanosystems at the diseased site [56, 57]. Active targeting is chiefly accomplished by powerful ligand-receptor attaching ability and additionally, this attachment also enhances the internalization of drug carriers by increasing cellular absorption. Cancer cells are featured by rapid proliferation with 24 hours doubling time as compared to healthy cells with days to weeks doubling time [58].

15.6.2 POLYAMIDOAMINE-BASED GENE ADMINISTRATION

Nucleic acids are administered to inhibit the expression of different genes, which are accountable for the production of various proteins. Changes in these proteins can perform an important function in fighting against many diseases like cancer. The successful administration of nucleic acid-based drugs like plasmid DNA, oligonucleotides, siRNA, and ribosomes into cells requires efficacious delivery agents, which should be safe and exhibit selectivity for target tissues [65–67].

Uncovered nucleic acids are certainly broken down by nucleases, having a short half-life. It is important to make carriers to save them from enzymatic breakdown. Furthermore prolonging their half-lives causes increased retention time, thereby increasing the likelihood of absorption into target tissues. Besides it is also cardinal to administer nucleic acid into suitable places inside the cell-like cytoplasm, mitochondria, and nucleus [10]. Viral carriers like adenoviruses and retroviruses have enough ability for the administration of a nucleic acid-based drug into the target tissues.

TABLE 15.1
PAMAM Bearing Ligand-Based Drug Administration

PAMAM	Receptor	Ligand	Drug	Target cell	Reference
G4	CD44	HA	Curcumin	MiaPaCa-2 cancer cell lines	[59]
G5	FA receptor	FA	Paclitaxel	KB cell line	[60]
G4	Somatostatin receptors	Octreotide	Methotrexate	MCF-7	[61]
G4	αvβ3	RGD	Doxorubicin	Glioma cell	[62]
G5	FA receptor	FA	Methotrexate	KB tumor cells	[63]
G4	VEGF	Flt-1	Gemcitabine	Pancreatic cancer	[64]

Notes: FA: Folic acid, αvβ3: Alpha-v beta-3, VEGF: Vascular endothelial growth factor, MiaPaCa- 2: hypotriploid human pancreatic cancer cell line, KB cell line: human epithelial carcinoma cells, MCF-7 (Michigan Cancer Foundation-7); breast cancer cell line.

Nevertheless, viral-based carriers also exhibit side effects like immunogenic reactions and the likelihood to develop cancer into the target cell DNA [68–70]. These crucial drawbacks have given rise to an investigation for non-viral carriers, which will not show immunogenicity and carcinogenicity [68]. The positive charge on the PAMAM surface and negative charge on the nucleic acid phosphate backbone link with each other, hence producing stable complexes like PAMAM-siRNA or PAMAM-DNA, also called dendriplexes. These dendriplexes exhibit strong effectiveness of transfection and strong capability to save the nucleic acid from breakdown [71, 72].

15.6.2.1 DNA Administration Utilizing Polyamidoamine Nanosystems

It was reported that folic acid (FA) was conjugated onto polyamidoamine dendrimer to serve as a DNA gene carrier administering genes in neck and head tumor cells (Table 15.2) [71].

15.6.2.2 RNA Administration Utilizing Polyamidoamine's Nanosystems

Small-interfering RNA (siRNA) exhibits a crucial function in inhibiting many cellular pathways through breakdown of mRNA, which codes for important genes. siRNA suppresses signaling pathways linked with tissue proliferation. Additionally, siRNA has an extraordinary ability to decrease the expression of different genes to enhance the function of anticancer medications against cancer [10].

15.6.3 POLYAMIDOAMINE-BASED CO-DELIVERY SYSTEM

Tumor normally evolves resistance to any anticancer drug that was originally successful giving rise to therapeutic failure. Hence combination treatment utilizing drug and drug or drug and gene are being investigated to reduce the resistance [77–79].

5.0G PAMAM was conjugated with HA for efficacious administration of DOX, in addition to siRNA targeting major vault protein (MVP). MVP-siRNA can decrease the expression of MVP and enhance the cytotoxicity of DOX. The outcomes of this research work described that cancer targeting, blood circulation, and cytotoxicity were increased by utilizing DOX-PAMAM-HA complex in comparison with DOX alone. Additionally, co-administration of DOX-PAMAM-HA along with MVP-siRNA exhibited adequate gene silencing, increased stability, and efficacious aggregation of siRNA, which give rise to elevated cytotoxicity [80].

15.6.3.1 Polyamidoamines for Treating Breast Cancer

Trastuzumab is a monoclonal antibody, which remarkably decreased the risk of recurrence and enhanced survival in females with metastatic tumors. It was the initial treatment accepted by the

TABLE 15.2
PAMAM Dendrimer-Based Gene Administration

PAMAM	Receptor	Ligand	Nucleic Acid	Target Cells	References
G5	αvβ3	RGD	siRNA	U87 glioma cells	[73]
G5	CD44	Thioaptamer	miRNA	breast cancer	[74]
G4	FA receptor	FA	siRNA-VEGFA	HN12 and HN12-YFP cells	[75]
G5	FA receptor	FA	DNA	KB cells	[76]

Notes: FA: Folic acid, αvβ3: αvβ3: Alpha-v beta-3, siRNA: Small-interfering RNA, miRNA: MicroRNAs, VEGFA: Vascular Endothelial Growth Factor A, CD44: cluster of differentiation 44; a non-kinase transmembrane glycoprotein, RGD: Arginylglycylaspartic acid, U87: human glioblastoma cell line.

Food and Drug Administration for the management of breast cancer [81, 82]. Trastuzumab was successfully used for the treatment of human epidermal growth factor receptor-2 (HER2) breast tumors. Unfortunately, this therapy was linked with many side effects including cardiotoxicity [83]. A remarkable number of people receiving anti-HER2-based treatment with trastuzumab exhibited resistance to therapy.

Therefore much research work has been carried out to develop combination therapies to reduce this resistance [84, 85]. Many studies have exhibited that neratinib combined with trastuzumab was efficacious in reducing the resistance, ameliorated the response rate, and causing a synergistic effect. Neratinib, is a kinase inhibitor used for treating HER2-overexpressed breast tumors [86].

Trastuzumab grafted G4 PAMAM dendrimer loaded with neratinib exhibited selectivity and increased antiproliferation activity against (HER2) cells in comparison with neratinib in plain or neratinib combined with G4 PAMAM dendrimer. Increased cellular absorption and higher cytotoxicity of trastazumab conjugated dendrimer loaded with neratinib was shown [82]. Increased chemotherapeutic effectiveness was noted.

Doxorubicin-loaded PAMAM-PF68 conjugates showed more anticancer activity than doxorubincin alone in MCF-7/ADR cells. Deeper penetration enhanced cancer inhibition, and enhanced drug accumulation with little cardiotoxicity was also observed in DOX-loaded PAMAM-n2 PF68 conjugates as compared to free doxorubicin [57]. MCF-7 (Michigan Cancer Foundation–7)/ADR cells have been extensively utilized as a multidrug-resistant breast tumor cell model in tumor research [57].

15.6.3.2 Polyamidiamine Drug Combinations for Treating Prostate Cancer

Cells treated with Paclitaxel (PTX) conjugated with PAMAM dendrimer showed significant morphological changes in cell size and shape and increased apoptosis in cultured prostate cancer cell line cells [87]. This could be on account of the enhanced solubility of the drug and cellular absorption of PTX-dendrimer conjugate by PC-3M cells. Paclitaxel is a chemotherapeutic agent, which has been accepted for the management of different types of cancers. A serious issue with developing Paclitaxel in cancer treatment is its inadequate aqueous solubility [88, 89].

Polyamidoamine G4 dendrimers have been investigated as transport vectors for many oligonucleotides like siRNAs for the previous two decades [90]. Doxorubicin shows adequate effectiveness as a commonly utilized antitumor drug. However, on account of its adverse effects remarkably a cardiomyopathy, polyamidoamine-based nanosystem has been developed to decrease the side effects of doxorubicin and maintain its effectiveness simultaneously [91, 92]. To inhibit the aggregation of the drug in the lung doxorubicin-dendrimer complexes were designed, decreasing the metastatic lung burden after its uptake [93]. In the complex doxorubicin is complexed with PAMAM via hydrazine bonds [94].

There are many examples of polyamidoamine dendrimers utilized in drug administration. The dendrimer 4 (G4) polyamidoamine has been suggested to complex paclitaxel via a glycinephenylalanine-leucine-glycine peptide linker. In agreement with experimental outcomes paclitaxel-dendrimer complex shows increased cytotoxicity in comparison with free paclitaxel. Using this approach it would be possible to deliver paclitaxel to renal tissues for renal tumor therapy [95].

In addition to PTX-dendrimer complex generation, 4 polyamidoamine can be used in active targeting therapy [95, 96]. In the paclitaxel administration for active targeting, polyethylene glycol is applied in the encapsulating procedure of docetaxel, changed with trastuzumab on the surface of polyamidoamine dendrimers [97]. Absorption of this molecule has been documented to be 70%, more than that observed with free docetaxel in cancers [96]. Polyamidoamine dendrimers can ameliorate the effects of drug delivery for tumor treatment after surface modifications with different kinds of molecules [91].

15.6.3.3 PAMAM Application in Malignant Gliomas

Most people who develop gliomas, the most common primary brain tumor, passed away within a few years. Despite the extensive use of surgery, radiation, and chemotherapy in the treatment of malignant gliomas, the therapeutic outcome is consistently poor. Therefore, the development of safe and effective drug and gene delivery systems is essential [98].

A unique family of macromolecules known as dendrimers has internal cavities, readily modifiable peripheral groups, and programmable nanoscale sizes. In particular, certain significant proteins and bio-assemblies substantially resemble the sizes and shapes of poly (amidoamine) (PAMAM) dendrimers [99].

It is widely recognized that controlling the number of anticancer medications that accumulate in tumors rather than permeate into healthy tissues in vivo is a significant challenge. This can result in dangerous side effects and even patient death. To investigate the targeting effects, a variety of targeting agents have been explored to conjugate on the surface of dendrimers. The receptors (FRs) of folic acid (FA) have received much research for therapeutic targeting since they are overexpressed on cancer cells and activated macrophages while having a restricted distribution in healthy tissues. The benefits of utilizing FA as a ligand are due to its high affinity for FRs, which was maintained even after FA was conjugated to other molecules via the g-carboxyl group, and its smaller size and lower molecular weight, which result in a deeper penetration effect than antibodies [100].

Mammen et al. present in a study a PAMAM dendrimer-based drug delivery system (G4-FA-PEG/DOX) with doxorubicin (DOX) enclosed in the interior and FA directly conjugated to the carrier's periphery to benefit from the "cluster" effect. DOX was a well-known and efficient anticancer medication that was also reported to be able to cure gliomas [101]. Moreover, the addition of free FA might impede cellular uptake, demonstrating the targeting function of FA in the delivery of medications specifically to glioma tumors [98].

15.6.3.4 Polyamidoamines in Gastric Cancer

The second most frequent primary cause of cancer-related mortality in gastric cancer (GC). The CD44-marked cancer stem cell (CSC) was crucial in the development of GC. Recombinant methioninase (rMETase) was extensively used as a GC chemotherapeutic alternative. Systems for synthetic polymer nanoparticle medication delivery have been widely employed in the treatment of cancer. Hyaluronic acid (HA), a CD44 receptor, is used to decorate nanoparticles, which enhances their biocompatibility and water solubility [102].

Most cancer cells require a higher amount of methionine (MET) for self-growth than normal cells do. *Clostridium*, *Aeromonas*, and *Pseudomonas putida* all have the high-efficiency MET depleting enzyme, L-methioninedeamino-mercaptomethane lyase (METase). In order to create recombinant methioninase (rMETase), which is utilized as a treatment for gastric cancer, the METase gene was cloned onto the pcDNA3.1(-) vector [103, 104].

The fifth-generation PAMAM (G5-PAMAM) was used to trap gold nanoparticles (AuNPs), which helped to preserve the dendrimers' 3D spherical form and increased the effectiveness of gene transfection. Moreover, PAMAM's surface was covered with HA to optimize its targeting of CD44+ gastric cancer stem cells and lessen its intrinsic toxicity, which increased the effectiveness of this nanoparticle's interaction with carrying METase [105].

15.6.3.5 Polyamidoamines Applications in Ovarian Cancer

Due to the development of drug resistance and expansion into the peritoneal cavity, which causes ascites, these later tumors typically do not respond to chemotherapy. For the effective treatment of these resistant tumors, targeted administration of large dosages of chemotherapeutics employing cancer cell-specific ligands may be a promising option [106].

A vital vitamin, biotin is found in high concentrations in rapidly multiplying cells like cancer cells. Biotin molecules are used in the manufacturing of poly(amido)amine dendrimers, which improve cancer cell-specific absorption [107].

Several innovative delivery systems employ the biotinylation technique as an appealing method to increase the system's targeting potential. It was demonstrated to be a very effective substitute for medications like Paclitaxel, which has certain cytotoxic effects and is only moderately soluble in water [108]. The overall findings supported the possibility of using biotinylated PAMAM dendrimer as a medication delivery system to specifically target ovarian cancer cells [109].

15.6.3.6 PAMAM Drug Combinations for Treating Brain Cancer

A commercially available PAMAM dendrimer was utilized with polyethylene glycol via binding of the amine group of PAMAM to the stimulated N-hydroxysuccinimide groups present on the surface of PEG [110]. The delivery vehicle formed by the binding of PAMAM with polyethylene glycol loaded with doxorubicin enhanced the development of glioma cells and enhanced the uptake of doxorubicin in vitro [111].

PAMAM dendrimers are important vectors for efficacious area-specific peptide targeting due to having the potential to enhance the bioavailability of drugs in addition to decreasing the dosing frequency [112, 113]. 3G polyamidoamine combined with PTX exhibited 12 times enhanced permeability of PTX in comparison with the drug administered alone [114]. The study showed a two times enhanced deposition of Pep-PEG-dendrimer in the target area in comparison with untargeted dendrimer. A biodistribution investigation also showed huge distribution in the target areas and quick excretion via liver due to its small size [115]. PAMAM dendrimers increased the retention time, which may enhance the efficacy of the transport system against brain cancer [116].

15.6.3.7 Polyamidiamine for Treating Cervical Cancer

Octa-arginine (R8) altered G4 poly (amidoamine) dendrimer was synthesized, PEGylated, and complexed with less soluble molecule paclitaxel (PTX). Cellular delivery in cervical tumor tissues showed that R8 changes noticeably ameliorated the cell association of complexes. R8-G4 PAMAM-PEG-PTX complex exhibited increased cytotoxicity and increased apoptosis as compared to free PTX. Increased intracellular transport of R8 altered PAMAM caused ameliorated anticancer effectiveness. That is why this novel transport system is effective for the intracellular transport of paclitaxel in tumor cells and possesses a potent ability to be used as an efficacious chemotherapeutic drug for cancer [117].

15.6.3.8 Polyamidiamine Applications in Retinal Tumor

Subconjunctival administration of PAMAM dendrimer nanosystem attached with carboplatin reduced the mean tumor load remarkably in the treated eyes as compared to untreated eyes in murine transgenic retinoblastoma. Only one injection of subconjunctival PAMAM carboplatin was efficacious in the management of transgenic murine retinoblastoma, free of any adverse effects. The increased dose of subconjunctival nanosystem carboplatin reduced the cancer load in the opposite eye [118].

15.6.3.9 Polyamidoamine for Treating Bone Cancer

3G PAMAM dendrimer has been complexed with carboxylic acids like aconitic acid, succinic acid, aspartic and glutamic acid and then PEGylated. In vitro investigations were done to analyze the binding of PAMAM complexes with calcium and hydroxyapatite. Bone accumulation was performed with PAMAM dendrimer radiolabeled with ^{111}Indium (^{111}In). Outcomes showed that PAMAM complexed with aspartic acid exhibited good results than others in bone deposition [119].

15.6.3.10 Polyamidoamine Therapy for Treating Myeloid Leukemia

One of the most important drugs for treating acute myeloid leukemia is 1-d-Arabinofuranosylcytosine (Cytarabine, Ara-C). There are a few drawbacks to Ara-C, including its quick deactivation by cytidine deaminase, which leads to the formation of the biologically inactive metabolite Ara-U (1-d-arabinofuranosyluracil), as well as its quick elimination from the body. To solve these issues, a conjugate in which the drug (Ara-C) was carried by PEG and hydroxyl-terminated PAMAM dendrimer G4-OH ["D,"] was designed. A covalent link was formed between the main hydroxyl group of Ara-C and dendrimer/PEG as a result of the effective multistep protection/deprotection conjugate synthesis technique.

The physicochemical characteristics, drug release kinetics, and structure were all thoroughly studied. Ten Ara-C molecules seemed to be covalently attached to the dendrimer, according to 1H NMR and MALDI-TOF mass spectrometry. Ara-C was released over 14 days in phosphate buffered saline (PBS), with the release speeding up in human plasma, according to the release profile in PBS buffer (pH 7.4) and human plasma. A549 human adenocarcinoma epithelial cells were used to assess how well dendrimer-Ara-C and PEG-Ara-C conjugates inhibited cancer growth. After 72 hours of treatment, free Ara-C was fourfold less efficient in inhibiting A549 cells than dendrimer or PEG-Ara-C conjugates [120].

15.7 CONCLUSION

Regular chemotherapies have been the foundation for treating cancer but are a long way from being fully up to the mark, on account of issues concerning their manufacturing, pharmacokinetics, and extreme adverse effects of such treatments. In recent decades, immense development has been carried out for an understanding of disease and the designing of novel targeted therapies. Unfortunately, effective therapy for various types of cancer remains a main question. Recently drugs and gene delivery based on dendrimers as a carrier have proved a good option to control the drawbacks of regular chemotherapy.

Recently, 50% of tumors are not treatable and nanovectors may assist to reduce the percentage. Nanomedicines represent one of the fastest developing research domains and are considered as one of the most hopeful ways of tumor therapy. Many solutions grounded on nanoparticles have been designed and various are used in clinical cancer care. Liposomes and polymer complexes were the primary nanovectors to be accepted by the Food and Drug Administration, although just five liposomal medicines, two dendrimers, and two protein-polymer complexes are on the market nowadays.

PAMAM dendrimers can be used in tumor treatment, like chemotherapy and gene therapy. Chemotherapies include anticancer drugs like doxorubicin and paclitaxel, which show high cytotoxicity to healthy cells in addition to cancer cells. The surfaces altered PAMAM dendrimers can complex anticancer drugs via chemical or physical interlinkage and transfer them specifically to the targeted area with decreased cytotoxicity and increased cellular absorption. Inhibition of nucleic acid breakdown during the administration of enhanced cellular absorption is the main concern relating to gene therapy. That is why new approaches have been designed to ameliorate PAMAM dendrimer performance as nucleic acid vectors. In conclusion, PAMAM dendrimers possess strong potential for treating tumors, while new changes can propel them more into clinical use.

REFERENCES

1. Lyu, Z., et al., *Poly (amidoamine) dendrimers: covalent and supramolecular synthesis. Materials Today Chemistry*, 2019. **13**: pp. 34–48.

2. Luong, D., et al., *PEGylated PAMAM dendrimers: Enhancing efficacy and mitigating toxicity for effective anticancer drug and gene delivery. Acta Biomaterialia*, 2016. **43**: pp. 14–29.

3. Surekha, B., et al., *PAMAM dendrimer as a talented multifunctional biomimetic nanocarrier for cancer diagnosis and therapy. Colloids and Surfaces B: Biointerfaces*, 2021. **204**: p. 111837.

4. Yellepeddi, V.K., A. Kumar, and S. Palakurthi, *Surface modified poly (amido) amine dendrimers as diverse nanomolecules for biomedical applications. Expert Opinion on Drug Delivery*, 2009. **6**(8): pp. 835–850.

5. Kharwade, R., et al., *Starburst pamam dendrimers: synthetic approaches, surface modifications, and biomedical applications. Arabian Journal of Chemistry*, 2020. **13**(7): pp. 6009–6039.

6. Florendo, M., et al., *Use of polyamidoamine dendrimers in brain diseases. Molecules*, 2018. **23**(9): p. 2238.

7. Taghavi Pourianazar, N., P. Mutlu, and U. Gunduz, *Bioapplications of poly (amidoamine)(PAMAM) dendrimers in nanomedicine. Journal of Nanoparticle Research*, 2014. **16**: pp. 1–38.

8. Dufès, C., I.F. Uchegbu, and A.G. Schätzlein, *Dendrimers in gene delivery. Advanced Drug Delivery Reviews*, 2005. **57**(15): pp. 2177–2202.

9. Bober, Z., D. Bartusik-Aebisher, and D. Aebisher, *Application of dendrimers in anticancer diagnostics and therapy. Molecules*, 2022. **27** (10): p. 3237.

10. Abedi-Gaballu, F., et al., *PAMAM dendrimers as efficient drug and gene delivery nanosystems for cancer therapy. Applied Materials Today*, 2018. **12**: pp. 177–190.

11. Lalwani, S., et al., *Mimicking PAMAM dendrimers with amphoteric, hybrid triazine dendrimers: a comparison of dispersity and stability. Macromolecules*, 2009. **42**(17): pp. 6723–6732.

12. Maiti, P.K. and W.A. Goddard, *Solvent quality changes the structure of G8 PAMAM dendrimer, a disagreement with some experimental interpretations. The Journal of Physical Chemistry B*, 2006. **110**(51): pp. 25628–25632.

13. Tarach, P. and A. Janaszewska, *Recent advances in preclinical research using PAMAM dendrimers for cancer gene therapy. International Journal of Molecular Sciences*, 2021. **22**(6): p. 2912.

14. Klajnert, B. and M. Bryszewska, *Dendrimers: properties and applications. Acta Biochimica Polonica*, 2001. **48**(1): pp. 199–208.

15. Santos, A., F. Veiga, and A. Figueiras, *Dendrimers as pharmaceutical excipients: synthesis, properties, toxicity and biomedical applications. Materials*, 2019. **13**(1): p. 65.

16. Pooresmaeil, M. and H. Namazi, *Advances in development of the dendrimers having natural saccharides in their structure for efficient and controlled drug delivery applications. European Polymer Journal*, 2021. **148**: p. 110356.

17. Boas, U., J. Christensen, and P.M. Heegaard, *Dendrimers: design, synthesis and chemical properties. Journal of Materials Chemistry*, 2006. **16**(38): pp. 3785–3798.

18. Eichman, J.D., et al., *The use of PAMAM dendrimers in the efficient transfer of genetic material into cells. Pharmaceutical Science & Technology Today*, 2000. **3**(7): pp. 232–245.

19. Vu, M.T., et al., *Modified carboxyl-terminated PAMAM dendrimers as great cytocompatible nano-based drug delivery system. International Journal of Molecular Sciences*, 2019. **20**(8): p. 2016.

20. Fana, M., et al., *PAMAM dendrimer nanomolecules utilized as drug delivery systems for potential treatment of glioblastoma: a systematic review. International Journal of Nanomedicine*, 2020. **15**: pp. 2789–2808.

21. Gupta, U., et al., *Dendrimers: novel polymeric nanoarchitectures for solubility enhancement. Biomacromolecules*, 2006. **7**(3): pp. 649–658.

22. Barraza, L.F., V.A. Jiménez, and J.B. Alderete, *Effect of PEGylation on the structure and drug loading capacity of PAMAM-G4 dendrimers: A molecular modeling approach on the complexation of 5-fluorouracil with native and PEGylated PAMAM-G4. Macromolecular Chemistry and Physics*, 2015. **216**(16): pp. 1689–1701.

23. Mait, P., Çagin, T.; Wang, G.; Goddard, WA, III. *Macromolecules*, 2004. **37**: pp. 6236–6254.

24. Voit, B., *New developments in hyperbranched polymers. Journal of Polymer Science Part A: Polymer Chemistry*, 2000. **38**(14): pp. 2505–2525.

25. Pittelkow, M. and J.B. Christensen, *Convergent Synthesis of Internally Branched PAMAM Dendrimers. Organic Letters*, 2005. **7**(7): pp. 1295–1298.

26. Medina, S.H. and M.E. El-Sayed, *Dendrimers as carriers for delivery of chemotherapeutic agents. Chemical Reviews*, 2009. **109**(7): pp. 3141–3157.

27. Tomalia, D.A., A.M. Naylor, and W.A. Goddard III, *Starburst dendrimers: molecular-level control of size, shape, surface chemistry, topology, and flexibility from atoms to macroscopic matter. Angewandte Chemie International Edition*, 1990. **29**(2): pp. 138–175.

28. Peterson, J., et al. *Synthesis and CZE analysis of PAMAM dendrimers with an ethylenediamine core.* In *Proceedings-Estonian Academy of Sciences Chemistry.* 2001. TRUEKITUD OU.

29. Martin, I.K. and L.J. Twyman, *The synthesis of unsymmetrical PAMAM dendrimers using a divergent/divergent approach. Tetrahedron Letters*, 2001. **42**(6): pp. 1119–1121.

30. Singh, J., et al., *Dendrimers in anticancer drug delivery: mechanism of interaction of drug and dendrimers. Artificial Cells, Nanomedicine, and Biotechnology*, 2016. **44**(7): pp. 1626–1634.

31. Astruc, D., et al., *Click dendrimers and triazole-related aspects: catalysts, mechanism, synthesis, and functions. A bridge between dendritic architectures and nanomaterials. Accounts of Chemical Research*, 2012. **45**(4): pp. 630–640.

32. Han, S.-C., J.-H. Kim, and J.-W. Lee, *Convergent synthesis of PAMAM dendrimers containing tetra (ethyleneoxide) at core using click chemistry. Bulletin of the Korean Chemical Society*, 2012. **33**(10): pp. 3501–3504.

33. Ferlay, J., et al., *Cancer incidence and mortality worldwide: sources, methods and major patterns in GLOBOCAN 2012. International Journal of Cancer*, 2015. **136**(5): pp. E359–E386.

34. Hoelder, S., P.A. Clarke, and P. Workman, *Discovery of small molecule cancer drugs: successes, challenges and opportunities. Molecular Oncology*, 2012. **6**(2): pp. 155–176.

35. Aslam, M.S., et al., *Side effects of chemotherapy in cancer patients and evaluation of patients opinion about starvation based differential chemotherapy. Journal of Cancer Therapy*, 2014. **5**: pp. 817–822.

36. Wang, Z., et al., *Antibody drug conjugates: The forefront of targeted chemotherapy for cancer treatment. Journal of Drug Design and Research*, 2015. **2**: pp. 2–9.

37. Wicki, A., et al., *Nanomedicine in cancer therapy: challenges, opportunities, and clinical applications. Journal of Controlled Release*, 2015. **200**: pp. 138–157.

38. Sievers, E.L. and P.D. Senter, *Antibody-drug conjugates in cancer therapy. Annual Review of Medicine*, 2013. **64**: pp. 15–29.

39. Sahoo, S.K. and V. Labhasetwar, *Nanotech approaches to drug delivery and imaging. Drug Discovery Today*, 2003. **8**(24): pp. 1112–1120.

40. Abeylath, S.C., et al., *Combinatorial-designed multifunctional polymeric nanosystems for tumor-targeted therapeutic delivery. Accounts of Chemical Research*, 2011. **44**(10): pp. 1009–1017.

41. Iyer, A.K., Z. Duan, and M.M. Amiji, *Nanodelivery systems for nucleic acid therapeutics in drug resistant tumors. Molecular Pharmaceutics*, 2014. **11**(8): pp. 2511–2526.

42. Dande, P., et al., *Improving RNA interference in mammalian cells by 4'-thio-modified small interfering RNA (siRNA): effect on siRNA activity and nuclease stability when used in combination with 2'-O-alkyl modifications. Journal of Medicinal Chemistry*, 2006. **49**(5): pp. 1624–1634.

43. Ferraresi, V., et al., *Toxicity and activity of docetaxel in anthracycline-pretreated breast cancer patients: A phase II study. American Journal of Clinical Oncology*, 2000. **23**(2): pp. 132–139.

44. Liu, Y., H. Miyoshi, and M. Nakamura, *Nanomedicine for drug delivery and imaging: a promising avenue for cancer therapy and diagnosis using targeted functional nanoparticles. International Journal of Cancer*, 2007. **120**(12): pp. 2527–2537.

45. Pauwels, E. and P. Erba, *Towards the use of nanoparticles in cancer therapy and imaging. Drug News & Perspectives*, 2007. **20**(4): pp. 213–220.

46. Thakur, S., et al., *The effect of polyethylene glycol spacer chain length on the tumor-targeting potential of folate-modified PPI dendrimers. Journal of Nanoparticle Research*, 2013. **15**: pp. 1–16.

47. Kannan, R., et al., *Emerging concepts in dendrimer-based nanomedicine: from design principles to clinical applications. Journal of Internal Medicine*, 2014. **276**(6): pp. 579–617.

48. Kesharwani, P., K. Jain, and N.K. Jain, *Dendrimer as nanocarrier for drug delivery. Progress in Polymer Science*, 2014. **39**(2): pp. 268–307.

49. Mignani, S., et al., *Anticancer copper (II) phosphorus dendrimers are potent proapoptotic Bax activators. European Journal of Medicinal Chemistry*, 2017. **132**: pp. 142–156.

50. Xiong, Z., M. Shen, and X. Shi, *Dendrimer-based strategies for cancer therapy: Recent advances and future perspectives. Sci. China mater*, 2018. **61**(11): pp. 1387–1403.

51. Das, M., C. Mohanty, and S.K. Sahoo, *Ligand-based targeted therapy for cancer tissue. Expert Opinion on Drug Delivery*, 2009. **6**(3): pp. 285–304.

52. Malik, N., E.G. Evagorou, and R. Duncan, *Dendrimer-platinate: a novel approach to cancer chemotherapy. Anti-Cancer Drugs,* 1999. **10**(8): pp. 767–776.

53. Mohammadifar, E., A.N. Kharat, and M. Adeli, *Polyamidoamine and polyglycerol; their linear, dendritic and linear–dendritic architectures as anticancer drug delivery systems. Journal of Materials Chemistry B,* 2015. **3**(19): pp. 3896–3921.

54. Maeda, H. and Y. Matsumura, *Tumoritropic and lymphotropic principles of macromolecular drugs. Critical Reviews in Therapeutic Drug Carrier Systems,* 1989. **6**(3): pp. 193–210.

55. Bazak, R., et al., *Passive targeting of nanoparticles to cancer: A comprehensive review of the literature. Molecular and Clinical Oncology,* 2014. **2**(6): pp. 904–908.

56. Adams, G.P., et al., *High affinity restricts the localization and tumor penetration of single-chain fv antibody molecules. Cancer Research,* 2001. **61**(12): pp. 4750–4755.

57. Kannagi, R., et al., *Carbohydrate-mediated cell adhesion in cancer metastasis and angiogenesis. Cancer Science,* 2004. **95**(5): pp. 377–384.

58. Cheung, A., et al., *Targeting folate receptor alpha for cancer treatment. Oncotarget,* 2016. **7**(32): p. 52553.

59. Kesharwani, P., et al., *Hyaluronic acid-conjugated polyamidoamine dendrimers for targeted delivery of 3, 4-difluorobenzylidene curcumin to CD44 overexpressing pancreatic cancer cells. Colloids and Surfaces B: Biointerfaces,* 2015. **136**: pp. 413–423.

60. Majoros, I.J., et al., *PAMAM dendrimer-based multifunctional conjugate for cancer therapy: synthesis, characterization, and functionality. Biomacromolecules,* 2006. **7**(2): pp. 572–579.

61. Peng, J., et al., *Octreotide-conjugated PAMAM for targeted delivery to somatostatin receptors overexpressed tumor cells. Journal of Drug Targeting,* 2014. **22**(5): pp. 428–438.

62. Zhang, L., et al., *RGD-modified PEG–PAMAM–DOX conjugates: In vitro and in vivo studies for glioma. European Journal of Pharmaceutics and Biopharmaceutics,* 2011. **79**(2): pp. 232–240.

63. Zong, H., et al., *Bifunctional PAMAM dendrimer conjugates of folic acid and methotrexate with defined ratio. Biomacromolecules,* 2012. **13**(4): pp. 982–991.

64. Öztürk, K., et al., *Effective targeting of gemcitabine to pancreatic cancer through PEG-cored Flt-1 antibody-conjugated dendrimers. International Journal of Pharmaceutics,* 2017. **517**(1–2): pp. 157–167.

65. Kurtoglu, Y.E., et al., *Drug release characteristics of PAMAM dendrimer–drug conjugates with different linkers. International Journal of Pharmaceutics,* 2010. **384**(1–2): pp. 189–194.

66. Wei, P., et al., *Dendrimer-Stabilized gold nanostars as a multifunctional theranostic nanoplatform for CT imaging, photothermal therapy, and gene silencing of tumors. Advanced Healthcare Materials,* 2016. **5**(24): pp. 3203–3213.

67. Kong, L., et al., *Dendrimer-modified MoS2 nanoflakes as a platform for combinational gene silencing and photothermal therapy of tumors. ACS Applied Materials & Interfaces,* 2017. **9**(19): pp. 15995–16005.

68. Hou, W., et al., *Partially PEGylated dendrimer-entrapped gold nanoparticles: A promising nanoplatform for highly efficient DNA and siRNA delivery. Journal of Materials Chemistry B,* 2016. **4**(17): pp. 2933–2943.

69. Qiu, J., et al., *Dendrimer-entrapped gold nanoparticles modified with β-cyclodextrin for enhanced gene delivery applications. RSC Advances,* 2016. **6**(31): pp. 25633–25640.

70. Kong, L., et al., *RGD peptide-modified dendrimer-entrapped gold nanoparticles enable highly efficient and specific gene delivery to stem cells. ACS Applied Materials & Interfaces,* 2015. **7**(8): pp. 4833–4843.

71. Hou, W., et al., *Partially acetylated dendrimer-entrapped gold nanoparticles with reduced cytotoxicity for gene delivery applications. Journal of Nanoscience and Nanotechnology,* 2015. **15**(6): pp. 4094–4105.

72. Qiu, J., et al., *Enhanced delivery of therapeutic siRNA into glioblastoma cells using dendrimer-entrapped gold nanoparticles conjugated with β-cyclodextrin. Nanomaterials,* 2018. **8**(3): p. 131.

73. Waite, C.L. and C.M. Roth, *PAMAM-RGD conjugates enhance siRNA delivery through a multicellular spheroid model of malignant glioma. Bioconjugate Chemistry,* 2009. **20**(10): pp. 1908–1916.

74. Fan, W., et al., *Thioaptamer-conjugated CD44-targeted delivery system for the treatment of breast cancer in vitro and in vivo. Journal of Drug Targeting,* 2016. **24**(4): pp. 359–371.

75. Xu, L., W.A. Yeudall, and H. Yang, *Folic acid-decorated polyamidoamine dendrimer exhibits high tumor uptake and sustained highly localized retention in solid tumors: Its utility for local siRNA delivery. Acta Biomaterialia,* 2017. **57**: pp. 251–261.

76. Choi, Y., et al., *Synthesis and functional evaluation of DNA-assembled polyamidoamine dendrimer clusters for cancer cell-specific targeting. Chemistry & Biology,* 2005. **12**(1): pp. 35–43.

77. Zhang, Y., et al., *Co-delivery of doxorubicin and paclitaxel with linear-dendritic block copolymer for enhanced anti-cancer efficacy. Science China Chemistry,* 2014. **57**: pp. 624–632.

78. Park, H.-K., et al., *Combination treatment with doxorubicin and gamitrinib synergistically augments anticancer activity through enhanced activation of Bim. BMC Cancer,* 2014. **14**(1): pp. 1–9.

79. Lin, L., et al., *UTMD-promoted co-delivery of gemcitabine and miR-21 inhibitor by dendrimer-entrapped gold nanoparticles for pancreatic cancer therapy. Theranostics,* 2018. **8**(7): p. 1923.

80. Han, M., et al., *Overcoming drug resistance of MCF-7/ADR cells by altering intracellular distribution of doxorubicin via MVP knockdown with a novel siRNA polyamidoamine-hyaluronic acid complex. Journal of Controlled Release,* 2012. **163**(2): pp. 136–144.

81. Arteaga, C.L., *Trastuzumab, an appropriate first-line single-agent therapy for HER2-overexpressing metastatic breast cancer. Breast Cancer Research,* 2003. **5**: pp. 1–5.

82. Aleanizy, F.S., et al., *Trastuzumab targeted neratinib loaded poly-amidoamine dendrimer nanocapsules for breast cancer therapy. International Journal of Nanomedicine,* 2020: pp. 5433–5443.

83. Guglin, M., R. Cutro, and J.D. Mishkin, *Trastuzumab-induced cardiomyopathy. Journal of Cardiac Failure,* 2008. **14**(5): pp. 437–444.

84. Nahta, R. and F.J. Esteva, *Herceptin: mechanisms of action and resistance. Cancer Letters,* 2006. **232**(2): pp. 123–138.

85. Valabrega, G., F. Montemurro, and M. Aglietta, *Trastuzumab: mechanism of action, resistance and future perspectives in HER2-overexpressing breast cancer. Annals of Oncology,* 2007. **18**(6): pp. 977–984.

86. Burstein, H.J., et al., *Neratinib, an irreversible ErbB receptor tyrosine kinase inhibitor, in patients with advanced ErbB2-positive breast cancer. Journal of Clinical Oncology,* 2010. **28**(8): pp. 1301–1307.

87. Devarakonda, B., et al., *The effect of polyamidoamine dendrimers on the in vitro cytotoxicity of paclitaxel in cultured prostate cancer (PC-3M) cells. Journal of Biomedical Nanotechnology,* 2007. **3**(4): pp. 384–393.

88. Aderibigbe, B., et al., *Polyamidoamine-drug conjugates containing metal-based anticancer compounds. Journal of Inorganic and Organometallic Polymers and Materials,* 2020. **30**: pp. 1503–1518.

89. Ooya, T., J. Lee, and K. Park, *Hydrotropic dendrimers of generations 4 and 5: synthesis, characterization, and hydrotropic solubilization of paclitaxel. Bioconjugate Chemistry,* 2004. **15**(6): pp. 1221–1229.

90. Pan, J., et al., *Polyamidoamine dendrimers-based nanomedicine for combination therapy with siRNA and chemotherapeutics to overcome multidrug resistance. European Journal of Pharmaceutics and Biopharmaceutics,* 2019. **136**: pp. 18–28.

91. Yan, X., Y. Yang, and Y. Sun. *Dendrimer applications for cancer therapies. In Journal of Physics: Conference Series.* 2021. IOP.

92. Carvalho, F.S., et al., *Doxorubicin-induced cardiotoxicity: From bioenergetic failure and cell death to cardiomyopathy. Medicinal Research Reviews,* 2014. **34**(1): pp. 106–135.

93. Zhong, Q., et al., *Conjugation to poly (amidoamine) dendrimers and pulmonary delivery reduce cardiac accumulation and enhance antitumor activity of doxorubicin in lung metastasis. Molecular Pharmaceutics,* 2016. **13**(7): pp. 2363–2375.

94. Kale, A.A. and V.P. Torchilin, *Design, synthesis, and characterization of pH-sensitive PEG–PE conjugates for stimuli-sensitive pharmaceutical nanocarriers: the effect of substitutes at the hydrazone linkage on the pH stability of PEG– PE conjugates. Bioconjugate Chemistry,* 2007. **18**(2): pp. 363–370.

95. Satsangi, A., et al., *Design of a paclitaxel prodrug conjugate for active targeting of an enzyme upregulated in breast cancer cells. Molecular Pharmaceutics,* 2014. **11**(6): pp. 1906–1918.

96. Kulhari, H., et al., *Trastuzumab-grafted PAMAM dendrimers for the selective delivery of anticancer drugs to HER2-positive breast cancer. Scientific Reports,* 2016. **6**(1): pp. 23179.

97. Chung, A., et al., *Current status of anti–human epidermal growth factor receptor 2 therapies: predicting and overcoming herceptin resistance. Clinical Breast Cancer,* 2013. **13**(4): pp. 223–232.

98. Li, Y., et al., *A poly (amidoamine) dendrimer-based drug carrier for delivering DOX to gliomas cells.* RSC Advances, 2017. **7**(25): pp. 15475–15481.

99. Mintzer, M.A. and M.W. Grinstaff, *Biomedical applications of dendrimers: a tutorial.* Chemical Society Reviews, 2011. **40**(1): pp. 173–190.

100. Hong, S., et al., *The binding avidity of a nanoparticle-based multivalent targeted drug delivery platform.* Chemistry & Biology, 2007. **14**(1): pp. 107–115.

101. Mammen, M., S.K. Choi, and G.M. Whitesides, *Polyvalent interactions in biological systems: implications for design and use of multivalent ligands and inhibitors.* Angewandte Chemie International Edition, 1998. **37**(20): pp. 2754–2794.

102. Lee, J.H., et al., *Current management and future strategies of gastric cancer.* Yonsei Medical Journal, 2012. **53**(2): pp. 248–257.

103. Yang, Z., et al., *PEGylation confers greatly extended half-life and attenuated immunogenicity to recombinant methioninase in primates.* Cancer Research, 2004. **64**(18): pp. 6673–6678.

104. Kokkinakis, D.M., et al., *Mitotic arrest, apoptosis, and sensitization to chemotherapy of melanomas by methionine deprivation stress.* Molecular Cancer Research, 2006. **4**(8): pp. 575–589.

105. Li, Y.-F., H.-T. Zhang, and L. Xin, *Hyaluronic acid-modified polyamidoamine dendrimer G5-entrapped gold nanoparticles delivering METase gene inhibits gastric tumor growth via targeting CD44+ gastric cancer cells.* Journal of Cancer Research and Clinical Oncology, 2018. **144**: pp. 1463–1473.

106. Agarwal, R. and S.B. Kaye, *Ovarian cancer: strategies for overcoming resistance to chemotherapy.* Nature Reviews Cancer, 2003. **3**(7): pp. 502–516.

107. Yellepeddi, V.K., A. Kumar, and S. Palakurthi, *Biotinylated poly (amido) amine (PAMAM) dendrimers as carriers for drug delivery to ovarian cancer cells in vitro.* Anticancer Research, 2009. **29**(8): pp. 2933–2943.

108. Ma, P. and R.J. Mumper, *Paclitaxel nano-delivery systems: a comprehensive review.* Journal of Nanomedicine & Nanotechnology, 2013. **4**(2): p. 1000164.

109. Ma, J. and H. Yao, *Dendrimer-paclitaxel complexes for efficient treatment in ovarian cancer: study on OVCAR-3 and HEK293T cells.* Acta Biochimica Polonica, 2018. **65**(2): pp. 219–225.

110. Meyers, J.D., et al., *Nanoparticles for imaging and treating brain cancer.* Nanomedicine, 2013. **8**(1): pp. 123–143.

111. He, H., et al., *PEGylated Poly (amidoamine) dendrimer-based dual-targeting carrier for treating brain tumors.* Biomaterials, 2011. **32**(2): pp. 478–487.

112. Gorain, B., et al., *Dendrimers as effective carriers for the treatment of brain tumor*, in Nanotechnology-based targeted drug delivery systems for brain tumors. 2018, Amsterdam: Elsevier. pp. 267–305.

113. Qin, W., et al., *Improved GFP gene transfection mediated by polyamidoamine dendrimer-functionalized multi-walled carbon nanotubes with high biocompatibility.* Colloids and Surfaces B: Biointerfaces, 2011. **84**(1): pp. 206–213.

114. Teow, H.M., et al., *Delivery of paclitaxel across cellular barriers using a dendrimer-based nanocarrier.* International Journal of Pharmaceutics, 2013. **441**(1–2): pp. 701–711.

115. Jiang, Y., et al., *PEGylated Polyamidoamine dendrimer conjugated with tumor homing peptide as a potential targeted delivery system for glioma.* Colloids and Surfaces B: Biointerfaces, 2016. **147**: pp. 242–249.

116. Zhao, J., et al., *CREKA peptide-conjugated dendrimer nanoparticles for glioblastoma multiforme delivery.* Journal of Colloid and Interface Science, 2015. **450**: pp. 396–403.

117. Rompicharla, S.V.K., et al., *Octa-arginine modified poly (amidoamine) dendrimers for improved delivery and cytotoxic effect of paclitaxel in cancer.* Artificial Cells, Nanomedicine, and Biotechnology, 2018. **46**(sup2): pp. 847–859.

118. Kang, S.J., et al., *Subconjunctival nanoparticle carboplatin in the treatment of murine retinoblastoma.* Archives of Ophthalmology, 2009. **127**(8): pp. 1043–1047.

119. Tunki, L., et al., *Dendrimer-based targeted drug delivery*, in Pharmaceutical Applications of Dendrimers. 2020, Amsterdam: Elsevier. pp. 107–129.

120. Sk, U.H., et al., *Enhancing the efficacy of Ara-C through conjugation with PAMAM dendrimer and linear PEG: a comparative study.* Biomacromolecules, 2013. **14**(3): pp. 801–810.

16 Photodynamic Therapies for Cancer Treatment

Ayesha Sadiqa, Saba Riaz, Azhar Rasul, Rabia Zara,
Khudeja Afroz, Zunaira Saeed, Gul Bushra Khan,
Khatereh Khorsandi, and Muhammad Yasir Ali

16.1 INTRODUCTION

Photodynamic therapy (PDT) is a non-invasive and emerging form of therapeutic procedure that involves treatment of the malignant and non-malignant diseases [1, 2]. The mechanism of action of PDT relies on singlet oxygen and particular excitation of photosensitizers (PS) by light at an appropriate wavelength, which leads to cell death [3]. PDT is also used to cure respiratory, pulmonary, and urinal tract cancers and chronic inflammation [2].

The preclinical applications of the PDT were accidentally discovered around the 1900s by a medical student, Oscar Raab. When he was studying the interaction of light and fluorescent dyes on infusaria, he found that the microorganisms were destroyed with the application of intense light applied to the dye [4]. However, many PSs have been used for PDT but with the great efforts of another medical specialist, Dougherty, hematoporphyrin received FDA approval for the clinical application of PDT [3, 5].

The field of PDT continues to further advance and today more than 2000 patients have been treated with this method. As it is shown, PDT is a painless method and is currently used in the treatment of various non-oncologic human diseases such as acne [6], photoaging [7], vascular malformation [8], dental diseases, rheumatoid arthritis [9], warts [10], and ophthalmologic diseases [11]. Also, it has been used in cancerous diseases including esophageal, skin, neck, breast, bladder, and lung cancers [12].

As cancer is one of the most life-threatening diseases in developed and developing countries the treatment of cancer with PDT can be considered an optimistic approach [13]. In this chapter, we will summarize the mechanism of cell death by PDT and later a brief on combinatorial therapy with PDT for the treatment of cancer.

16.2 PRINCIPLE OF PHOTODYNAMIC THERAPY

The principle of photodynamic therapy (PDT) is based on the use of a photosensitizing agent that is selectively taken up by abnormal cells, such as cancer cells, and then activated by light of a specific wavelength. This activation leads to the production of reactive oxygen species (ROS), such as singlet oxygen and free radicals, which can cause damage to the abnormal cells, leading to their destruction [14].

The photosensitizing agent is typically administered either topically or systemically, and it preferentially accumulates in the abnormal cells. The light source used to activate the photosensitizing agent is typically a laser or light-emitting diode (LED) of a specific wavelength that matches the absorption spectrum of the photosensitizing agent.

DOI: 10.1201/9781003363958-19

Once activated, the photosensitizing agent generates ROS, which can induce cell death by various mechanisms, such as oxidative stress, apoptosis, and necrosis. ROS can also damage the blood vessels that supply the abnormal cells, leading to their destruction [15, 16].

PDT is a selective and minimally invasive treatment that can be repeated as needed. The selectivity of PDT allows for the preservation of healthy tissue, and the minimally invasive nature of the treatment makes it an attractive option for many patients.

As it said the principle of PDT depends on dynamic interactions of PS with specific light in the presence of molecular oxygen leading to the production of ROS and consequently enhancing the death rate of targeted cells [17]. The accepted molecular changes that take place on the illumination of light are the formation of free radicals of PS and neighboring molecules [14]. Exposure to a specific wavelength excites the PS from its ground state (S_0) to the excited state (S_1). This unstable state through intersystem crossing reaches the excited triplet state (T_1), which is a key state for radical formation which have a maximum half-life duration [18–21].

At T_1 state, PS releases extra energy through phosphorescence or transfers it to neighboring molecules through simple collisions that give rise to reactive particles as a byproduct of two types of reactions [14, 15]. During this collision, when PS donates its electron to surrounding biomolecules (nucleic acids, amino acids, or fatty acids) to generate ROS (superoxide radical, hydrogen peroxide, or hydroxyl anion) it follows the type I mechanism. PS can react directly with diffused oxygen molecules in the type II mechanism and convert ground-state oxygen ($^3O_2$) into singlet oxygen ($^1O_2$), which is a highly unstable molecule as compared to other ROS species [15, 16]. The ROS generated by either mechanism will ultimately create cytotoxicity [22].

ROS produced by the type I mechanism directly damages biological compartments and can also contribute to the reaction for hydrogen peroxide formation [23]. Singlet oxygen that is produced by the type II mechanism can cause oxidative damage in target cells. For example, when singlet oxygen interacts with amino acids later the vital proteins will lose their function and ultimately cause cell death as elaborated in Figure 16.1 [24].

16.3 CELL DEATH MECHANISM INDUCED VIA PDT

Cancer treatment by PDT can perform through the involvement of three primary cell death mechanisms [26]. ROS created by PDT photochemical responses can straightforwardly annihilate growing cells by prompting apoptosis, necrosis, and autophagy. PDT can initiate an inflammatory reaction against the cancer cells [27].

16.3.1 PDT-MEDIATED APOPTOSIS

Apoptosis can be defined as a mechanism of genetically encoded programmed cell death that requires energy. During apoptosis, cells shrink and wrinkle, the DNA molecule breaks down into internucleosomal fragments, chromatin condenses and apoptotic bodies form without disruption of the plasma membrane [18, 28]. For controlled cell death, apoptosis is a highly modulated process [29], which can start in a variety of ways after PDT damages several organelles [30]. The most likely PSs to cause apoptosis are those that localize to mitochondria [31, 32]. Multiple apoptotic signaling pathways are activated in response to photodamage [33].

The extrinsic/death receptor route and intrinsic pathway are the two primary apoptosis processes [34]. When mitochondria are exposed to light, their membranes become permeable, allowing cytochrome c to seep into the cytosol [35]. When the Bcl-2 family is regulated, allowing cytochrome c is released through mitochondrial porin channels, which results in cell death by triggering a cascade of caspases [36].

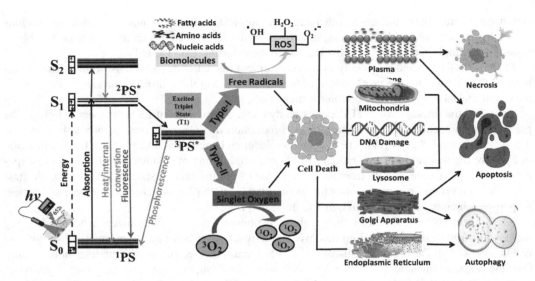

FIGURE 16.1 Mechanism of photosensitizer activation upon illumination in PDT by following type I and type II reactions and cell death pathways [25].

Through intrinsic pathway, different PSs including chlorin e6 (Ce6) induces apoptosis in SW480 [37], berberin in BxPC-3 and HPDE-E6E7c7 [38], methyl pyropheophorbide a (MPPa) in MG-63 [39], photofrin in ASTC-a-1 [40] and 5-ALA in A431 and COLO-13 [41]. Endoplasmic reticulum stress also activated the apoptotic reactions by increasing the amount of CCAAT-enhancer-binding protein homologous protein (CHOP) when different PS were exposed to specific wavelengths as elaborated in Figure 16.2 [42].

PTEN, a tumor suppressor gene that is frequently mutated, regulates complex cellular networks like the mitogen-activated protein kinase (MAPK) and PI3K/Akt pathways, preserving cellular homeostasis and promoting growth and development. MAP kinase-1, c-Jun N terminal kinase (JNK), MAPK/ERK family and p38 MAPK are the four primary signaling domains that make up the MAPK (Table 16.1). These kinases transmit the extracellular cues, which control cell death, proliferation, migration, and differentiation when they are activated [43].

Phosphatidylinositol 3-kinase (P13K)/Akt signaling cascade is considered as an important anti-tumor target [44] and targeting P13K/Akt and MAPK pathways is a promising strategy for the treatment of cancer [45].

16.3.2 PDT-MEDIATED AUTOPHAGY

Through the process of autophagy, a cell has the potential to recycle cytoplasmic elements and damaged organelles. An autophagosome is a double-membrane structure that engulfs damaged particles and unites with lysosomes to break down its contents [46]. Autophagy has been seen as a cell death mechanism in response to PDT, although it is thought to be a cytoprotective mechanism [47].

PDT-mediated autophagy is thought to occur as a response to the cellular stress caused by the production of reactive oxygen species (ROS) during PDT. ROS can trigger the activation of several cellular pathways, including the mTOR (mammalian target of rapamycin) pathway, which is involved in regulating autophagy. PDT-induced autophagy has been observed in various types of cancer cells, including those of the breast, lung, and colon (Table 16.2). Studies have suggested that autophagy induced by PDT may play a role in the antitumor effects of PDT by enhancing the destruction of cancer cells.

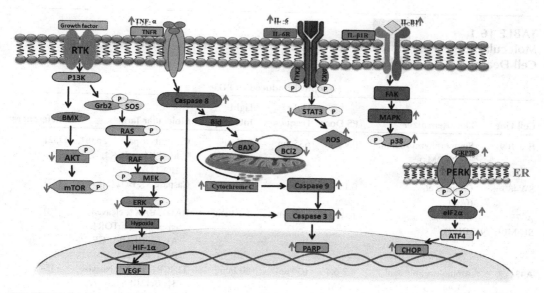

FIGURE 16.2 Schematic illustration of the plasma membrane, cytoplasmic and nuclear targets of numerous photosensitizers that result in anticancer activity in different cancer types [42].

However, the role of autophagy in PDT-mediated cell death is complex and not fully understood. In some cases, autophagy may promote cell survival, while in other cases it may contribute to cell death. Further research is needed to better understand the relationship between PDT-induced autophagy and the therapeutic effects of PDT.

When apoptosis is compromised, autophagy seems to be the primary mechanism causing cell death [48]. Autophagy appears to act as a protective mechanism at lower PDT doses (with less damage), however, at higher PDT levels, apoptotic cell death can be induced [49, 50]. Localization of PS is crucial because PS that are targeted to the endoplasmic reticulum cause an autophagic reaction that is a pro-survival strategy. PS that is directed at lysosomes can stop autophagy [51].

16.3.3 PDT-MEDIATED NECROSIS

A local inflammatory response is caused by the release of cytoplasmic content and pro-inflammatory mediators into the extracellular medium during necrosis [17]. The components of apoptotic pathway components may be disrupted in cells that have sustained significant damage, making apoptosis unable to be complete [59].

When the plasma membrane is the site for the action of PS, necrosis is also more frequently seen. For example, photofrin promotes apoptotic cell death when it is activated in the cytoplasm. On the other hand, it causes increased necrotic cell death when it is activated in the plasma membrane by changing the incubation technique [60].

Inflammation can be on by induced by the release of intracellular substances into the immediate environment caused by photodamage to the plasma membrane. The tumor cells are quickly ablated by necrosis when high light intensity is used [44].

16.3.4 VASCULAR MECHANISMS

The use of PDT frequently results in the devastation of the tumor microvasculature. When stimulated by the right light irradiation, vascular endothelial cells can concentrate PS to produce free radicals.

TABLE 16.1
Molecular Targets in Numerous Cancer Cell Lines after PDT to Induce Apoptotic Cell Death

Cell Line	Photosensitizer	PS Dose	Apoptosis Induced by PDT		Molecular Targets	References
			Light Frequency	Light Intensity		
Eca-109	Sinoporphyrin sodium (DVDMs)	0.9 μM	635 nm	3 J/cm^2	Cleaved caspase 3↑, p38↑, MAPK↑, p-JNK↑, HO-1↑	[52]
SW480	Chlorine e6 (Ce6)	0.125-8 μg	650 nm	6 J/cm^2	Caspase 3↑, Bcl2↓, β actin↑	[37]
A375 SK-MEL-19	Berberine (BBR)	10 μM	354 nm	7.2 J/cm^2	BAD↑, BAX↑, cleaved caspase 3↑, mTOR↓, AKT↓, CHOP↑, GRP78/BIP↑, PERK^{Act}	[53]
A431	Aminolevulinic acid (ALA)	0.2-6.4 mM	630 nm	80 J/cm^2	TINCR↑, BAX↑, caspase 3↑, Bcl2↓, ERK1/2↓, Sp3↓	• [54]
HeLa cell line, C33A	Berberine (BBR-F)	1 μg- 50 μg	405 nm	1.8 J/cm^2	Kits use	[42]
HEK293 SMCC-7721	Berberine (BBR)	----	----	----	VEGFR2↓, AKT↓, ERK1/2↓, MMP2↓, MMP9↓	[42]
ZR-75-30 BxPC-3 HPDE-E6E7c7	Berberine (BBR)	10 μM	570–650 nm	----	Caspase 3↑, Caspase 7↑	[38]
THP-1	Methylene Blue (MB)	5 μM	660 nm	40 J/cm^2	Caspase 3↑, Caspase 9↑, Cleaved PARP↑, TNFα↑, IL-6↓, IL-1β↑	[55]
MG-63	Pyropheophorbide-α methyl ester (MPPa)	0.25–1.5 μM	630 nm	40 mW/cm^2	Cytochrome c↑, Bax↑, Bcl$_2$↓, β actin↑	[39]
FaDu cell line	Hematoporphyrin (HP)	1–2 μM	635 nm	4.5 mW/cm^2	Caspase 8↑, Caspase 3↑, Bcl$_2$↓, mTOR↓, PARP-1^{Act}	[56]
A431	5-ethylamino-9-diethylaminobenzo [a] phenoselenazinium (EtNBSe)	400 nM	635 nm	2.8 J/cm^2	PERK^{Act}, GRP78↑, eIF$_2$α↑, ATF4↑, CHOP↑, Caspase 9↑, Caspase 3↑, cleaved PARP↑	[42]
ASTC-a-1	Photofrin	10 μg/ml	632.8 nm	10 J/cm2	Caspase 3^{Act}, Bim↑, Bax↑	[40]
HCT116	Sinoporphyrin sodium (DVDMs)	1 μg/ml	630 nm	19.1 mW/cm^2	CD133↓, cleaved caspase 3↑, Bax↑	[57]
A431 COLO-16	Aminolevulinic acid (ALA)		630 nm	10 mW/cm^2	Bcl2↓, STAT 3↓, Bax↑	[41]

TABLE 16.2
Molecular Targets in PDT-Mediated Autophagic Cell Death of Various Cancer Types

Cancer Type	Cell Line	Photosensitizer	Dose	Light Frequency	Light Intensity	Autophagy Induced by PDT Molecular Targets	References
Esophageal Cancer	Eca-109	Sinoporphyrin sodium (DVDMs)	0.9 µM	635 nm	3 J/cm^2	LC3 II ↑	[52]
Human Colon Cancer	SW480	Chlorine e6 (Ce6)	0.125–8 µg	650 nm	6 J/cm^2	LC3B II↑	[37]
Malignant Melanoma	A375 SK-MEL-19	Berberine (BBR)	30–34 µM	354 nm	7.2 J/cm^2	CHOP↑, mTOR↓, AKT↓, LC3B II↑	[53]
Cutaneous Squamous Cell Carcinoma (CSCC)	A431	Aminolevulinic acid (ALA)	0.2–6.4 mM	630 nm	80 J/cm^2	Beclin-1↑, LC3 II↑	[54]
Human Osteosarcoma	MG-63	Pyropheophorbide-α methyl ester (MPPa)	0.2–1.5 µM	630 nm	40 mW/cm^2	Beclin-1↑, LC3- II↑,Jnk↑	[39]
Human Oral Cancer	FaDu cell line	Hematoporphyrin (HP)	1–2 µM	635 nm	4.5 mW/cm^2	mTOR↓, LC3-II↑, PARP-1^{Act}	[56]
Squameous Cell Carcinoma (SCC)	A431	5-ethylamino-9-diethylaminobenzo [a] phenoselenazinium (EtNBSe)	400 nM	635 nm	2.8 J/cm^2	IRE1^{Act}, PERK^{Act}, GRP78↑, GADD153↑,eIF$_2$α↑, ATF4↑, cleaved PARP↑, LC3-II/LC3-I↑, Lamp↑, Beclin-1↑	[58]
Colorectal Cancer	HCT116	Sinoporphyrin sodium (DVDMs)	1 µg/ml	630 nm	19.1 mW/cm^2	LC3-II↑,ATG7↑, Bcl$_2$↓, P62↓	[57]

When the vascular walls are damaged, the supply of oxygen and nutrients is cut off to tumor cells, which results in tumor cell death [61].

The vascular effect of PDT has several important advantages; it uses PSs that are cleared from the body quickly and reduce skin photosensitivity. It has higher long-term efficacy and it can be completed in a single brief session [62].

16.3.5 IMMUNOLOGICAL MECHANISMS

Recent research has shown that PDT can dramatically affect the adaptive immune response in a variety of ways, including stimulating or suppressing the immunological response. The direct effects of PDT on the lesion and its vasculature combined with immune system stimulation provide long-term tumor treatment [44].

16.4 SOME IMPORTANT COMPONENTS OF PDT

Mainly there are three components of photodynamic therapy, which include photosensitizers, light, and oxygen as shown in Figure 16.3.

16.4.1 PHOTOSENSITIZERS

A PS is a light-sensitive drug that enables ROS production upon energy transfer in its excited state to molecular oxygen [63]. PS experienced an energy state transition from a low ground state to the excited singlet state upon irradiation with light of a specific wavelength [30]. There are two main mechanisms by which a PS may act: type-I and type-II (Figure 16.1).

The type-I mechanism involves direct transfer of electron or hydrogen from PS resulting in the removal of hydrogen or electron from a biomolecule establishing radical species. These radicals further react with the oxygen, which results in the formation of highly reactive oxygen species such as S_2O_2, H_2O_2 and OH^-. In the case of type-II reactions, the excited triplet PS state reacts with O_2 to generate singlet oxygen, i.e., $^1O_2$ [30, 64]. Kochevar and co-authors reported that cell death via necrosis is significantly associated with type-I photoreactions while type II has a better association with cell death via apoptosis [65]. Various tetrapyrrole structures such as porphyrins, bacteriochlorins, chlorins, and phthalocyanines having proper functions have been examined in PDT, and on these bases, many compounds have been approved clinically [66]. Nanotechnology played a significant role in PDT and gave rise to new methods like fullerene-based PSs, nanoparticle delivery, and titania photocatalysis [67].

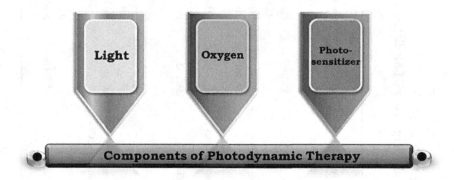

FIGURE 16.3   Three basic components of photodynamic therapy; light, oxygen, and photosensitizer.

The characteristics of an ideal photosensitizer have been discussed by various authors in the literature [68, 69].

- They should have a low level of dark toxicity to both human and experimental animals and should have a low incidence of administrative toxicity.
- They should absorb light in the red or infrared wavelengths to penetrate the tissue as the absorption bands at shorter wavelengths have less tissue penetration and are more likely to lead to skin photosensitivity (the power in the sunlight drops off at $\lambda > 600$ nm) while the absorption bands at the wavelength (> 800 nm) means that the photons will not have sufficient energy for the PS triplet state to transfer energy to the ground state oxygen molecule to excite it to the singlet state.
- They should have relatively high absorption bands ($> 20,000–30,000$ M-1cm-1) to minimize the dose of photosensitizer needed to achieve the desired effect.
- They should have high selectivity for the tumor tissue as compared to the healthy tissue.
- The synthesis of the PS should be relatively easy and the starting materials readily available to make large-scale production feasible.
- The photosensitizer should be a pure compound with constant composition and stable shelf life and be ideally water-soluble or soluble in the harmless aqueous solvent mixture. It should not aggregate in the biological environment as this reduces its photochemical efficiency.
- The pharmacokinetic elimination from the patient should be rapid, i.e., less than one day to avoid the necessity for post-treatment protection from light exposure and prolonged skin sensitivity.
- A short interval between injection and illumination is desirable to facilitate outpatient treatment that is both patient-friendly and cost-effective [10, 11].

In the past few decades, photosensitizers have been vastly studied and used in clinical settings to gain approval. However, due to their photochemistry and uptake efficiency, only a few have been approved. Some of the approved photosensitizers for PDT in cancer are ALA, foscan, photofrin, verteporfin, talaporfin sodium, tookad, etc. (Table 16.3). Antrin, purlytin, and liposomal zinc pthalocyanine were denied approval in their first or second phase of clinical trial either due to an increase in serum prostate-specific antigen (PSA) or their instability. Various other compounds like photochlor, redaporfin, fimaporfin, PC4, TLD1433, etc., are still under clinical study in order to be granted approval. While some of the photosensitizers like photodithiazine, photolon, radachlorin, photosens, hemoporfin, etc., have so far only been approved in non-Western countries [28].

16.4.2 SINGLET OXYGEN

PDT works on the basis of the formation of singlet oxygen through the reaction of oxygen, PS, and light. Singlet oxygen is a highly reactive and primary cytotoxic agent in PDT. PDT dose is based on the amount of oxygen that reacts [80]. For the efficient generation of singlet oxygen target-specific, PS agents should be delivered into sub-cellular compartments like the nucleus, plasma membrane, mitochondria, and cytoskeleton [81].

An explicit dosimetry model can be used to determine the amount of singlet oxygen produced during the process of illumination [82]. Photodynamic therapy directly affects the cells that are near the area of production of singlet oxygen. Because of this property, healthy cells are less affected by PDT than chemotherapy. PDT outcomes can be predicted by evaluating dose matrices such as reacting singlet oxygen, PDT dose, total light influence, and photobleaching ratio. Death of a cancer cell can be caused by singlet oxygen when it interacts with cellular components such as DNA, proteins, and lipids [83].

TABLE 16.3
Examples of Photosensitizers along with their Clinical Status

Sr. No.	Photosensitizer	Chemical Family	Cancer Type	Activation Wavelength	Clinical Status	Reference
1.	5-ALA	Porphyrin precursor	Brain, bladder, esophagus, skin	630 nm	Approved	[70, 71]
2.	Photofrin	Porphyrin	Brain, breast, bladder, lung, esophagus, bile duct, ovarian, skin	630 nm	Approved	[72]
3.	Foscan or Temoporfin	Chlorin	Brain, breast lungs, head, neck, pancreas, skin	652 nm	Approved	[73]
4.	Verteporfin or visudyne	Porphyrin	Esophagus, prostate	689 nm	Approved	[74]
5.	Lutex or motexafin lutetium	Texaphyrin	Breast	732 nm	Rejected	[28]
6.	Photochlor	Chlorin	Lung, neck, head, esophagus	665 nm	Under trials	[75]
7.	Redaporfin or LUZ11	Chlorin	Head, neck	750 nm	Under trials	[76]
8.	Fimaporfin	Chlorin	Liver, colon, breast	652 nm	Under trials	[77]
9.	Metvix or methyl-aminolevulinate (MAL)	Porphyrin precursor	Skin	630 nm	Approved	[78]
10.	Tin ethyl etiopurpurin (SnET2)	Chlorin	Skin, breast	660 nm	Rejected	[79]

16.4.3 FLUENCE RATE

In PDT, for treatment planning, a light fluence rate should be determined for the effective treatment of diseases. Cell death and tissue necrosis can be carried out by light at a certain wavelength in PDT. The efficiency of the treatment can be determined by light fluence, which is sent to the tumor [84]. PDT in combination with surgery of a tumor can remove disease residuals that are not considered resectable because of their small size or their location near vital structures. For example, after the removal of the brain tumor, light is delivered to the resection cavity for getting rid of residual disease [85].

A lower fluence rate of illumination poses fewer harms than a higher fluence rate. Multiple studies have reported that low fluence rates (5 or 30 mW/cm^2) prolong the regrowth of HT29 human colon adenocarcinoma, which was xenografted with (mTHPC)-PDT (meta-tetra hydroxyphenyl chlorin-PDT). While high fluence rates (90 or 160 mW/cm^2) light delivery does not delay tumor regrowth for a longer period [86]. Different fluence rate treatments can exert different biological effects. During photodynamic therapy, less hypoxia is related to a lower fluence rate and can result in more treatment-associated cytotoxicity. Low fluence rate at sub-curative doses induces inflammatory responses [85].

16.5 DELIVERY STRATEGY FOR PS IN PDT

Different nanoparticles have been developed for the delivery of PSs to specific targets in PDT, some of them will be discussed below.

16.5.1 POLYMERIC NANOPARTICLES (PNPs)

Nano drug delivery systems are affected by the size, hydrophobicity, and charge of nanoparticles [87]. They are allowed to circulate the body and capillaries. Nanocapsules and nanospheres come under one term called nanoparticle. Nanocapsules are vascular in structure with solidified polymeric shells. Pharmaceutical drugs are reserved in a core that lies within the vascular cavity of the nanocapsule. Nanospheres can retain the drug inside or adsorb on the surface and have a continuous polymeric network [88].

Once nanoparticles get inside the body, they interact with blood and disrupt its function. Blood can aggregate, the cell membrane can get porous and hemolysis can take place due to the administration of nanoparticles. Blood components can engulf nanoparticles on adhesion [89]. Nanoparticles are usually made from metals, polymers, silica, protein, and lipids [90, 91]. Polymeric nanoparticles (NPs) are particles with a size of 1 to 1000 nm. They have attracted attention over past years because of their small size. Polymeric nanoparticles can be synthesized by a solvent evaporation method, spontaneous emulsification/solvent diffusion method, nanoprecipitation/solvent displacement method and salting out method [92].

16.5.2 Polymeric Micelles (PMs)

In the last 5 years, various research papers published on the use of polymeric micelles for drug administration through different routes [93]. They are spherical in shape and possess block co-polymers that are amphiphilic and self-assembled. These block co-polymers consist of core and corona, which are hydrophobic and hydrophilic, respectively. They range in diameter from 10–100 nm. The hydrophobic drug can board into the core of the micelle [94].

Polymeric micelles have a simple architecture that can be prepared easily and can provide stability, biodistribution, pharmacokinetics, and biocompatibility to the drug. Genexol®-PM is a polymeric micelle load paclitaxel (PTX) used for the treatment of breast cancer and ovarian cancer [95]. The drug binds to the nano-carrier with some force of attraction, it enters the cell through the endosome, releases the drug in the cytoplasm, and gets accumulated in tumor tissue [96].

The drug released by polymeric micelle must maintain a balance between efficacy and toxicity [94]. Polymeric micelles are commonly developed by polystyrene, poloxamers, polyethylene glycol, graft, poly(vinyl pyrrolidone), poly (trimethylene carbonate), and poly (acryloylmorpholine) [93]. In active tumor targeting, tumor drug is directly released at the tumor site leading to the death of cells by ischemia and necrosis [96].

16.5.3 Liposomes

Liposomes are lipid nano-particles with an aqueous core surrounded by a lipid bilayer [97]. This diverse structure makes it possible for liposomes to select, load, and send molecules depending on their solubility. Their core loads hydrophilic molecules, lipid bilayer loads hydrophobic molecules, and amphiphilic molecules get loaded at the interface of the core and lipid bi-layer [98]. Drugs can be encapsulated in the lipid bi-layer or can be incorporated in the core. Targeted bioconjugates are formed by altering the liposome with protein and are delivered to destined tissues or cells [99]. The drug incorporated within the liposome cannot target the tumor until unless it is released [88].

Drug delivery with liposomes has some disadvantages. Mono-nuclear phagocyte system ingests liposomes and decreases the level of drug within the blood [89]. Liposomal drugs are mostly incorporated intravenously. Drugs can also be administered by intranasal delivery, intra-tumor delivery, dermal and trans-dermal delivery, and ocular delivery [90]. Liposomal drugs are also being used as vaccines, antibacterial, and for severe pain management [91].

16.5.4 Metallic Nanoparticles (MNPs)

Metallic nanoparticles serve as a drug carrier for the treatment of cancer. Pathophysiology of tumor cells is used by metallic nanoparticles for the impactful delivery of drugs for cancer treatment [100].

The mononuclear phagocyte system (MPS) and reticuloendothelial system (RES) can remove the drug from circulation by phagocytic cells. Nanoparticles must avoid this removal [101]. Polyethylene glycol (PEG) can be used to protect metallic nanoparticles from the effect of the reticuloendothelial system (RES) [100].

Metallic nanoparticles can decrease the rate of drug excretion by the kidney to increase their circulation time in blood and increase the solubility of hydrophobic drugs [102]. Gold is a metal that can be prepared in a wide range of sizes ranging from 1–150 nm. It is preferred as a potential drug carrier because of its non-toxic nature and biocompatibility [103]. Platinum is a metal with strong anticancer activity. Platinum nanoparticles enter the cell by endocytosis and result in DNA damage leading to inhibited replication and apoptosis [104].

Cancer treatment can be carried out by active or passive targeting of tumor cells. Leaky blood vessels form during passive targeting due to the rapid growth of tumor cells that facilitate the better accumulation of MNPs. While, during active targeting, MNPs and ligands are conjugated that bind to specific receptors and release drugs [102].

16.6   COMBINED THERAPY

Nowadays, PDT is mostly used to treat many cancers, which include neck, head, brain, prostate, pancreas, lung, breast, intraperitoneal cavity, and skin cancer [27]. Weakness of the laser penetration [105] and toxicity of the PSs may affect the usage of PDT to treat tumors clinically [106]. A combination of PDT along with other therapies exhibits anticancer efficiency and excellent drug-loading ability as compared to monotherapy [107, 108]. An increasing number of approaches have been made to combine PDT with other conventional cancer treatments, such as chemotherapy, immunotherapy, radiotherapy, and enzyme inhibitors to enhance the therapeutic efficacy of PDT [109]. Some of them are discussed below.

16.6.1   PDT AND CHEMOTHERAPY

Chemotherapy is mostly used for the treatment of many tumors. It is thought that the anti-tumor mechanism of chemotherapy medications involves binding to the DNA of the tumor cells to impede cell division and so halt DNA replication, ultimately causing the death of cancer cells [110]. Chemotherapy has serious adverse effects on the entire body due to the non-specificity of medications and drug resistance [109]. PDT has been suggested for usage in conjunction with chemotherapy for cancer to maximize any additional antitumor effects. The impact of PDT and anticlastic medications together demonstrated a very additive anticancer effect [111, 112].

16.6.2   PDT COMBINED WITH RADIOTHERAPY

Patients with early-stage and advanced-stage breast cancer continue to benefit from radiotherapy, which is typically given in addition to chemotherapy, hormone treatment, or surgery. Despite the curative ability of radiotherapy, metastatic progression restricts its use to treat cancer. TGF-β, is a protein that controls the epithelial-mesenchymal transition. Radioactive resistance is elicited by ionizing radiation, which increases cancer cells' capacity to metastasize [113]. PDT-coupled radiotherapy can dramatically enhance the quality of life, ease pain, reduce the symptoms, and increase survival in patients with advanced cancers [114]. Yi-shan Wang [115] examined the impact of PDT in conjunction with radiotherapy and these findings demonstrated that intensity-modulated radiation (IMRT) in conjunction with PDT significantly reduced symptoms and consequently improved quality of the life for patients having intermediate and advanced-stage malignant tumors [116].

16.6.3 PDT COMBINED WITH IMMUNOTHERAPY

PDT combined with immunotherapy can be an effective means, not only to eliminate primary tumors but also to initiate an antitumor immunogenic response. That immune response can be utilized as a potential tool to outwit the emergence of secondary disease, i.e., cancer recurrence or metastasis. PDT is also capable of triggering some systemic effects like reinstallation of the immunosurveillance [117].

In contrast to traditional therapies, anti-tumor immunity can be induced by low-dose PDT regimens and can be combined with high-dose PDT to control local tumors along with immune suppression [118]. The PDT mechanisms include immune stimulation, i.e., acute inflammatory response just after PDT, which activates dendritic cells (DC) by enhancing the tumor antigens' presentation, and their localization to local and peripheral lymph nodes, ultimately causing the activation of CD8+ cytotoxic T cells and natural killer (NK) cells, the development of immunological memory, and the prevention of any recurrent tumor growth in response to a subsequent challenge. According to reports, the degree of PDT-induced acute inflammation varies depending on the regimen and is correlated with the severity of the vascular damage. PDT regimens that cause the most tissue damage and quick cell death (within 1 hour of treatment) were shown to cause the least acute inflammation. This is probably because vascular closure prevents neutrophil infiltration and the release of cytokines into the bloodstream. Contrarily, protocols that result in diffuse tumor damage ought to permit neutrophil infiltration, followed by the stimulation of production and release of inflammatory mediators important for boosting anti-tumor immunity [119].

An anti-tumor combination PDT treatment regimen that limits primary and metastatic tumor growth and improves anti-tumor immunity of both colon and mammary carcinomas has recently been discovered, according to results from a preclinical study [118]. The goal of ongoing research is to identify the ideal conditions for PDT that will stimulate systemic immunity. Recent studies have demonstrated that PDT can be a successful postoperative therapy that increases the likelihood of long-term local disease control [120]. It was only recently that PDT using the photosensitizer hypericin (Hyp-PDT) was recognized as the first PDT technique capable of generating immunogenic cell death (ICD) [121]. Even if the immunogenic potential of all PS has not yet been investigated, the current discoveries involving hypericin represent a significant accomplishment because they have allowed PDT to be categorized as a treatment that can cause ICD [122].

Overall, mounting evidence suggests that the therapeutic effectiveness of PDT depends on its ability to affect the tumor–host interaction, tipping the scales in favor of the activation of an immune response specific for malignant cells, particularly for cancer that has spread to other organs. Hence, both of these mechanisms combined can not only improve the quality of the patient's life but also subside the mortality rate associated with cancer.

16.6.4 PDT COMBINED WITH OTHER DRUGS AND SURGERIES

Excision and topical PDT can be applied repeatedly without causing resistance, or serious adverse effects [123]. It was proven that PDT alone was less effective than ALA-PDT (twice a week for 16 weeks). In the 12th month, patients receiving combined treatment had a median lesion reduction of 89.9% as compared to PDT alone, which had a lesion reduction of 74.5% [124].

16.7 CONCLUSION

PDT is a harmless and effective therapeutic technique for the treatment of numerous cancer and non-cancer diseases. The most significant feature of this technique is its targeted accumulation only in diseased tissues with low toxic effects on healthy cells. Enormous progress has been made in the science of PDT with the development of improved PS and with a better understanding of its working principle. Regardless of scientific advances, the clinical application of PDT is quite limited to the small number of excellence centers and individual practitioners partly due to its vicious cycle of high PS cost. Therefore, PDT needs to come out of the shadow and into the light of its common use with a more cost-effective approach.

REFERENCES

1. Awan, M. and S. Tarin, *Review of photodynamic therapy. The Surgeon*, 2006. **4**(4): pp. 231–236.
2. Kwiatkowski, S., et al., *Photodynamic therapy–mechanisms, photosensitizers and combinations. Biomedicine & Pharmacotherapy*, 2018. **106**: pp. 1098–1107.
3. Gunaydin, G., M.E. Gedik, and S. Ayan, *Photodynamic therapy—current limitations and novel approaches. Frontiers in Chemistry*, 2021. **9**: pp. 691697.
4. Allison, R.R. and K. Moghissi, *Photodynamic therapy (PDT): PDT mechanisms. Clinical Endoscopy*, 2013. **46**(1): pp. 24–29.
5. Rkein, A.M. and D.M. Ozog, *Photodynamic therapy. Dermatologic Clinics*, 2014. **32**(3): pp. 415–425.
6. Calzavara-Pinton, P.G., et al., *A retrospective analysis of real-life practice of off-label photodynamic therapy using methyl aminolevulinate (MAL-PDT) in 20 Italian dermatology departments. Part 1: Inflammatory and aesthetic indications. Photochemical & Photobiological Sciences*, 2012. **12**(1): pp. 148–157.
7. Shin, H.T., et al., *Photodynamic therapy using a new formulation of 5-aminolevulinic acid for wrinkles in Asian skin: A randomized controlled split face study. Journal of Dermatological Treatment*, 2015. **26**(3): pp. 246–251.
8. Jerjes, W., et al., *Interstitial PDT for vascular anomalies. Lasers in Surgery and Medicine*, 2011. **43**(5): pp. 357–365.
9. Gallardo-Villagrán, M., et al., *Photosensitizers used in the photodynamic therapy of rheumatoid arthritis. International Journal of Molecular Sciences*, 2019. **20**(13): p. 3339.
10. Stender, I.-M., et al., *Photodynamic therapy with 5-aminolaevulinic acid or placebo for recalcitrant foot and hand warts: Randomised double-blind trial. The Lancet*, 2000. **355**(9208): pp. 963–966.
11. Yoo, S.W., et al., *Non-oncologic applications of nanomedicine-based photo-therapy. Biomedicines*, 2021. **9**(2): p. 113.
12. Plaetzer, K., et al., *New applications of photodynamic therapy in biomedicine and biotechnology*. 2013, Hindawi.
13. Muniyandi, K., et al., *Role of photoactive phytocompounds in photodynamic therapy of cancer. Molecules*, 2020. **25**(18): p. 4102.
14. Henderson, B.W. and T.J. Dougherty, *How does photodynamic therapy work? Photochemistry and Photobiology*, 1992. **55**(1): pp. 145–157.
15. Foote, C.S., *Definition of Type I and Type II Photosensitized Oxidation*. 1991, Hoboken: Wiley Online Library. pp. 659–659.
16. Bacellar, I.O., et al., *Photodynamic efficiency: From molecular photochemistry to cell death. International Journal of Molecular Sciences*, 2015. **16**(9): pp. 20523–20559.
17. Correia, J.H., et al., *Photodynamic therapy review: Principles, photosensitizers, applications, and future directions. Pharmaceutics*, 2021. **13**(9): p. 1332.
18. Lee, C.-N., et al., *Daylight photodynamic therapy: An update. Molecules*, 2020. **25**(21): p. 5195.
19. Wagnieres, G.A., W.M. Star, and B.C. Wilson, *In vivo fluorescence spectroscopy and imaging for oncological applications. Photochemistry and Photobiology*, 1998. **68**(5): p. 603.
20. Dobson, J., G.F. de Queiroz, and J.P. Golding, *Photodynamic therapy and diagnosis: Principles and comparative aspects. The Veterinary Journal*, 2018. **233**: pp. 8–18.
21. Dougherty, T.J., et al., *Photodynamic therapy. JNCI: Journal of the National Cancer Institute*, 1998. **90**(12): pp. 889–905.
22. Jensen, T.J., et al., *Effect of overall charge and charge distribution on cellular uptake, distribution and phototoxicity of cationic porphyrins in HEp2 cells. Journal of Photochemistry and Photobiology B: Biology*, 2010. **100**(2): pp. 100–111.
23. Sharman, W.M., C.M. Allen, and J.E. van Lier, *Role of activated oxygen species in photodynamic therapy. Methods in Enzymology*, 2000. **319**: pp. 376–400.

24. Moan, J. and K. Berg, *The photodegradation of porphyrins in cells can be used to estimate the lifetime of singlet oxygen. Photochemistry and Photobiology*, 1991. **53**(4): pp. 549–553.

25. Amor, T.B. and G. Jori, *Sunlight-activated insecticides: historical background and mechanisms of phototoxic activity. Insect Biochemistry and Molecular Biology*, 2000. **30**(10): pp. 915–925.

26. Ackroyd, R., et al., *The history of photodetection and photodynamic therapy¶. Photochemistry and Photobiology*, 2001. **74**(5): pp. 656–669.

27. Dolmans, D.E., D. Fukumura, and R.K. Jain, *Photodynamic therapy for cancer. Nature Reviews Cancer*, 2003. **3**(5): pp. 380–387.

28. Hamblin, M.R., *Photodynamic therapy for cancer: what's past is prologue. Photochemistry and Photobiology*, 2020. **96**(3): pp. 506–516.

29. Igney, F.H. and P.H. Krammer, *Death and anti-death: tumour resistance to apoptosis. Nature Reviews Cancer*, 2002. **2**(4): pp. 277–288.

30. Oleinick, N.L., R.L. Morris, and I. Belichenko, *The role of apoptosis in response to photodynamic therapy: what, where, why, and how. Photochemical & Photobiological Sciences*, 2002. **1**(1): pp. 1–21.

31. Kessel, D. and J.J. Reiners Jr, *Apoptosis and autophagy after mitochondrial or endoplasmic reticulum photodamage. Photochemistry and Photobiology*, 2007. **83**(5): pp. 1024–1028.

32. Khorsandi, K., R. Hosseinzadeh, and E. Chamani, *Molecular interaction and cellular studies on combination photodynamic therapy with rutoside for melanoma A375 cancer cells: an in vitro study. Cancer Cell International*, 2020. **20**(1): pp. 1–15.

33. Buytaert, E., M. Dewaele, and P. Agostinis, *Molecular effectors of multiple cell death pathways initiated by photodynamic therapy. Biochimica et Biophysica Acta (BBA)-Reviews on Cancer*, 2007. **1776**(1): pp. 86–107.

34. Rasul, A., et al., *Targeting apoptosis pathways in cancer with alantolactone and isoalantolactone. The Scientific World Journal*, 2013. **2013**: p. 248532.

35. Wu, S. and D. Xing, *Mechanism of mitochondrial membrane permeabilization during apoptosis under photofrin-mediated photodynamic therapy. Journal of X-Ray Science and Technology*, 2012. **20**(3): pp. 363–372.

36. Zafar, M., et al., *Tubeimoside-1, triterpenoid saponin, as a potential natural cancer killer. Natural Product Communications*, 2018. **13**(5): p. 1934578X1801300530.

37. Luo, M., et al., *Inhibition of autophagy enhances apoptosis induced by Ce6-photodynamic therapy in human colon cancer cells. Photodiagnosis and Photodynamic Therapy*, 2021. **36**: p. 102605.

38. Hashim, A., et al., *Exploration of cassava plant xylem for water treatment: preparation, characterization and filtration capability. Water Science & Technology*, 2022. **86**(5): pp. 1055–1065.

39. Huang, Q., et al., *Apoptosis and autophagy induced by pyropheophorbide-α methyl ester-mediated photodynamic therapy in human osteosarcoma MG-63 cells. Apoptosis*, 2016. **21**(6): pp. 749–760.

40. Wang, X., et al., *Involvement of bim in photofrin-mediated photodynamically induced apoptosis. Cellular Physiology and Biochemistry*, 2015. **35**(4): pp. 1527–1536.

41. Qiao, L., et al., *ALA-PDT inhibits proliferation and promotes apoptosis of SCC cells through STAT3 signal pathway. Photodiagnosis and Photodynamic Therapy*, 2016. **14**: pp. 66–73.

42. Sacks, D., et al., *Multisociety consensus quality improvement revised consensus statement for endovascular therapy of acute ischemic stroke. International Journal of Stroke*, 2018. **13**(6): pp. 612–632.

43. Burotto, M., et al., *The MAPK pathway across different malignancies: a new perspective. Cancer*, 2014. **120**(22): pp. 3446–3456.

44. Fitzgerald, F., *Photodynamic Therapy (PDT)*. 2017, New York: Nova Science.

45. Faes, S. and O. Dormond, *PI3K and AKT: unfaithful partners in cancer. International Journal of Molecular Sciences*, 2015. **16**(9): pp. 21138–21152.

46. Levine, B. and D.J. Klionsky, *Development by self-digestion: molecular mechanisms and biological functions of autophagy. Developmental Cell*, 2004. **6**(4): pp. 463–477.

47. Kessel, D., M.G.H. Vicente, and J.J. Reiners Jr, *Initiation of apoptosis and autophagy by photodynamic therapy. Lasers in Surgery and Medicine: The Official Journal of the American Society for Laser Medicine and Surgery*, 2006. **38**(5): pp. 482–488.

48. Xue, L.y., et al., *The death of human cancer cells following photodynamic therapy: Apoptosis competence is necessary for Bcl-2 protection but not for induction of autophagy. Photochemistry and Photobiology*, 2007. **83**(5): pp. 1016–1023.
49. Inguscio, V., E. Panzarini, and L. Dini, *Autophagy contributes to the death/survival balance in cancer photodynamic therapy. Cells*, 2012. **1**(3): pp. 464–491.
50. Khorsandi, K., R. Hosseinzadeh, and F.K. Shahidi, *Photodynamic treatment with anionic nanoclays containing curcumin on human triple-negative breast cancer cells: Cellular and biochemical studies. Journal of Cellular Biochemistry*, 2019. **120**(4): pp. 4998–5009.
51. Kessel, D.H., M. Price, and J. Reiners, John J, *ATG7 deficiency suppresses apoptosis and cell death induced by lysosomal photodamage. Autophagy*, 2012. **8**(9): pp. 1333–1341.
52. Shi, Y., et al., *Apoptosis and autophagy induced by DVDMs-PDT on human esophageal cancer Eca-109 cells. Photodiagnosis and Photodynamic Therapy*, 2018. **24**: pp. 198–205.
53. Fang, J., et al., *Berberine-photodynamic induced apoptosis by activating endoplasmic reticulum stress-autophagy pathway involving CHOP in human malignant melanoma cells. Biochemical and Biophysical Research Communications*, 2021. **552**: pp. 183–190.
54. Zhou, W., et al., *lncRNA TINCR participates in ALA-PDT-induced apoptosis and autophagy in cutaneous squamous cell carcinoma. Journal of Cellular Biochemistry*, 2019. **120**(8): pp. 13893–13902.
55. Jiang, C., et al., *Methylene blue-mediated photodynamic therapy induces macrophage apoptosis via ROS and reduces bone resorption in periodontitis. Oxidative Medicine and Cellular Longevity*, 2019. **2019**: p. 1529520.
56. Kim, J., et al., *Photodynamic therapy (PDT) resistance by PARP 1 regulation on PDT-induced apoptosis with autophagy in head and neck cancer cells. Journal of Oral Pathology & Medicine*, 2014. **43**(9): pp. 675–684.
57. Zhu, B., et al., *Inhibition of autophagy with chloroquine enhanced sinoporphyrin sodium mediated photodynamic therapy-induced apoptosis in human colorectal cancer cells. International Journal of Biological Sciences*, 2019. **15**(1): p. 12.
58. Chen, J., et al., *Endoplasmic reticulum stress-mediated autophagy contributes to 5-ethylamino-9-diethylaminobenzo [a] phenoselenazinium-mediated photodynamic therapy via the PERK–eIF2α pathway. Oncotargets and Therapy*, 2018. **11**: p. 4315.
59. Luo, Y. and D. Kessel, *Initiation of apoptosis versus necrosis by photodynamic therapy with chloroaluminum phthalocyanine. Photochemistry and Photobiology*, 1997. **66**(4): pp. 479–483.
60. Hsieh, Y.J., et al., *Subcellular localization of Photofrin® determines the death phenotype of human epidermoid carcinoma A431 cells triggered by photodynamic therapy: when plasma membranes are the main targets. Journal of Cellular Physiology*, 2003. **194**(3): pp. 363–375.
61. Hamblin, M.R. and Y. Huang, *Imaging in Photodynamic Therapy*. 2017, Boca Raton: CRC Press.
62. Dąbrowski, J.M. and L.G. Arnaut, *Photodynamic therapy (PDT) of cancer: from local to systemic treatment. Photochemical & Photobiological Sciences*, 2015. **14**(10): pp. 1765–1780.
63. Tada, D.B. and M.S. Baptista, *Photosensitizing nanoparticles and the modulation of ROS generation. Frontiers in Chemistry*, 2015. **3**: p. 33.
64. Zhu, T.C. and J.C. Finlay, *The role of photodynamic therapy (PDT) physics. Medical Physics*, 2008. **35**(7Part1): pp. 3127–3136.
65. Kochevar, I.E. and R.W. Redmond, *[2] Photosensitized production of singlet oxygen*, in *Methods in Enzymology*. 2000, Amsterdam: Elsevier. pp. 20–28.
66. Battersby, A.R., *Tetrapyrroles: The pigments of life. Natural Product Reports*, 2000. **17**(6): pp. 507–526.
67. Abrahamse, H. and M.R. Hamblin, *New photosensitizers for photodynamic therapy. Biochemical Journal*, 2016. **473**(4): pp. 347–364.
68. Detty, M.R., S.L. Gibson, and S.J. Wagner, *Current clinical and preclinical photosensitizers for use in photodynamic therapy. Journal of Medicinal Chemistry*, 2004. **47**(16): pp. 3897–3915.
69. Allison, R., H. Mota, and C. Sibata, *Clinical PD/PDT in North America: an historical review. Photodiagnosis and Photodynamic Therapy*, 2004. **1**(4): p. 263–277.
70. Mahmoudi, K., et al., *5-aminolevulinic acid photodynamic therapy for the treatment of high-grade gliomas. Journal of Neuro-Oncology*, 2019. **141**: p. 595–607.

71. Fargnoli, M.C. and K. Peris, *Photodynamic therapy for basal cell carcinoma. Future Oncology*, 2015. **11**(22): pp. 2991–2996.

72. Baskaran, R., J. Lee, and S.-G. Yang, *Clinical development of photodynamic agents and therapeutic applications. Biomaterials Research*, 2018. **22**(1): p. 1–8.

73. Yakavets, I., et al., *Current state of the nanoscale delivery systems for temoporfin-based photodynamic therapy: Advanced delivery strategies. Journal of Controlled Release*, 2019. **304**: pp. 268–287.

74. Gao, Y., et al., *Anti-VEGF monotherapy versus photodynamic therapy and anti-VEGF combination treatment for neovascular age-related macular degeneration: a meta-analysis. Investigative Ophthalmology & Visual Science*, 2018. **59**(10): pp. 4307–4317.

75. Bellnier, D.A., et al., *Mild skin photosensitivity in cancer patients following injection of Photochlor (2-[1-hexyloxyethyl]-2-devinyl pyropheophorbide-a; HPPH) for photodynamic therapy. Cancer Chemotherapy and Pharmacology*, 2006. **57**: pp. 40–45.

76. Santos, L.L., et al., *Treatment of head and neck cancer with photodynamic therapy with redaporfin: A clinical case report. Case Reports in Oncology*, 2018. **11**(3): pp. 769–776.

77. Wong, J.J.W., S. Lorenz, and P.K. Selbo, *All-trans retinoic acid enhances the anti-tumour effects of fimaporfin-based photodynamic therapy. Biomedicine & Pharmacotherapy*, 2022. **155**: p. 113678.

78. Cohen, D.K. and P.K. Lee, *Photodynamic therapy for non-melanoma skin cancers. Cancers*, 2016. **8**(10): p. 90.

79. Yawalkar, M.M., et al., *Fundamentals of photodynamic therapy*, in *Photophysics and Nanophysics in Therapeutics*. 2022, Elsevier. pp. 51–88.

80. Jarvi, M.T., M.S. Patterson, and B.C. Wilson, *Insights into photodynamic therapy dosimetry: simultaneous singlet oxygen luminescence and photosensitizer photobleaching measurements. Biophysical Journal*, 2012. **102**(3): pp. 661–671.

81. Zhang, H., *Pyro-Gly-Asp-Glu-Val-Asp-Gly-Ser-Gly-Lys (BHQ3) PPB*. In Molecular Imaging and Contrast Agent Database (MICAD) [Internet]. 2008, Bethesda (MD): National Center for Biotechnology Information.

82. Kim, M.M., et al., *A comparison of singlet oxygen explicit dosimetry (SOED) and singlet oxygen luminescence dosimetry (SOLD) for photofrin-mediated photodynamic therapy. Cancers*, 2016. **8**(12): p. 109.

83. Nasr, S., et al., *A naturally derived carrier for photodynamic treatment of squamous cell carcinoma: in vitro and in vivo models. Pharmaceutics*, 2020. **12**(6): p. 494.

84. Li, J., T.C. Zhu, and J.C. Finlay. *Study of light fluence rate distribution in photodynamic therapy using finite-element method*. In *Optical Methods for Tumor Treatment and Detection: Mechanisms and Techniques in Photodynamic Therapy XV*. 2006. SPIE.

85. Grossman, C.E., et al., *Fluence rate differences in photodynamic therapy efficacy and activation of epidermal growth factor receptor after treatment of the tumor-involved murine thoracic cavity. International Journal of Molecular Sciences*, 2016. **17**(1): p. 101.

86. Busch, T.M., et al., *Fluence rate-dependent intratumor heterogeneity in physiologic and cytotoxic responses to photofrin photodynamic therapy. Photochemical & Photobiological Sciences*, 2009. **8**(12): pp. 1683–1693.

87. Severino, P., et al., *Alginate nanoparticles for drug delivery and targeting. Current Pharmaceutical Design*, 2019. **25**(11): pp. 1312–1334.

88. Khalid, M. and H.S. El-Sawy, *Polymeric nanoparticles: Promising platform for drug delivery. International Journal of Pharmaceutics*, 2017. **528**(1–2): pp. 675–691.

89. Ahmed, A., et al., *Surface-modified polymeric nanoparticles for drug delivery to cancer cells. Expert Opinion on Drug Delivery*, 2021. **18**(1): pp. 1–24.

90. Abd Ellah, N.H. and S.A. Abouelmagd, *Surface functionalization of polymeric nanoparticles for tumor drug delivery: approaches and challenges. Expert Opinion on Drug Delivery*, 2017. **14**(2): pp. 201–214.

91. Ghazaeian, M., et al., *Curcumin–silica nanocomplex preparation, hemoglobin and DNA interaction and photocytotoxicity against melanoma cancer cells. Journal of Biomolecular Structure and Dynamics*, 2021. **39**(17): pp. 6606–6616.

92. Ahlawat, J., G. Henriquez, and M. Narayan, *Enhancing the delivery of chemotherapeutics: role of biodegradable polymeric nanoparticles. Molecules*, 2018. **23**(9): p. 2157.

93. Ghezzi, M., et al., *Polymeric micelles in drug delivery: an insight of the techniques for their characterization and assessment in biorelevant conditions. Journal of Controlled Release,* 2021. **332**: pp. 312–336.

94. Majumder, N., N. G Das, and S.K. Das, *Polymeric micelles for anticancer drug delivery. Therapeutic Delivery,* 2020. **11**(10): pp. 613–635.

95. Zhou, Q., et al., *Stimuli-responsive polymeric micelles for drug delivery and cancer therapy. International Journal of Nanomedicine,* 2018. **13**: p. 2921.

96. Jeetah, R., A. Bhaw-Luximon, and D. Jhurry, *Polymeric nanomicelles for sustained delivery of anticancer drugs. Mutation Research/Fundamental and Molecular Mechanisms of Mutagenesis,* 2014. **768**: pp. 47–59.

97. Fan, Y., M. Marioli, and K. Zhang, *Analytical characterization of liposomes and other lipid nanoparticles for drug delivery. Journal of Pharmaceutical and Biomedical Analysis,* 2021. **192**: p. 113642.

98. Guimarães, D., A. Cavaco-Paulo, and E. Nogueira, *Design of liposomes as drug delivery system for therapeutic applications. International Journal of Pharmaceutics,* 2021. **601**: p. 120571.

99. Almeida, B., et al., *Recent progress in bioconjugation strategies for liposome-mediated drug delivery. Molecules,* 2020. **25**(23): p. 5672.

100. Desai, N., et al., *Metallic nanoparticles as drug delivery system for the treatment of cancer. Expert Opinion on Drug Delivery,* 2021. **18**(9): pp. 1261–1290.

101. Ahmad, M.Z., et al., *Metallic nanoparticles: technology overview & drug delivery applications in oncology. Expert Opinion on Drug Delivery,* 2010. **7**(8): pp. 927–942.

102. Chandrakala, V., V. Aruna, and G. Angajala, *Review on metal nanoparticles as nanocarriers: Current challenges and perspectives in drug delivery systems. Emergent Materials,* 2022: pp. 1–23.

103. Singh, P., et al., *Gold nanoparticles in diagnostics and therapeutics for human cancer. International Journal of Molecular Sciences,* 2018. **19**(7): p. 1979.

104. Abed, A., et al., *Platinum nanoparticles in biomedicine: preparation, anti-cancer activity, and drug delivery vehicles. Frontiers in Pharmacology,* 2022. **13**: p. 797804.

105. Josefsen, L.B. and R.W. Boyle, *Photodynamic therapy and the development of metal-based photosensitisers. Metal-Based Drugs,* 2008. **2008**.

106. Pantiushenko, I., et al., *Development of bacteriochlorophyll a-based near-infrared photosensitizers conjugated to gold nanoparticles for photodynamic therapy of cancer. Biochemistry (Moscow),* 2015. **80**(6): pp. 752–762.

107. Wang, X., et al., *A reactive 1O2-responsive combined treatment system of photodynamic and chemotherapy for cancer. Scientific Reports,* 2016. **6**(1): pp. 1–9.

108. Khorsandi, K., et al., *Comparative study of photodynamic activity of methylene blue in the presence of salicylic acid and curcumin phenolic compounds on human breast cancer. Lasers in Medical Science,* 2019. **34**(2): pp. 239–246.

109. Zhang, Q. and L. Li, *Photodynamic combinational therapy in cancer treatment. J. BUON,* 2018. **23**(3): pp. 561–567.

110. Faber, M., et al., *Lipid peroxidation products, and vitamin and trace element status in patients with cancer before and after chemotherapy, including adriamycin. Biological Trace Element Research,* 1995. **47**(1): pp. 117–123.

111. Canti, G., et al., *Antitumor efficacy of the combination of photodynamic therapy and chemotherapy in murine tumors. Cancer Letters,* 1998. **125**(1–2): pp. 39–44.

112. Khorsandi, K. and Z. Kianmehr, *Synergistic effect of photodynamic treatment and doxorubicin on triple negative breast cancer cells. Photochemical & Photobiological Sciences: Official Journal of the European Photochemistry Association and the European Society for Photobiology,* 2020.

113. Aumeeruddy, M.Z. and M.F. Mahomoodally, *Combating breast cancer using combination therapy with 3 phytochemicals: Piperine, sulforaphane, and thymoquinone. Cancer,* 2019. **125**(10): pp. 1600–1611.

114. Nakano, A., et al., *Treatment efficiency of combining photodynamic therapy and ionizing radiation for Bowen's disease. Journal of the European Academy of Dermatology and Venereology,* 2011. **25**(4): pp. 475–478.

115. Wang, Y., et al., *Photodynamic therapy combined with IMCRT for cancer: a clinical study. Chinese Journal of Laser Medicine and Surgery,* 2009. **18**: pp. 82–87.

116. Ghoodarzi, R., et al., *Assessing of integration of ionizing radiation with Radachlorin-PDT on MCF-7 breast cancer cell treatment. Lasers in Medical Science*, 2016. **31**(2): pp. 213–219.

117. dos Santos, A.l.F., et al., *Photodynamic therapy in cancer treatment-an update review. Journal of Cancer Metastasis and Treatment*, 2019. **5**: p. 25.

118. Shams, M., et al., *Development of photodynamic therapy regimens that control primary tumor growth and inhibit secondary disease. Cancer Immunology, Immunotherapy*, 2015. **64**: pp. 287–297.

119. Henderson, B.W., et al., *Choice of oxygen-conserving treatment regimen determines the inflammatory response and outcome of photodynamic therapy of tumors. Cancer Research*, 2004. **64**(6): pp. 2120–2126.

120. Agostinis, P., et al., *Photodynamic therapy of cancer: An update. CA: A Cancer Journal for Clinicians*, 2011. **61**(4): p. 250–281.

121. Garg, A.D., et al., *Hypericin-based photodynamic therapy induces surface exposure of damage-associated molecular patterns like HSP70 and calreticulin. Cancer Immunology, Immunotherapy*, 2012. **61**: pp. 215–221.

122. Tanaka, M., et al., *Immunogenic cell death due to a new photodynamic therapy (PDT) with glycoconjugated chlorin (G-chlorin). Oncotarget*, 2016. **7**(30): p. 47242.

123. Li, X., et al., *Ocular preservation through limited tumor excision combined with ALA-PDT in patients with periocular basal cell carcinoma. Photodiagnosis and Photodynamic Therapy*, 2019. **27**: pp. 291–294.

124. Shaffelburg, M., *Treatment of actinic keratoses with sequential use of photodynamic therapy; and imiquimod 5% cream. Journal of Drugs in Dermatology: JDD*, 2009. **8**(1): pp. 35–39.

Index

Note: Page numbers in **bold** refer to tables and those in *italic* refer to figures.

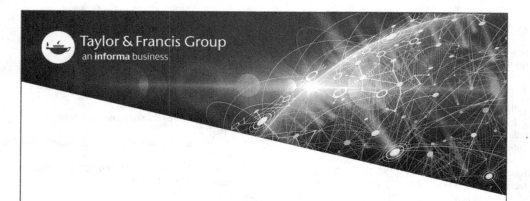
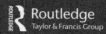
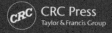